Selecting
the Right Acupoints

— A Handbook on Acupuncture Therapy

Written by:
Geng Junying, Huang Wenquan, and Sun Yongping

Assisted by:
Dong Xiang, and Du Wei

NEW WORLD PRESS, BEIJING, CHINA

First Edition 1995

ISBN 7-80005-181-1/R.014

Published by
NEW WORLD PRESS
24 Baiwanzhuang Road, Beijing 100037, China

Distributed by
CHINA INTERNATIONAL BOOK TRADING CORPORATION
35 Chegongzhuang Xilu, Beijing 100044, China
P.O. Box 399, Beijing, China

Printed in the People's Republic of China

CONTENTS

Foreword

Acupuncture therapy, a shining pearl in Chinese medicine, has spread throughout the world in recent years. The rest of the world is beginning to see the value of acupuncture which the Chinese have known for thousands of years. Unlike Western medical treatments, acupuncture utilizes simple tools and boasts a low instance of adverse side effect. Combined with marked efficacy, it has been widely accepted and welcomed by both doctors and patients.

Selection of acupoints is one of the decisive factors of the therapy, and experience accumulated by Chinese acupuncturists in ancient and modern times is important to its successful practice. Most of this knowledge is scattered throughout acupuncture classics, modern books and magazines, or is possessed by practicing physicians.

In an effort to spread the knowledge of acupoints, and to bring together this vast array of methods in one concise and useful tool, we have compiled *Selecting the Right Acupoints — A Handbook on Acupuncture Therapy*. The content of this book reflects current practices in the selection of acupoints, and methods newly developing in clinical research. Primarily, this book is meant to provide easy access to reference material for acupuncture practitioners who possess a certain level of knowledge of acupuncture science. But it may also serve as a useful guide for beginners.

Chapter I

General Introduction
to Methods of Selection of Acupoints

There are a variety of needling techniques involved in acupuncture therapy. Those commonly used are body acupuncture, ear acupuncture, head acupuncture, hand acupuncture, foot acupuncture, wrist-and-ankle acupuncture and eye acupuncture.

1. Body Acupuncture

The needle used for body acupuncture is the filiform or fine needle. This is the most popular technique, having a long history of use. Based on the theories of *zang-fu* organs, body acupuncture is used to prevent and treat diseases by puncturing points located along 14 channels, the extraordinary points and the Ashi points with needles.

There are a few basic principles for the selection of acupoints in body acupuncture. The practitioner selects symmetrical points, specific points, Ashi points, and points according to the time table, to the course of the channel or to the courses of externally and internally related channels.

1) Selection of acupoints according to the course of the channel

Select local points and remote points along the involved channel for treatment. For example, for epigastric pain: channels of stomach, pericardium and Ren are involved. The remote points, Zusanli (St. 36) and Neiguan (P. 6), and the local point, Zhongwan (Ren 12), could be selected for treatment. As another example, for a one-side headache: the three *yang* channels of hand and foot are involved. The selection of remote points, Foot-Qiaoyin (G.B. 44), Qiuxu (G.B. 40), Zhiyin (U.B.

67), Lidui (St. 45), Neiting (St. 44), Waiguan (S.J. 5), Hegu (L.I. 4), Houxi (S.I. 3), Yanggu (S.I. 5), and local points, Fengchi (G.B. 20), Head-Linqi (G.B. 15), Qubin (G.B. 7), Shuaigu (G.B. 8), Sizhukong (S.J. 23), Jiaosun (S.J. 20), Yifeng (S.J. 17), Quanliao (S.I. 18), Nose-Juliao (St. 3), Xiaguan (St. 7), Jiache (St. 6) and Zanzhu (U.B. 2), should be considered to relieve the pain.

2) Selection of acupoints according to externally and internally related channels

Determine points of the affected channel as well as points of respective externally and internally related channels. For instance, for abdominal pain: Zusanli (St. 36) and Sanyinjiao (Sp. 6) are recommended for treatment; for hypochondriac pain: Taichong (Liv. 3) and Yanglingquan (G.B. 34) can additionally be used.

3) Selection of symmetrical points

The use of symmetrical points is a crossing method, selecting points on the right side to treat disorders crossing on the left, and vice versa. For instance, Yanglingquan (G.B. 34) on the right side may be chosen for a one-side headache on the left side; Hegu (L.I. 4) on the right side may be punctured for facial paralysis on the left side; for hemiplegia affecting the left side, Hegu (L.I. 4), Huantiao (G.B. 30), Yanglingquan (G.B. 34) and Fengshi (G.B. 31) on the healthy side (right side) are used for treatment. In general, puncturing points on the left and right sides, in turn, provides better results than needling points on one side only.

4) Selection of specific points

Specific points include five Shu points, Yuan (source) points, Luo (connecting) points, Back-Shu points, Front-Mu points, eight influential points, eight confluent points, lower He-Sea points and Xi (cleft) points.

a. Application of the five Shu points

The five Shu points are Jing-Well, Ying-Spring, Shu-Stream, Jing-River and He-Sea. In general, the therapeutic properties of the five Shu points are in the treatment of any *zang-fu* organ disorders. Two principles of selection apply to the five Shu points. First, point selection is based on their therapeutic properties. For example, Jing-Well points are used for a stifling sensation in the chest, Ying-Spring points for febrile diseases, Shu-Stream points for soreness, a heavy sensation and painful joints, Jing-River points for asthma, cough, chills and fever, and He-Sea points for vomiting and diarrhea. Second, point selection is determined according to the category of the five elements. The five Shu points are at-

12

tributed to the five elements. Parts of points share the relationship of "mother" and "son." Reinforce the "mother" to treat deficiencies, and reduce the "son" for excesses. For example, reducing the point of Xingjian (Liv. 2, fire point) for excess syndrome of the liver; reinforcing the point of Ququan (Liv. 8, water point) for deficiency of the liver. Another example, reducing the point of Shaofu (H. 8, fire point) is used for excess syndrome of the liver, while reinforcing Yingu (K. 10, water point) is used to treat deficiency of the liver. The first example shows the application of "reinforcing the 'mother'" and "reducing the 'son'" to the involved channel. The second example shows the same method can also be applied to the related channel.

Five Shu Points

TABLE I. THE FIVE SHU POINTS OF THE *YANG* CHANNELS

| Channel | Points | | | | |
	Jing-Well (Metal)	Ying-Spring (Water)	Shu-Stream (Wood)	Jing-River (Fire)	He-Sea (Earth)
Large Intestine (Metal)	Shangyang (L.I. 1)	Erjian (L.I. 2)	Sanjian (L.I. 3)	Yangxi (L.I. 5)	Quchi (L.I. 11)
Stomach (Earth)	Lidui (St. 45)	Neiting (St. 44)	Xiangu (St. 43)	Jiexi (St. 41)	Zusanli (St. 36)
Small Intestine (Fire)	Shaoze (S.I. 1)	Qiangu (S.I. 2)	Houxi (S.I. 3)	Yanggu (S.I. 5)	Xiaohai (S.I. 8)
Urinary Bladder (Water)	Zhiyin (U.B. 67)	Foot-Tonggu (U.B. 66)	Shugu (U.B. 65)	Kunlun (U.B. 60)	Weizhong (U.B. 40)
Sanjiao (Minister-fire)	Guanchong (S.J. 1)	Yemen (S.J. 2)	Hand-Zhongzhu (S.J. 3)	Zhigou (S.J. 6)	Tianjing (S.J. 10)
Gall Bladder (Wood)	Foot-Qiaoyin (G.B. 44)	Xiaxi (G.B. 43)	Foot-Linqi (G.B. 41)	Yangfu (G.B. 38)	Yangling-quan (G.B. 34)

TABLE II. THE FIVE SHU POINTS OF THE *YIN* CHANNELS

Channel	Points				
	Jing-Well (Wood)	Ying-Spring (Fire)	Shu-Stream (Earth)	Jing-River (Metal)	He-Sea (Water)
Lung (Metal)	Shaoshang (Lu. 11)	Yuji (Lu. 10)	Taiyuan (Lu. 9)	Jingqu (Lu. 8)	Chize (Lu. 5)
Spleen (Earth)	Yinbai (Sp. 1)	Dadu (Sp. 2)	Taibai (Sp. 3)	Shangqiu (Sp. 5)	Yinlingquan (Sp. 9)
Heart (Fire)	Shaochong (H. 9)	Shaofu (H. 8)	Shenmen (H. 7)	Lingdao (H. 4)	Shaohai (H. 3)
Kidney (Water)	Yongquan (K. 1)	Rangu (K. 2)	Taixi (K. 3)	Fuliu (K. 7)	Yingu (K. 10)
Pericardium (Minister-fire)	Zhongchong (P. 9)	Laogong (P. 8)	Daling (P. 7)	Jianshi (P. 5)	Quze (P. 3)
Liver (Wood)	Dadun (Liv. 1)	Xingjian (Liv. 2)	Taichong (Liv. 3)	Zhongfeng (Liv. 4)	Ququan (Liv. 8)

b. The application of the Back-Shu and Front-Mu points

The combination of the Back-Shu and Front-Mu points is recommended when internal organs are affected. Normally, whenever an internal organ is diseased, the corresponding Back-Shu point and Front-Mu point of that organ may be used for treatment. For instance, Feishu (U.B. 13), Back-Shu point of the lung, and Zhongfu (Lu. 1), Front-Mu point of the lung, can be selected for disorders of the lung; Weishu (U.B. 21), Back-Shu point of the stomach, and Zhongwan (Ren 12), Front-Mu point of the stomach, may be used for gastric disorders; Dachangshu (U.B. 25), Back-Shu point of the large intestine, and Tianshu (St. 25), Front-Mu point of the large intestine, can be needled for large intestine disorders. The Back-Shu points and Front-Mu points can also be used separately.

14

BACK-SHU AND FRONT-MU POINTS

Internal Organ	Back-Shu Point	Front-Mu Point
Liver	Ganshu (U.B. 18)	Qimen (Liv. 14)
Heart	Xinshu (U.B. 15)	Juque (Ren 14)
Pericardium	Jueyinshu (U.B. 14)	Shanzhong (Ren 17)
Lung	Feishu (U.B. 13)	Zhongfu (Lu. 1)
Spleen	Pishu (U.B. 20)	Zhangmen (Liv. 13)
Kidney	Shenshu (U.B. 23)	Jingmen (G.B. 25)
Gall Bladder	Danshu (U.B. 19)	Riyue (G.B. 24)
Small Intestine	Xiaochangshu (U.B. 27)	Guanyuan (Ren 4)
Sanjiao	Sanjiaoshu (U.B. 22)	Shimen (Ren 5)
Large Intestine	Dachangshu (U.B. 25)	Tianshu (St. 25)
Stomach	Weishu (U.B. 21)	Zhongwan (Ren 12)
Urinary Bladder	Pangguangshu (U.B. 28)	Zhongji (Ren 3)

c. The application of the Yuan (source) points and the Luo (connecting) points

The Yuan (source) points are used in the treatment of syndromes affecting their related organs. The Luo (connecting) points are used in the treatment of syndromes affecting their externally-internally related channels. When an internal organ is affected, the Yuan (source) point of that involved channel can be chosen in combination with the Luo (connecting) point of its externally-internally related channel for treatment. For instance, if the lung channel is diseased, Taiyuan (Lu. 9), the Yuan (source) point of the lung channel, and Pianli (L.I. 6), the Luo (connecting) point of the large intestine channel, may be prescribed to treat the disease; or, if the large intestine channel is disfunctional, Hegu (L.I. 4), the Yuan (source) point of the large intestine channel, and Lieque (Lu. 7), the Luo (connecting) point of the lung channel, may be selected for treatment of the disease.

THE YUAN (SOURCE) POINTS
AND THE LUO (CONNECTING) POINTS

Internal Organ	Yuan (Source) Point	Luo (Connecting) Point
Lung	Taiyuan (Lu. 9)	Lieque (Lu. 7)
Large Intestine	Hegu (L.I. 4)	Pianli (L.I. 6)
Stomach	Chongyang (St. 42)	Fenglong (St. 40)

THE YUAN (SOURCE) POINTS
AND THE LUO (CONNECTING) POINTS

(Continued)

Internal Organ	Yuan (Source) Point	Luo (Connecting) Point
Spleen	Taibai (Sp. 3)	Gongsun (Sp. 4)
Heart	Shenmen (H. 7)	Tongli (H. 5)
Small Intestine	Hand-Wangu (S.I. 4)	Zhizheng (S.I. 7)
Urinary Bladder	Jinggu (U.B. 64)	Feiyang (U.B. 58)
Kidney	Taixi (K. 3)	Dazhong (K. 4)
Pericardium	Daling (P. 7)	Neiguan (P. 6)
Sanjiao	Yangchi (S.J. 4)	Waiguan (S.J. 5)
Gall Bladder	Qiuxu (G.B. 40)	Guangming (G.B. 37)
Liver	Taichong (Liv. 3)	Ligou (Liv. 5)

d. The application of the eight influential points

There are eight influential points. Each has an effect on diseases of certain tissue. For disorders of *qi*, blood, pulse, tendon, bone, marrow, *zang* organ and *fu* organ, the corresponding points can be determined for treatment.

EIGHT INFLUENTIAL POINTS

Tissue	Influential Point
Qi	Shanzhong (Ren 17)
Blood	Geshu (U.B. 17)
Pulse (Vessels)	Taiyuan (Lu. 9)
Bone	Dazhu (U.B. 11)
Tendon	Yanglingquan (G.B. 34)
Marrow	Xuanzhong (G.B. 39)
Zang Organ	Zhangmen (Liv. 13)
Fu Organ	Zhongwan (Ren 12)

e. The application of the eight confluent points

The eight confluent points are points on the twelve regular channels which provide connections with the eight extra channels. These points have therapeutic properties for the treatment of diseases of the extra channels and their related regular channels. One point on the upper extremity is often used in combination with another point on the lower extremity. In this way, two points are paired for treatment. For example, Neiguan (P. 6) combined with Gongsun (Sp. 4) is suggested in treating distention and a sensation of fullness in the chest, epigastric pain, poor appetite, etc. This is because Neiguan (P. 6) connects the Yinwei Extra Channel, while Gongsun (Sp. 4) connects the Chong Extra Channel; both the Yinwei and Chong Extra channels are confluent to areas of the heart, chest and stomach. Another example, Lieque (Lu. 7) and Zhaohai (K. 6) in combination are recommended for the treatment of a sore throat, fullness in the chest and cough. Lieque (Lu. 7) connects the Ren Extra Channel, while Zhaohai (K. 6) connects the Yinqiao Extra Channel. Both the extra channels reach areas of the lung system, throat, chest and diaphragm.

EIGHT CONFLUENT POINTS WITH EXTRA CHANNELS

Confluent Point	Extra Channel	Indication (Portion of the Body)
Gongsun (Sp. 4)	Chong	Heart, chest, stomach
Neiguan (P. 6)	Yinwei	
Foot-Linqi (G.B. 41)	Dai	Outer canthus, retroauricle
Waiguan (S.J. 5)	Yangwei	cheek, shoulder, neck
Houxi (S.I. 3)	Du	Inner canthus,
Shenmai (U.B. 62)	Yangqiao	shoulder, nape, ear
Lieque (Lu. 7)	Ren	Lung, throat, chest,
Zhaohai (K. 6)	Yingqiao	diaphragm

f. The application of the lower He-Sea points

There are six lower He-Sea points including three points on the three *yang* channels of hand, as well as three points on the three *yang* channels of foot. These points are used to treat disorders of the six *fu* organs. Each can be used to treat its corresponding *fu*-organ disease. For example, Shangjuxu (St. 37) may be chosen to treat appendicitis.

17

LOWER HE-SEA POINTS

	Fu Organ	Lower He-Sea Point
Yang Channel of Hand	Sanjiao	Weiyang (U.B. 39)
	Large intestine	Shangjuxu (St. 37)
	Small intestine	Xiajuxu (St. 39)
Yang Channel of Foot	Gall bladder	Yanglingquan (G.B. 34)
	Urinary bladder	Weizhong (U.B. 40)
	Stomach	Zusanli (St. 36)

g. The application of the Xi (cleft) points

There is a Xi (cleft) point in each of the 12 regular channels plus another in each of the extra channels of Yinwei, Yangwei, Yinqiao and Yangqiao, totaling 16 in all. The therapeutic properties of the Xi (cleft) points are for the treatment of acute disorders and pain. For example, Kongzui (Lu. 6) may be chosen for hemoptysis, and Ximen (P. 4) may be selected to relieve chest pain.

XI (CLEFT) POINTS

Channel	Xi (Cleft) Point
Lung	Kongzui (Lu. 6)
Heart	Yinxi (H. 6)
Liver	Foot-Zhongdu (Liv. 6)
Spleen	Diji (Sp. 8)
Kidney	Shuiquan (K. 5)
Pericardium	Ximen (P. 4)
Large Intestine	Wenliu (L.I. 7)
Small Intestine	Yanglao (S.I. 6)
Gall Bladder	Waiqiu (G.B. 36)
Stomach	Liangqiu (St. 34)
Urinary Bladder	Jinmen (U.B. 63)
Sanjiao	Huizong (S.J. 7)
Yangqiao	Fuyang (U.B. 59)
Yinqiao	Jiaoxin (K. 8)
Yangwei	Yangjiao (G.B. 35)
Yinwei	Zhubin (K. 9)

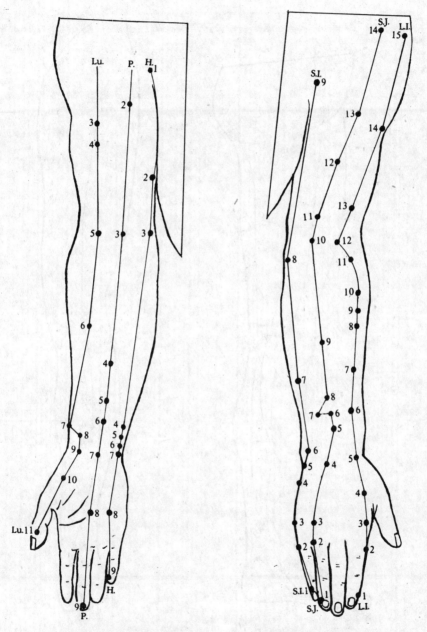

Fig. 1-1 The Points at the Upper Extremities.

19

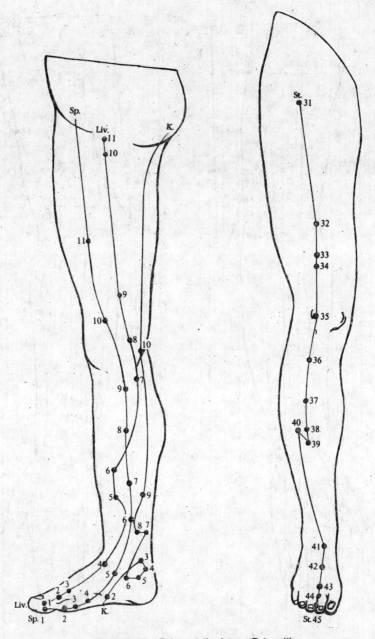

Fig. 1-2 The Points at the Lower Extremities.

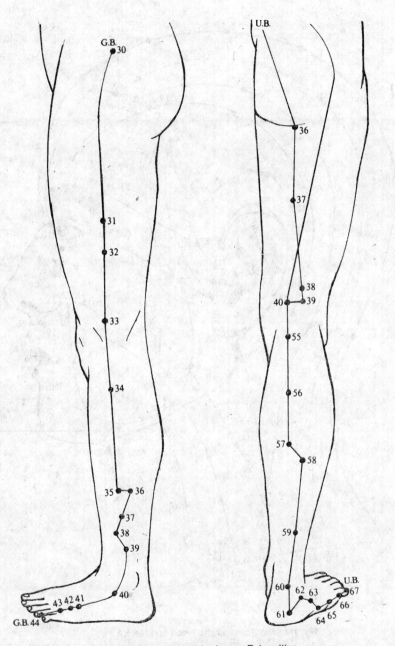

Fig. 1-3 The Points at the Lower Extremities.

21

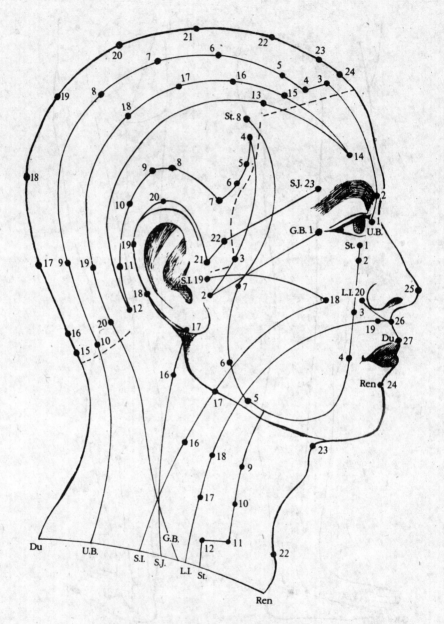

Fig. 1-4 The Points at the Head and Neck.

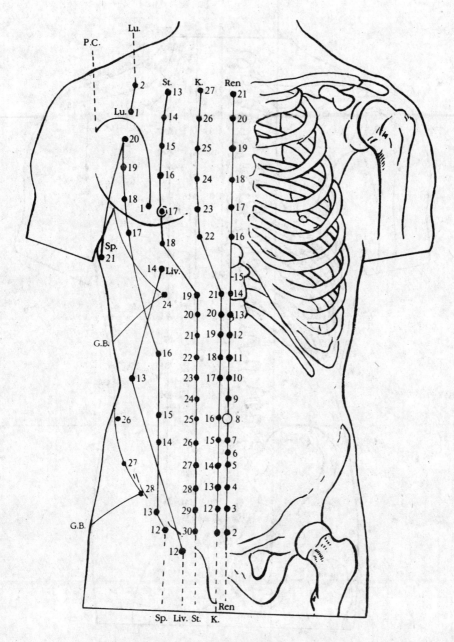

Fig. 1-5 The Points at the Chest and Abdominal Region.

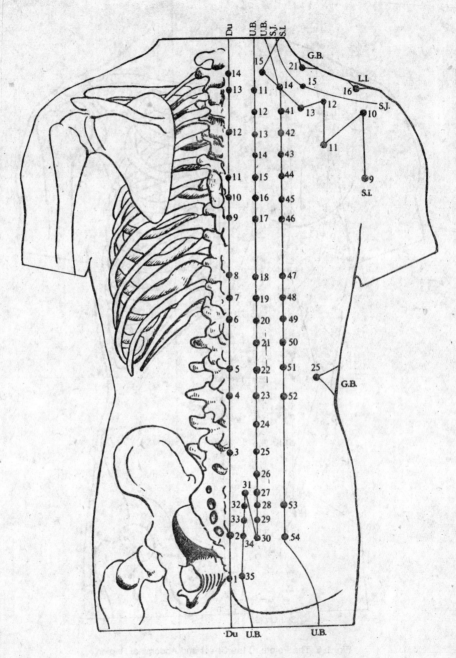

Fig. 1-6 The Points at the Back.

5) The application of Ashi points

When a human body is diseased, some abnormal phenomena, such as tenderness, morphological changes or discoloration, may appear at the corresponding parts of the body. Therapeutic results can be obtained by applying moxibustion or needling the tender spots. For instance, for a patient with asthma, tenderness or soreness is sometimes found at the point of Feishu (U.B. 13); or, for a patient with a disorder of the large intestine, Dachangshu (U.B. 25) is often the tender spot. Pain will be quickly checked by needling the designated spot.

6) Selection of acupoints according to the time table

This is a selection method for acupoints based on equal divisions of time. This method is complicated, and is not often used in clinics. So no details are given here.

2. Ear Acupuncture

Ear acupuncture is the treatment of diseases by needling points of the auricle, as the auricle surface is closely related to various parts of the body. Diseases can be cured by treating the corresponding auricular points. The main principles of point selection are:

1) Selection of points according to the diseased area. For example, Pt. Eye for eye disorders, Pt. Stomach for gastralgia, Pt. Large Intestine for diarrhea or constipation.

2) Selection of points based on the sensitive sites, or spots with morphological changes, or discoloration.

3) Selection of points according to the theories of modern medicine. For instance, Pt. Intertragicus is chosen for irregular menstruation, Pt. End of Inferior Helix Crus for abdominal diseases.

4) Selection of points according to the theories of traditional Chinese medicine. For example, Pt. Liver for eye disorders, Pt. Kidney for ear disease, Pt. Lung for skin disease.

5) Selection of points according to clinic experience. For instance, Pt. Hypertension for hypertension, Pt. Ear Apex for acute conjunctivitis.

TABLE OF EAR POINTS

Auricular Area	Name of Point	Location	Indication
Helix crus	Middle of Ear	On the helix crus	Hiccup, skin diseases
Helix	Lower Portion of Rectum	On end of helix, near supratragic notch	Constipation, prolapsed rectum, tenesmus
	Urethra	On helix, at level of lower border of inferior antihelix crus	Frequency, urgency or retention of urine
	External Genitalia	On helix, at level of upper border of inferior antihelix crus	Orchitis, vaginitis, impotence
	Ear Apex	At tip of auricle when folded towards tragus	Acute conjunctivities, fever, hypertension
	Helix 1-6	Region from lower border of auricular tubercle (Helix 1) to mid-point of lower border of lobule (Helix 6) is divided into five equal parts. The points marking the divisions are respectively Helix 2, 3, 4 and 5	Fever, upper respiratory tract infection
Scapha	Finger	In scapha, superior to auricular tubercle	Pain at corresponding part of body
	Wrist	In scapha, level with auricular tubercle	Pain at corresponding part of body
	Elbow	Between Pt. Wrist and Pt. Shoulder	Pain at corresponding part of body
	Urticaria	Between Pt. Wrist and Pt. Finger	Itching, allergic diseases

Auricular Area	Name of Point	Location	Indication
	Shoulder	In scapha, level with supratragic notch	Stiff neck, periarthritis of shoulder
	Clavicle	In scapha, level with notch between antitragus and antihelix, slightly lateral to helix cauda	Pain at corresponding part of body
	Shoulder Joint	Between Pt. Shoulder and Pt. Clavicle	Periarthritis of shoulder
Superior antihelix crus	Toe	At posterior upper corner of superior antihelix crus	Pain of the toes, paronychia
	Ankle	At anterior upper corner of superior antihelix crus	Injury or pain of the ankle
	Knee	At origin of superior antihelix crus, level with upper border of inferior antihelix crus	Injury or pain of the knee
Inferior antihelix crus	Buttocks	Posterior half of upper border of inferior antihelix crus	Sciatica
	Sciatic Nerve	Anterior half of upper border of inferior antihelix crus	Sciatica
Triangular fossa	Shenmen	At bifurcating point of superior antihelix crus and inferior antihelix crus	Insomnia, dream-disturbed sleep, inflammation, pain
	Uterus (Seminal Vesicle)	In triangular fossa, at mid-point inferior to border of helix	Irregular menstruation, leukorrhea, dysmenorrhea, impotence, nocturnal emission

27

Auricular Area	Name of Point	Location	Indication
	End of Inferior Helix Crus	At junction of inferior antihelix crus and medial border of helix	Antispasmotism and analgesia for internal organs
Antihelix	Abdomen	On antihelix, level with lower border of inferior antihelix crus	Abdominal pain, dysmenorrhea
	Chest	On antihelix, level with supratragic notch	Chest pain, intercostal neuralgia, mastitis
	Neck	At junction of antihelix and antitragus, near scapha	Strained neck
	Lumbosacral Vertebrae	Curved line of medial border of antihelix corresponds to vertebral column. The line is divided into three parts by drawing two horizontal lines respectively from Pt. Lower Portion of Rectum and Pt. Shoulder Joint. The upper, middle and lower parts are respectively locations of Lumbosacral, Thoracic and Cervical Vertebrae.	Pain at corresponding part of body
	Thoracic Vertebrae		Pain at corresponding part of body
	Cervical Vertebrae		Pain at corresponding part of body
Tragus	External Nose	In center of lateral aspect of tragus	Rhinitis, allergic rhinitis
	Pharynx and Larynx	Upper half of medial aspect of tragus	Pharyngitis, laryngitis, tonsillitis
	Internal Nose	Lower half of medial aspect of tragus	Rhinitis, maxillary sinusitis

Auricular Area	Name of Point	Location	Indication
	Upper Apex of Tragus	At upper tubercle on border of tragus	Toothache, strabismus
	Lower Apex of Tragus	At lower tubercle on border of tragus	Hypotension, allergic diseases
Notch between antitragus and antihelix	Brain Stem	At junction of antitragus and antihelix	Headache, vertigo
Antitragus	Asthma	At apex of antitragus	Asthma, bronchitis, mumps
	Central Rim	At mid-point of line connecting Pt. Asthma and Pt. Stem	Enuresis, insomnia
	Brain	On interior wall of antitragus	Restlessness, pain
	Testis (Ovary)	A part of Pt. Brain, at lower part of interior wall of antitragus	Epididymitis, irregular menstruation
	Forehead	At anterior inferior corner of lateral aspect of antitragus	Headache, dizziness, insomnia
	Occiput	At posterior superior corner of lateral aspect of antitragus	Headache, neurasthenia
	Temple	At mid-point of line connecting Pt. Forehead and Pt. Occiput	Migraine, headache
Periphery of helix crus	Esophagus	At anterior two-thirds of inferior aspect of helix crus	Dysphagia
	Cardiac Orifice	At posterior third of inferior aspect of helix crus	Nausea, vomiting

TABLE OF EAR POINTS

Auricular Area	Name of Point	Location	Indication
	Stomach	At area where helix crus terminates	Gastralgia, vomiting, dyspepsia
	Duodenum	At posterior third of superior aspect of helix crus	Duodenal ulcer, phlorospasm
	Small Intestine	At middle third of superior aspect of helix crus	Dyspepsia, palpitation
	Large Intestine	At anterior third of superior aspect of helix crus	Diarrhea, constipation
	Appendix	Between Pt. Large Intestine and Pt. Small Intestine	Acute simple appendicitis
Cymba conchae	Urinary Bladder	On lower border of inferior antihelix crus, directly above Pt. Large Intestine	Enuresis, retention of urine
	Kidney	On lower border of inferior antihelix crus, directly above Pt. Small Intestine	Lumbago, tinnitus, impaired hearing
	Ureter	Between Pt. Kidney and Pt. Urinary Bladder	Urethra disorders
	Liver	Posterior to Pt. Stomach and Pt. Duodenum	Hypochondriac pain, eye diseases
	Spleen	Inferior to Pt. Liver, close to border of antihelix	Abdominal distention, dyspepsia
	Pancreas and Gall Bladder	Between Pt. Liver and Pt. Kidney	Pancreatitis, dyspepsia, diseases of bile duct

Auricular Area	Name of Point	Location	Indication
		(Pt. Pancreas on the left ear; Pt. Gall Bladder on the right ear)	
Cavum conchae	Mouth	Close to posterior wall of orifice of external auditory meatus	Facial paralysis, ulceration of the mouth
	Heart	In center of cavum conchae	Hysteria, palpitation, arrhythmia
	Lung	A U-shaped area superior, inferior and posterior to Pt. Heart	Cough, asthma, urticaria, skin diseases
	Trachea	Between Pt. Mouth and Pt. Heart	Cough, asthma
	Intertragicus	In cavum conchae, near intertragic notch	Dysmenorrhea, irregular menstruation
	Sanjiao	In middle of four points of Mouth, Intertragicus, Brain and Lung	Constipation, edema
Lobule	Eye 1	On both sides of intertragic notch, the anterior being	Glaucoma, myopia, hordeolum
	Eye 2	Eye 1 and the posterior Eye 2	Glaucoma, myopia, hordeolum
	Toothache 1	At posterior-inferior corner of first section of lobule*	Toothache, anaesthetic for tooth extraction, periodontitis

* In order to facilitate locating the points, the lobule must be divided into nine sections. First, draw a horizontal line at the cartilage border of the intertragic notch. Draw two parallel lines below it to divide the lobule into three equal parts transversely, then mark the second parallel line into three equal parts with points and draw two vertical lines from the points crossing the three horizontal lines to divide the lobule into nine sections. These sections are numbered anteroposteriorly and superoinferiorly in the order of 1, 2, 3, 4, 5, 6, 7, 8, and 9.

Auricular Area	Name of Point	Location	Indication
	Toothache 2	In center of fourth section of lobule	Toothache, anaesthetic for tooth extraction, periodontitis
	Eye	In center of fifth section of lobule	Eye diseases
	Jaw	In center of third section of lobule	Toothache, submandibular arthritis
	Internal Ear	In center of sixth section of lobule	Tinnitus, impaired hearing
	Tonsil	In center of eighth section of lobule	Tonsillitis
	Cheek	At junction of fifth and sixth sections of lobule	Facial paralysis
Back of auricle	Lowering Blood Pressure Groove	At back of ear, in groove between lateral border of protuberance of cartilage and helix	Hypertension
	Yangwei	Superior to Pt. Vagus Root where the auricle intersects the mastoid process	Tinnitus, deafness
	Vagus Root	Level with the helix crus where the auricle intersects the mastoid process	Headache, nasal obstruction, biliary ascariasis
	Upper Portion of Back of Auricle	On protuberance of cartilage at upper portion of back of auricle	Back and lower back pain, skin diseases
	Middle Portion of Back of Auricle	At mid-point of line connecting the two points of upper and	Back and lower back pain, skin diseases

Auricular Area	Name of Point	Location	Indication
		lower portions of back of auricle	
	Lower Portion of Back of Auricle	On protuberance of cartilage at lower portion of back of auricle	Back and lower back pain, skin diseases
	Upper Root of Auricle	At upper border of auricle	Pain, paralysis
	Lower Root of Auricle	At lower border of auricle	Pain, paralysis

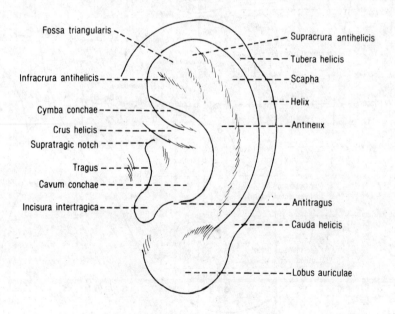

Fig. 2-1 The Anatomy of the Auricle.

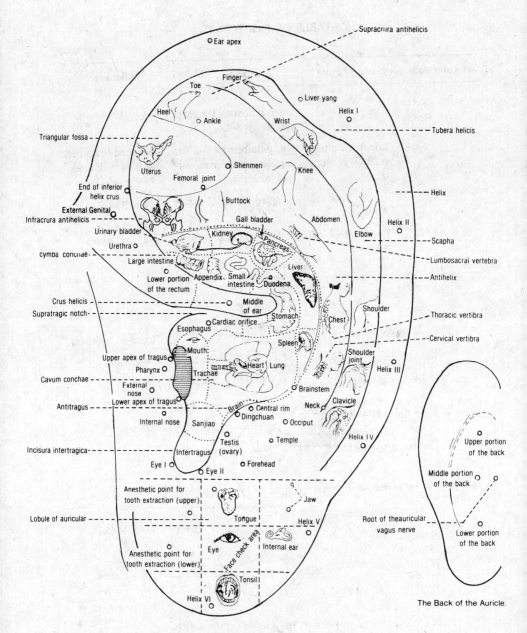

Fig. 2-2 Distribution of Ear Points.

34

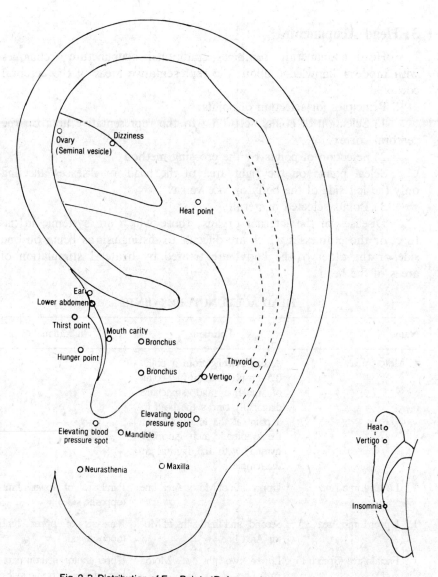

Fig. 2-3 Distribution of Ear Points (Reference).

35

3. Head Acupuncture

Head acupuncture combines traditional acupuncture techniques with modern knowledge about the representative areas of the cerebral cortex.

Principles for selection of points:

1) Selection of points according to the representative area on the cerebral cortex

2) Selection of points by the crossing method

Select points on the right area of the head for diseases affecting only the left side of the body or vice versa.

3) Points selected bilaterally

Diseases of the internal organs, those which are systemic in nature, or those illnesses which are difficult to distinguish as being on one side or the other of the body, are treated by bilateral stimulation of areas of the head.

HEAD ACUPUNCTURE POINTS

Name	Location	Indication
1. Motor Area	A line starting from a point 0.5 cm posterior to mid-point of mid-line and stretching diagonally across the head to a point at the intersection of the zygomatic arch (superior margin) with the hairline at the temple	
1.1 Lower Limb Area	Upper fifth of Motor Area line	Paralysis of lower limb (opposite side)
1.2 Upper Limb Area	Second- and third-fifths of Motor Area line	Paralysis of upper limb (opposite side)
1.3 Facial Area (Speech 1)	Lower two-fifths of Motor Area line	Upper motor neuron paralysis of face (opposite side), motor
2. Sensory Area	A line parallel and 1.5 cm posterior to the Motor Area line	

Name	Location	Indication
2.1 Lower Limb, Head and Trunk Area	Upper fifth of Sensory Area line	Lower back pain (opposite side), numbness or paresthesia in that area, occipital headache, stiff neck, vertigo
2.2 Upper Limb Area	Second- and third-fifths of Sensory Area line	Pain, numbness or other paresthesia of upper limb (opposite side)
2.3 Facial Area	Lower two-fifths of Sensory Area line	Migraine headache, trigeminal neuralgia, toothache (opposite side), arthritis of the temporomandibular joint
3. Chorea and Tremor Control Area	Parallel with and 1.5 cm anterior to Motor Area line	Syndenham's chorea, tremors, palsy and related syndromes
4. Blood Vessel Dilation and Constriction Area	Parallel with and 1.5 cm to Chorea and Tremor Control Area	Superficial edema, hypertension
5. Vertigo and Hearing Area	Horizontal line 1.5 cm above and centered on the apex of ear, 4 cm in length	Tinnitus, vertigo, diminished hearing, Menier's syndrome
6. Speech 2	Vertical line 2 cm beside tuber parietale on back of head, 3 cm in length	Nominal aphasia
7. Speech 3	Overlaps Vertigo and Hearing Area at mid-point and continues 3 cm posteriorly	Receptive aphasia
8. Voluntary Movement Area	With a tuber parietale origin, three needles can be inserted inferiorly, anteriorly and posteriorly to a length of 3 cm. Between them, the three lines will form a 40 ° angle	Apraxia

Name	Location	Indication
9. Leg Motor and Sensory Area	Parallel with mid-line of head, 1 cm beside mid-point (bilaterally), about 3 cm long	Paralysis, pain, or numbness of lower limb, acute lower back sprain, nocturnal urination, prolapsed uterus
10. Vision Area	1 cm lateral to external occipital protuberance, parallel to mid-line of head, 4 cm in length, extending upward	Cortical blindness
11. Balance Area	3 cm lateral to external occipital protuberance, parallel to mid-line of head, 4 cm in length, extending downward	Loss of balance due to cerebellar disorders
12. Stomach Area	Beginning at the hairline directly above pupil of eye, parallel with mid-line of head, 2 cm in length, extending posteriorly	Discomfort in upper abdomen
13. Thoracic Cavity Area	Midway between and parallel with Stomach Area and midline of head, bilaterally, 2 cm in length	Asthma, chest pain, intermittent supraventricular tachycardia
14. Reproduction Area	Parallel and lateral to the Stomach Area at a distance equal to that between Stomach Area and Thoracic Cavity Area, 2 cm in length	Abnormal uterine bleeding, combined with Leg Motor Area for prolapsed uterus

4. Eye Acupuncture

Eye acupuncture, based on the close relationship between the eyes and internal organs, is due stimulation of points on the skin around the eyes. The skin around the eye is divided into eight regions in which there are 13 points: Lung, Large Intestine, Kidney, Urinary Bladder,

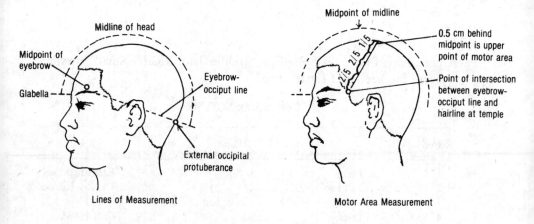

Lines of Measurement

Midline of head
Midpoint of eyebrow
Glabella
Eyebrow-occiput line
External occipital protuberance

Motor Area Measurement

Midpoint of midline
2/5 2/5 1/5
0.5 cm behind midpoint is upper point of motor area
Point of intersection between eyebrow-occiput line and hairline at temple

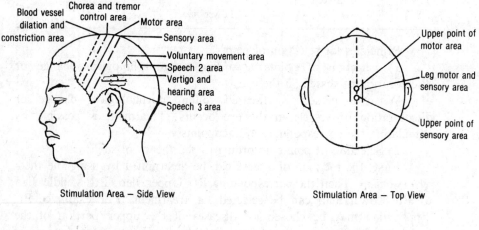

Stimulation Area – Side View

Blood vessel dilation and constriction area
Chorea and tremor control area
Motor area
Sensory area
Voluntary movement area
Speech 2 area
Vertigo and hearing area
Speech 3 area

Stimulation Area – Top View

Upper point of motor area
Leg motor and sensory area
Upper point of sensory area

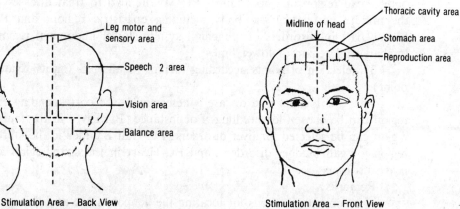

Stimulation Area – Back View

Leg motor and sensory area
Speech 2 area
Vision area
Balance area

Stimulation Area – Front View

Midline of head
Thoracic cavity area
Stomach area
Reproduction area

Fig. 3 Head-acupuncture Areas.

39

Upper Jiao, Liver, Gall Bladder, Middle Jiao, Heart, Small Intestine, Spleen, Stomach and Lower Jiao.

EYE ACUPUNCTURE

Region	Point		
1	Lung		Large Intestine
2	Kidney		Urinary Bladder
3		Upper Jiao	
4	Liver		Gall Bladder
5		Middle Jiao	
6	Heart		Small Intestine
7	Spleen		Stomach
8		Lower Jiao	

Principles for selection of points:

1) Selection of points according to morphological change or discoloration of vessels in the eye

When a person is diseased, often morphological change or discoloration of vessels in the eye occurs. Treatment is possible by stimulating the corresponding eye acupoints.

2) Selection of points according to the theory of *sanjiao*

First, the location of disease can be determined by using the theory of *sanjiao*. Then the corresponding Pt. Upper Jiao, Pt. Middle Jiao or Pt. Lower Jiao can be selected for treatment. For example, Pt. Upper Jiao may be chosen for diseases of the upper portion of the body, head region or upper limbs, Pt. Middle Jiao to treat diseases of the middle portion of the body including epigastric region, and Pt. Lower Jiao for disorders of urogenital system, lower abdominal region, lumbarsacral region or lower limbs.

3) Selection of points according to regions affected (or its related point)

After the locality of a disease is determined, the corresponding eye region can be chosen for needling. For instance, Pt. Liver in the fourth region can be selected for liver disorders, Pt. Gall Bladder in the fourth region for gall bladder disorders, and Pt. Heart in the sixth region for heart disorders.

Remarks:

The concrete methods for locating the acupoints are as follows:

1) The sensitive spot in the region can be used as an acupoint.

2) A spot in the region probed by electro-apparatus can be used as an acupoint for the application of stimuli.

3) In the region, the needle is punctured subcutaneously, parallel with the orbital ridge or inserted perpendicularly and superficially.

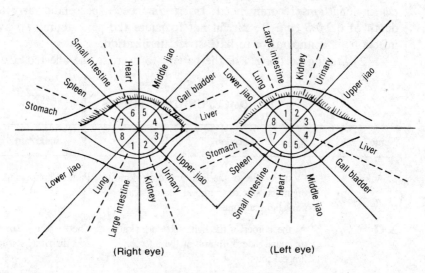

(Right eye)   (Left eye)

Fig. 4 Eye-acupuncture Points.

5. Hand Acupuncture

Hand acupuncture is the stimulation of points on the hands. Principles for selection of points:

1) Selection of points according to the therapeutic properties of the point

For example, if bedwetting is the problem, Pt. Kidney and Pt. Bedwetting may be selected. For fever, Pt. Reduce Fever can be used for relief. When asthma or a cough is the ailment, Pt. Asthma, Pt. Cough or Pt. Lung may be chosen.

2) Selection of points according to the crossing method

A disease affecting the left side of the body is treated by inserting

41

needles in the right hand, and vice versa.

3) Selection of points bilaterally

Diseases of the internal organs with general manifestations, or illnesses difficult to distinguish as affecting only one side or the other of the body, are treated by stimulating bilateral points on the hands.

Remarks:

1) Ask the patient to relax his hands. A gauge 28-30 needle, 0.5 *cun* in length, is recommended. Insert the needle perpendicularly to a depth of 0.3-0.5 *cun*. Be careful not to injure the periosteum. To avoid infection, it is imperative to have strict sterilization.

2) During needling, ask the patient to exercise the affected part.

HAND-ACUPUNCTURE POINTS

Name	Location	Indication
1. Ankle	At the border of the light and dark skin on radial side of thumb at the metacarpophalangeal joint	Pain of ankle joint
2. Chest	At the border of the light and dark skin on radial side of thumb at the interphalangeal joint	Chest pain, vomiting and diarrhea, seizures
3. Eye	At the border of the light and dark skin on ulnar side of thumb at the interphalangeal joint	Eye pain, eye diseases
4. Shoulder	At the border of the light and dark skin on radial side of index finger at the metacarpophalangeal joint	Shoulder pain
5. Forehead	At the border of the light and dark skin on radial side of index finger at the first interphalangeal joint	Frontal headache, stomach spasms, acute gastro-enteritis, acute, uncomplicated appendicitis, pain of knee joint
6. Vertex	At the border of the light and dark flesh on radial side of middle finger at the first interphalangeal joint	Nervous headache, headache at vertex

Name	Location	Indication
7. Side of Head	At the border of the light and dark flesh on ulnar side of fourth finger at the first interphalangeal joint	Migraine headache, pain of chest and ribs, pain in region of spleen and liver, colic of the gall bladder
8. Perineum	At the border of the light and dark skin on radial side of little finger at the first interphalangeal joint	Pain in perineal region
9. Occiput	At the border of the light and dark skin on ulnar side of little finger at the first interphalangeal joint	Occipital headache, acute tonsillitis, arm pain, jaw pain, hiccoughs
10. Vertebrae	At the border of the light and dark skin on ulnar side of little finger at metacarpophalangeal joint	Acute sprain of interspinous ligaments, slipped disk, postoperative lower back pain, coccygeal pain, tinnitus, occluded nose
11. Sciatic Nerve	At the ulnar margin of fourth metacarpophalangeal joint on dorsum of hand	Sciatica, pain of hip joint and buttocks
12. Throat and Toothache	At the ulnar margin of third metacarpophalangeal joint on dorsum of hand	Acute tonsillitis, pharyngitis, trigeminal neuralgia, toothache
13. Neck	At the ulnar margin of second metacarpophalangeal joint on dorsum of hand	Stiff or sprained neck
14. Lumbar	1.5 *cun* anterior to transverse crease on dorsum of wrist, at radial side of the tendon of the second extensor digitorum manus (first point), and the ulnar side of fourth (second point)	Pain of lower back and leg, lower back sprain
15. Gastrointestinal	Midway between Laogong (P. 8) and Daling (P. 7) on the palm	Chronic gastritis, ulcers, indigestion, round worm in bile duct

Name	Location	Indication
16. Cough and Wheeze	On the ulnar side of index finger at metacarpophalangeal joint on the palm	Bronchitis, brochial asthma, tension headache
17. Bedwetting	At the mid-point of transverse crease on the second interphalangeal joint of the little finger, palmar surface	Bedwetting, frequent urination
18. Heel	At the mid-point of the connecting line between Pt. Gastrointestinal and Daling (P. 7)	Heel pain
19. Raise Pressure	At the mid-point of transverse crease on dorsum of wrist	Low blood pressure
20. Hiccup	At the mid-point of transverse crease on dorsum of middle finger at the second interphalangeal joint	Hiccups
21. Reduce Fever	In the web at radial side of middle finger on dorsum of hand	Fever, impaired vision
22. Diarrhea	1 *cun* proximal to the mid-point of a line between the third and fourth metacarpophalangeal joints on the dorsum of hand	Diarrhea
23. Malaria	At the articulation of the first metacarpal bone with the wrist (trapezium), on the radial margin of the thenar eminence	Malaria
24. Tonsil	At the mid-point of ulnar side of first metacarpal bone on the palm	Tonsillitis, pharyngitis
25. Revive	At the tip of middle finger, about 0.2 *cun* from finger nail	Revive from coma
26. Stop Convulsions	At the mid-point of the intersection of the thenar and the hypothenar, palmar surface	Convulsions due to high fever
27. Spleen	At the mid-point of transverse crease of thumb on palmar surface	Stomach problems, edema

Name	Location	Indication
28. Small Intestine	On the palm of hand, at the mid-point of transverse crease of the first interphalangeal joint of the index finger	Small intestinal disorders
29. Large Intestine	At the mid-point of transverse crease of the second interphalangeal joint of the index finger on the palm	Large intestinal disorders
30. Sanjiao	At the mid-point of transverse crease of the first interphalangeal joint of the middle finger on the palm	Diseases of the chest, abdomen and pelvis
31. Heart	At the mid-point of transverse crease of the second interphalangeal joint of the middle finger on the palm	Cardiovascular diseases
32. Liver	At the mid-point of transverse crease of the first interphalangeal joint of the ring finger on the palm	Liver and gall bladder disorders
33. Lung	At the mid-point of transverse crease of the second interphalangeal joint of the ring finger on the palm	Respiratory disorders
34. Life Gate	At the mid-point of transverse crease of the first interphalangeal joint of the little finger on the palm	Genetic system problems
35. Kidney	Same as Pt. Bedwetting	

6. Foot Acupuncture

Foot acupuncture involves the needling of points along the foot.

Principles for selection of points:

1) Selection of points based on the therapeutic properties of the points

For example, Pt. No. 2 should be selected for trigeminal neuralgia, Pt. No. 5 for sciatica, Pts. No. 6 and 19 for disorders of the stom-

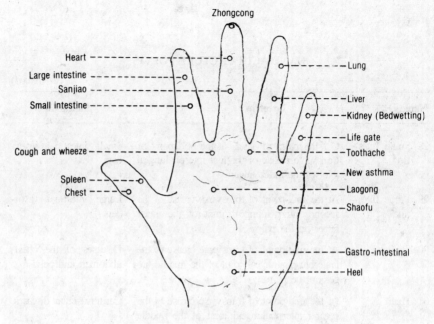

Fig. 5-1 Palmar Aspect.

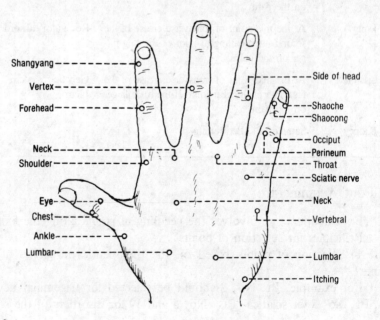

Fig. 5-2 Dorsal Aspect.

ach and intestines.

2) Selection of points based on the crossing method

A disease affecting the left side of the body is treated by inserting needles in the right foot, and vice versa.

3) Selection of points bilaterally

A disease with general manifestations, or which is difficult to distinguish as affecting only one side or the other side of the body, should be needled at bilateral points on the feet.

Remarks:

1) Treat once a day, or once every other day. Seven to ten treatments constitute one course.

2) If required, electro-acupuncture may be added.

3) While needling is in progress, ask the patient to exercise his affected part.

4) Strict sterilization is a must and care must be taken not to damage the periosteum.

FOOT-ACUPUNCTURE POINTS

Pt. No.	Location	Indication	Needling Method
1	1 *cun* above the mid-point at base of heel, posterior aspect	Common cold, headache, sinusitis, rhinitis	Straight insertion, 0.5 *cun*
2	1 *cun* medial to the point which is 3 *cun* directly above the mid-point of posterior border of heel	Trigeminal neuralgia	Straight insertion or slanted insertion, 0.5-1.5 *cun*
3	3 *cun* directly above the mid-point of posterior of heel (The mid-point of the connecting line between the lateral malleolus and the medial malleolus on the bottom of foot)	Neurasthenia, hysteria, insomnia, hypotension	Straight insertion or slanted downward, 0.5-1 *cun*
4	1 *cun* lateral to the place which is 3 *cun* directly above the mid-point of posterior border of heel	Intercostal neuralgia, chest pain, stifling sensation in chest	Straight insertion, 0.5 *cun*

(Continued)

Pt. No.	Location	Indication	Needling Method
5	1.5 *cun* lateral to middle line and 4 *cun* directly above heel	Sciatica, chest pain, appendisitis	Straight insertion or slanted downward, 1-1.5 *cun*
6	1 *cun* medial to middle line and 5 *cun* directly above heel	Dysentery, diarrhea, duodenal ulcer	Straight or slanted insertion, 0.5-1.5 *cun*
7	5 *cun* directly above the mid-point of posterior border of heel	Asthma, incomplete maturation of brain	Straight or slanted insertion, 0.5-1.5 *cun*
8	1 *cun* lateral to Pt. No. 2	Neurasthenia, seizures, neurosis	Straight insertion or slanted medially, 0.5-1 *cun*
9	4 *cun* posteriorly to the junction between the first toe and the second toe	Dysentery, diarrhea, uteritis	Straight insertion or slanted medially, 0.5-1 *cun*
10	1 *cun* medial to Yongquan (K. 1)	Chronic gastroenteritis, gastrospasm	Straight insertion, 1 *cun*
11	2 *cun* lateral to Yongquan (K. 1)	Shoulder pain, urticaria	Straight insertion or slanted downward, 0.5-1 *cun*
12	1 *cun* posterior to the junction between the first toe and the second toe	Toothache	Straight insertion, 0.5-1 *cun*
13	1 *cun* posterior to mid-point of transverse crease of the fifth toe	Toothache	Straight insertion or slanted downward, 0.5-1 *cun*
14	At mid-point of transverse crease of the fifth toe	Incontinence, frequent urination	Straight insertion or slanted downward, 0.5 *cun*
15	In depression on either side, 0.5 *cun* inferior to mid-point of transverse crease of ankle joint	Lower back pain, leg pain, gastrocnemius spasm	Joining insertion or slanted upward, 1.5-2 *cun*

(Continued)

Pt. No.	Location	Indication	Needling Method
16	In depression above the tubercle of the navicular on medial aspect of foot	Hypertension, mumps, acute tonsillitis	Straight insertion, 0.5 *cun*
17	2.5 *cun* inferior to mid-point of transverse crease of the ankle joint	Angina pectoris, asthma, common cold	Pricking or straight insertion, 0.5-1 *cun*
18	In depression medial and anterior to the first metatarsal bone on dorsum of foot	Acute lumbar sprain, chest pain, stifling sensation of the chest	Straight or slanted insertion, 1-2 *cun*
19	3 *cun* posterior to the junction between the second toe and the third toe on dorsum of foot	Headache, otitis media, acute or chronic gastroenteritis, gastro-duodenal ulcer	Straight insertion or slanted upward, 2 *cun*
20	2 *cun* posterior to the junction between the third toe and the fourth toe on dorsum of foot	Stiff neck	Straight insertion or slanted upward, 1.5 *cun*
21	0.5 *cun* posterior to the junction between the fourth toe and the fifth toe on dorsum of foot	Sciatica, mumps, tonsillitis	Straight or slanted insertion, 0.5-1 *cun*
22	1 *cun* posterior to the junction between the first toe and the second toe on dorsum of foot	Acute tonsillitis, mumps, hypertension	Straight insertion or slanted upward, 1-2 *cun*
23	At metacarpophalangeal joint on medial aspect of extensor hallucis longus tendon on dorsum of foot	Acute tonsillitis, mumps, hypertension, nodularis, eczema, urticaria	Pricking or shallow insertion, 0.5-1 *cun*
24	At border of light and dark skin on medial aspect of the second interphalangeal joint of the second toe	Headache, otitis media	Pricking, 0.1-0.3 *cun*

(Continued)

Pt. No.	Location	Indication	Needling Method
25	At border of light and dark skin on medial aspect of the second interphalangeal joint of the third toe	Headache	Pricking, 0.1-0.3 *cun*
26	At border of light and dark skin on medial aspect of the second interphalangeal joint of the fourth toe	Headache, hypertension	Pricking, 0.1-0.3 *cun*
27	At mid-point of the connecting line between Taibai (Sp. 3) and Gongsun (Sp. 4)	Seizures, hysteria, abdominal pain	Transverse insertion, 0.3-1 *cun*
28	In depression posterior and inferior to the tubercle of navicular on medial aspect of foot	Dysmenorrhea, functional uterine bleeding, adnexitis	Straight insertion, 2 *cun*
29	2 *cun* directly below middle of medial malleolus	Functional uterine bleeding, bronchitis, asthma	Straight insertion or transverse insertion, 1-3 *cun*
30	1.5 *cun* above posterior border of lateral malleolus	Sciatica, lumbar pain, headache	Transverse insertion or slanted upward, 1-2 *cun*

7. Wrist-and-ankle Acupuncture

Stimulation of points on the wrist or ankle can be used to relieve diseases.

Principles for selection of points:

1) Selection of points according to the therapeutic properties of the points

For example, Pt. Lower 1 may be chosen for dysmenorrhea, Pt. Upper 1 for stomach pain, Pt. Upper 2 for chest pain, Pt. Lower 2 for hypochondriac pain, etc.

2) Selection of points unilaterally, on the affected side

3) Selection of points bilaterally, to deal with a disease with gener-

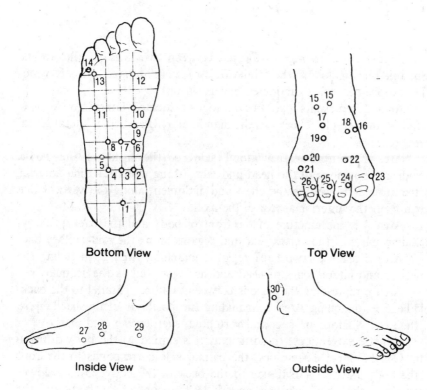

Bottom View

Top View

Inside View

Outside View

Fig. 6 Foot-acupuncture Points.

Measurement:

1)The distance from mid-point of toe posterior border of heel to the web between the second toe and the third toe is measured as 10 *cun*.

2)The distance between every two parallel lines is 1 *cun*.

3)The distance from the top of lateral malleolus (or medial malleolus) to the lateral border of foot (or the medial border of foot) is measured as 3 *cun*.

al manifestations

4) Selection of points according to the disease's locality Select points on the wrist for treatment of a disease located above the diaphragm, or points on the ankle for treatment of a disease located below the diaphragm.

Remarks

Insert the needle subcutaneously and upwardly, 1-1.5 *cun* in depth. If hands or feet are affected, point the tip of the needle downward. Retain the needles for 20-30 minutes.

Distribution of areas of the body:

The body is divided into six areas.

Area 1 refers to regions located between two lines parallel to the front mid-line, including the forehead, eyes, nose, tongue, throat, windpipe, esophagus, heart, abdomen and perineum.

Area 2 represents two frontal regions located lateral to Area 1, including the temple, cheek, teeth, mandibular, breast and lateral abdomen.

Area 3 comprises the lateral sides of the front of the body, including the regions of the head and face, along a vertical line anterior to the auricle, as well as the chest and abdomen, along the vertical line down from the anterior aspect of the axilla.

Area 4 is the juncture of the front of body and the back of body, including parts of the vertex, ear and regions along the mid-axillary line.

Area 5 refers to two back regions, matching Area 2, including the posterior and lateral sides of head and neck, as well as the scapulae.

Area 6 represents the regions between two lines parallel to the back-middle line, matching Area 1, including the posterior of the head, nape of the neck, spinous process and vertebrae, sacrococcyx and anus.

For the extremities, the distribution is similar to the body distribution. On the upper extremities, the palmar side corresponds to the front of the body and the dorsal side to the back of the body. On the lower extremities, the tibial side corresponds to the front of the body and the fibular side to the back of the body.

Using the diaphragm as a dividing line, the six areas, mentioned above, can also be subdivided into upper and lower areas.

WRIST-AND-ANKLE ACUPUNCTURE POINTS

Area	Point	Location	Indication
1	Upper 1	In depression anterior to border of ulnar bone on the ulnar side of the little finger	Front headache, eye and nose disorders, facial nerveritis, toothache, sore-throat, cough, asthma, palpitation, dizziness, night sweating, insomnia, depression, mania, seizures

WRIST-AND-ANKLE ACUPUNCTURE POINTS

(Continued)

Area	Point	Location	Indication
	Lower 1	Near the medial border of tendo calcaneus	Epigastric distention and pain, pain around navel, dysmenorrhea, leukorrhagia, enuresis, pruritus, heel pain
2	Upper 2	Also Neiguan (P. 6), 2 *cun* above the transverse crease of the wrist, between the tendons of M. palmaris longus and M. flexor carpi radialis	Submandibular pain and swelling, stifling sensation in the chest, chest pain, asthma, delactation
	Lower 2	Near the posterior border of tibia bone in the center of medial aspect	Hypochondriac pain, abdominal pain, allergic enteritis
3	Upper 3	Near the lateral aspect of radial nerve	Hypertension, chest pain
	Lower 3	1 cm medial to the anterior border of the tibia bone	Knee joint pain
4	Upper 4	On the border of the radius, on dorsum aspect	Vertical headache, ear disorders, inflammation of temporomandibular joint, periarthritis of shoulder, chest pain
	Lower 4	At mid-point between the anterior border of the fibula and the anterior border of the tibia	Pain of quadriceps femoris, gonarthritis, flaccidity and pain of the lower limbs, paralysis of the lower limbs, pain of phalangeal joint
5	Upper 5	Also Waiguan (S.J. 5), on the dorsum of hand between the radius and ulna	Pain of posterior temples, periarthritis of shoulder, numbness of upper limbs, motor impairment of upper limbs, joint pain of elbow, wrist and finger
	Lower 5	In the center of lateral aspect of leg	Pain of hip joint, sprain of ankle joint

WRIST-AND-ANKLE ACUPUNCTURE POINTS

(Continued)

Area	Point	Location	Indication
6	Upper 6	On the border of the ulna	Occipital headache, pain of nape, pain along the cervical vertebrae and the thoracic vertebrae
	Lower 6	Near the lateral border of tendo calcaneus	Acute lumbar sprain, lumbar muscle sprain, pain of sacroiliac articulation, sciatica, spasm of gastrocnemius muscle, dorsal digital pain of foot

Note:
1. Points Upper 1-6 are located 2 *cun* above the transverse crease of the wrist.
2. Points Lower 1-6 are located 3 *cun* above the ankle.

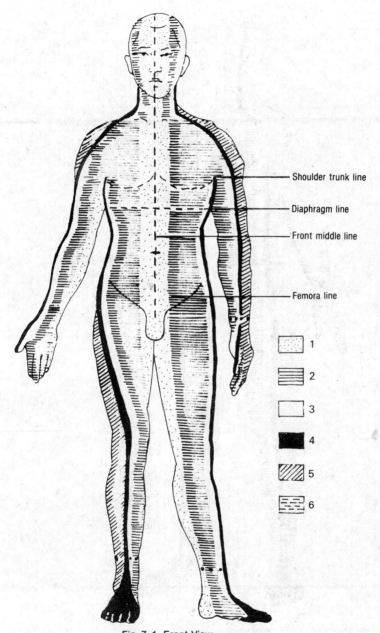

Shoulder trunk line

Diaphragm line

Front middle line

Femora line

1
2
3
4
5
6

Fig. 7-1 Front View

Fig. 7 Distribution of Wrist-and-Ankle Acupuncture Area.

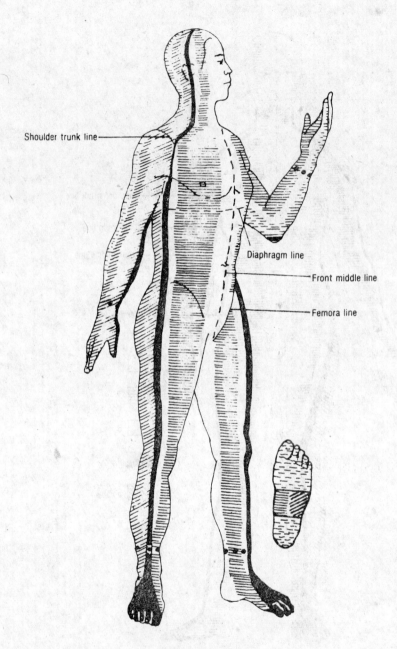

Shoulder trunk line

Diaphragm line

Front middle line

Femora line

Fig. 7-2 Side View

56

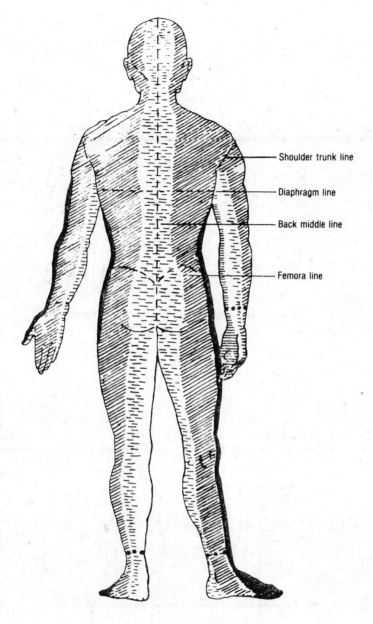

Fig. 7-3 Back View

57

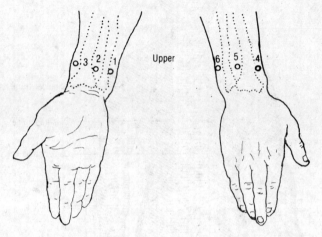

Fig. 7-4 Palmar Aspect

Fig. 7-5 Dorsal Aspect

Upper

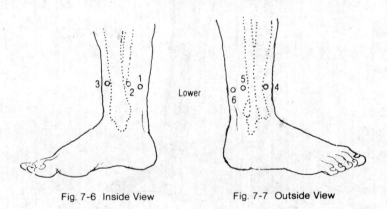

Fig. 7-6 Inside View

Fig. 7-7 Outside View

Lower

58

Chapter II

Acupuncture Therapies

1. Syncope

Principal points: Renzhong (Du 26), Neiguan (P. 6), Yongquan (K. 1), Suliao (Du 25), Zhongchong (P. 9), Zusanli (St. 36)

Method: When needling Renzhong (Du 26), point the tip of the needle upward with slanted insertion to a depth of 0.5-0.7 *cun.* Apply slanted and upward insertion to Neiguan (P. 6). Deep insertion is needed for Suliao (Du 25). Puncture Zhongchong (P. 9) shallowly and withdraw the needle quickly. The needle can be inserted into Zusanli (St. 36) to a depth of 2 *cun.* Apply continuous manipulation and strong stimulation to each point until the blood pressure becomes stable. Then periodic manipulation is needed.

Other therapies:

1. Moxibustion

Points: Baihui (Du 20), Shenque (Ren 8), Guanyuan (Ren 4), Qihai (Ren 6)

Method: Use moxibustion with a moxa stick or moxa cone. Indirect moxibustion with salt is applied at Shenque (Ren 8). The number of cones is determined by the restoration of pulse or sweating stopped.

2. Ear acupuncture

Points: Heart, Shenmen, End of Inferior Helix Crus, Lower Apex of Tragus, Brain

Method: Puncture bilaterally with moderate stimulation and periodic manipulation. The needles remain in position for 1-2 hours.

Remarks: Acupuncture and moxibustion are first-aid treatments which must be combined with other medications.

REFERENCE:
Seven emergency methods of acupuncture and moxibustion in the treatment of syncope

1) Clear heat for resuscitation: Dazhui (Du 14), Shixuan (Extra)

2) Remove phlegm obstruction for resuscitation: Neiguan (P. 6), Zhongwan (Ren 12)

3) Raise *yang* and promote *qi* circulation for resuscitation: Renzhong (Du 26), Guanyuan (Ren 4)

4) Bring down blood pressure for resuscitation: Weizhong (U.B. 40), Zhiyin (U.B. 67), Changqiang (Du 1)

5) Calm the liver and lower the endogenous wind: Dadun (Liv. 1), Sanyinjiao (Sp. 6)

6) Recapture *yang* and avert the collapsing state: Guanyuan (Ren 4), Qihai (Ren 6)

7) Soothe *qi* for resuscitation: Shanzhong (Ren 17), Zhongwan (Ren 12)

(*Source:* Zhejiang Journal of Traditional Chinese Medicine, 15(8):370, 1980)

2. Headache

Principal points: Baihui (Du 20), Taiyang (Extra), Fengchi (G.B. 20)

Method: Fengchi (G.B. 20) is punctured first. Let the needling sensation extend to the temple. The needles remain inserted for 20-30 minutes with periodic manipulation. Treat daily. Ten treatments constitute one course.

Supplementary points:

Frontal headache: Shangxing (Du 23), Touwei (St. 8), Yintang (Extra), Hegu (L.I. 4)

Parietal headache: Qianding (Du 21), Taichong (Liv. 3), Yongquan (K. 1)

One-side headache: Shuaigu (G.B. 8), Hand-Zhongzhu (S.J. 3), Taiyang (Extra) joining to Shuaigu (G.B. 8)

Occipital headache: Houding (Du 19), Tianzhu (U.B. 10), Houxi (S.I. 3)

Invasion by exogenous pathogenic factors: Hegu (L.I. 4), Lieque (Lu. 7)

Deficiency of *qi* and blood: Zusanli (St. 36), Xuehai (Sp. 10)

Upward disturbance of wind-phlegm: Fenglong (St. 40), Taichong (Liv. 3), Taixi (K. 3)

Blood stagnation: Hegu (L.I. 4), Sanyinjiao (Sp. 6)

Other therapies:

1. Cutaneous acupuncture

Points: Taiyang (Extra), Yintang (Extra), Ashi point

Method: Use cutaneous needles to tap until the local skin becomes congested. Then apply cupping. This method is applicable to the treatment of headaches due to an invasion by exogenous pathogenic wind or a hyperfunction of the *yang* of the liver.

2. Ear acupuncture

Points: Occiput, Forehead, Brain, Shenmen

Method: 2-3 points are usually chosen during one session. Use filiform needles, applying moderate stimulation. The needles are left in place for 20-30 minutes, with periodic manipulation once every five minutes. Also needle-embedding may be used for 3-7 days. As to the stubborn headache, the venous bleeding method applied to the back of the ear can be used.

3. Hydro-acupuncture

Point: Fengchi (G.B. 20)

Method: For stubborn headache, a 3.5 ml of 0.25% procaine and 0.5 ml of caffeine solution is injected into Fengchi (G.B. 20), (0.5-1 ml of solution each application), or 0.1 ml is injected into Ashi point.

Remarks: Acupuncture is quite effective in relieving pain in the treatment of headaches.

REFERENCES:

1. Results of needling Taichong (Liv. 3) in the treatment of 30 cases of vascular headache

Points: Taichong (Liv. 3), Yangfu (G.B. 38), Ashi point, all on the affected side

Method: First, a needle is rapidly inserted into Taichong (Liv. 3) to a depth of 1 *cun*. Apply a high degree of lifting, thrusting, twirling and rotating, with a large range of movement tolerable to the patient. After manipulating the needle for 3-5 minutes, puncture Yangfu (G.B. 38) and Ashi point with periodic manipulation, approximately once every 10 minutes. The needles remain inserted for 30-60 minutes. Treat daily.

Results: In 22 cases, the pain was completely checked with no short-term relapse. The pain was reduced in 7 cases, while there was no effect in only 1 case.

(*Source:* Shaanxi Journal of Traditional Chinese Medicine, 4(2):27, 1983)

2. Observation of therapeutic results in 34 cases of vascular headaches treated with head acupuncture

Points: Lower two-fifths of Sensory Area, bilateral

Method: Reinforcing method, twirling and rotating are used with a frequency of 100 times per minute, with 90-180-degree periodic manipulation, once every five minutes. Try to get soreness, distention and a sensation of numbness. The needles are left in place for 15 minutes. Treat once every other day. Seven treatments constitute one course.

Results: Six cases showed a marked effect. Improvement was seen in 23 cases, while no effect was observed in 5 cases. The total effective rate reached 85.3 percent.

(*Source:* Shanghai Journal of Acupuncture and Moxibustion, 4(15), 1987)

3. Observed results of acupuncture in the treatment of 123 cases of headache

Points:

Taiyang headache: Kunlun (U.B. 60), Houxi (S.I. 3), Fengchi (G.B. 20)

Shaoyang headache: Xuanzhong (G.B. 39), Fengchi (G.B. 20), Taiyang (Extra)

Yangming headache: Zhongwan (Ren 12), Hegu (L.I. 4), Neiting (St. 44)

Jueyin headache: Xingjian (Liv. 2), Neiguan (P. 6), Foot-Qiaoyin (G.B. 44)

Method: Treat daily. Seven treatments constitute one course. Normally, effective treatment requires 1-2 courses.

Results: The number of cases which showed total recovery was 67. There was a marked effect in 38 cases, some level of improvement in 11 cases, and no effect in 7 cases.

(*Source:* Liaoning Journal of Traditional Chinese Medicine, (11):34, 1983)

4. Clinical observation on the application of hand acupuncture in the treatment of 102 cases of headache

Points:

Yangming headache: Yintang (Extra), Forehead (on the radial side of the index finger, close to the phalangeal joint at the junction of the white and red skin)

Shaoyang headache: Taiyang (Extra), Side of Head (on the ulnar side of the ring finger, close to the phalangeal joint at the junction of the white and red skin)

Jueyin headache: Baihui (Du 20), Vertex (on the radial side of the middle finger, close to the phalangeal joint, at the junction of the white and red skin)

Taiyang headache: Fengchi (G.B. 20), Occiput (on the ulnar side of the little finger, close to the phalangeal joint, at the junction of the white and red skin)

Method: Use gauge 28 needles at an acute angle, inserting to a depth of 0.5 *cun*. Lift and rotate the needles for 30 seconds. Remain the needles for 30 minutes. Treat daily. Ten treatments constitute one course.

Results: Of 102 cases treated, 39 cases were cured, 36 cases showed marked effects, 20 cases showed some improvement, and 7 cases displayed no effect. The total effective rate reached 93.1 percent.

(*Source:* Shaanxi Journal of Traditional Chinese Medicine, (7):326, 1988)

5. Observation of the application of three needles in treating 34 cases of one-side headache

Principal points: Taiyang (Extra) and Taichong (Liv. 3) on the affected side, Hegu (L.I. 4) on the healthy side

Supplementary points:

Chronic severe headache: Fengchi (G.B. 20), Shuaigu (G.B. 8)

Method: Taiyang (Extra) is inserted at an acute angle towards Quanliao (S.I. 18), penetrating through the medial aspect of the zygomatic arch, enabling the needling sensation to extend to the mandible on the affected side. The needles are left in place for 30 minutes with periodic manipulation.

Results: All cases were cured after 1-3 treatments, with the exception of 1 unpursued case.

(*Source:* Jiangsu Journal of Traditional Chinese Medicine, 9(8):27, 1988)

6. Observations of the therapeutic results of acupuncture in the treatment of 90 cases of postconcussion syndrome

Points:

Deficient *yin* of the liver and kidney: a) Fengchi (G.B. 20), Xuanlu (G.B. 5), Baihui (Du 20) joining to Sishencong (Extra); b) Hegu (L.I. 4), Taichong (Liv. 3), moxi Yongquan (K. 1), Yamen (Du 15), Changqiang (Du 1), Ear points (Liver, Central Rim, Brain)

Qi deficiency and accumulation of phlegm: a) Taiyang (Extra), Houxi (S.I. 3); b) Fengfu (Du 16), Shenting (Du 24), Zusanli (St. 36), Moxi Fenglong (St. 40), Qihai (Ren 6), Baihui (Du 20), Ear points (Spleen, Shenmen, Brain Stem)

Method: Treat daily, retaining the position of the needles for 30 minutes. Twelve treatments constitute one course. The interval between courses is one week.

Results: A complete reversal was observed in 47 cases, with marked effects observed in an additional 18 cases. Improvement was shown in 17 cases, and no effect was seen in 8 cases.

(*Source:* Chinese Acupuncture & Moxibustion, 5(6):13, 1985)

3. Cerebrovascular Accident (Apoplexy)

I. Acute condition

1) Tense syndrome

Principal points: Renzhong (Du 26), Baihui (Du 20), Yongquan (K. 1), Taichong (Liv. 3), the 12 Jing-Well points of both hands (Lu. 11, H. 9, P. 9, L.I. 1, S.J. 1, S.I. 1), Laogong (P. 8)

Method: Strong stimulation is used. When needling Renzhong (Du 26), the needle is deeply inserted, angling upward, and repeated lift-thrust stimulation is required to strengthen the needling sensation. Cause bleeding at the 12 Jing-Well points (Lu. 11, H. 9, P. 9, L.I. 1, S.J. 1, S.I. 1). The other points are punctured with continued manipulation. The needles are not left inserted.

Supplementary points:

Clenched jaws: Jiache (St. 6), Hegu (L.I. 4)

Fever: Quchi (L.I. 11)

2) Flaccid syndrome

Principal points: Guanyuan (Ren 4), Shenque (Ren 8)

Method: Moxibustion, using large moxa cones, is used for both points, plus salt insulated cones on Shenque (Ren 8). Continue the moxibustion until warmth is regained in the limbs and a pulse is restored.

Supplementary points:

Sweating: Yinxi (H. 6), Houxi (S.I. 3)

Incontinence of urine: Zhongji (Ren 3), Sanyinjiao (Sp. 6)

II. Mild condition and its sequelae

1) Paralysis

Principal points:

Paralysis of upper limbs: Jianyu (L.I. 15), Jianliao (S.J. 14), Quchi (L.I. 11), Shousanli (L.I. 10), Waiguan (S.J. 5), Hegu (L.I. 4)

Paralysis of lower limbs: Huantiao (G.B. 30), Fengshi (G.B. 31), Yanglingquan (G.B. 34), Zusanli (St. 36), Jiexi (St. 41), Weizhong (U.B. 40), Sanyinjiao (Sp. 6), Yinlingquan (Sp. 9), Kunlun (U.B. 60)

Method: During one session, 5-7 points on the paralyzed area are used. Puncture with moderate stimulation, and electro-acupuncture can be combined with moderate stimulation. Needle the affected side first, then the healthy side can be needled with mild stimulation. For a chronic case, moxibustion can be applied after withdrawal of the needles.

Supplementary points:

Convulsion at the elbow: Quze (P. 3)

Convulsion at the wrist: Daling (P. 7)

Convulsion at the knee: Ququan (Liv. 8)

Convulsion at the ankle: Taixi (K. 3)

2) Facial paralysis

Principal points: Dicang (St. 4), Jiache (St. 6), Yangbai (G.B. 14), Zanzhu (U.B. 2), Yingxiang (L.I. 20), Xiaguan (St. 7), Hegu (L.I. 4), Neiting (St. 44), Qianzhen (Extra)

Method: For an acute case, the points on the affected side can be needled. For a chronic case, the points on both the affected and healthy sides can be needled. Bilateral Hegu (L.I. 4) and Neiguan (P. 6) are always selected for the treatment. Puncture with moderate stimulation. Treat daily or once every other day. Moxibustion can also be combined with needling.

Supplementary points:

Salivation: Chengjiang (Ren 24)

3) Aphasia

Principal points: Lianquan (Ren 23), Yamen (Du 15), Tongli (H. 5)

Method: Puncture Yamen (Du 15) to a depth of 1 *cun*, rotating but not lifting and thrusting. Withdraw the needle right after the needling sensation is obtained. Leave the needles inserted in Lianquan (Ren 23) and Tongli (H. 5) for 20-30 minutes, with moderate stimulation.

Supplementary points:

Stiffness of the tongue: Jinjin-Yuye (Extra), with 1 *cun* insertion; the needle is removed immediately.

4) Dysphagia

Points: Lianquan (Ren 23), Neck-Futu (L.I. 18), Fengchi (G.B. 20), Hegu (L.I. 4)

Method: Neck-Futu (L.I. 18) should be punctured shallowly. Insert at Fengchi (G.B. 20) to a depth of 1 *cun*, and rotate. Slanted insertion to the left and right can be used when needling Lianquan (Ren 23). Treatment is given daily or once every other day. Leave the needles in place for 15 minutes.

Other therapies:

1. Ear acupuncture

Principal points: Kidney, Lower Apex of Tragus, Spleen, Heart, Liver, Gall Bladder, Shenmen, Brain, Central Rim, ear points corresponding to the portion suffering paralysis

Supplementary points:

Dysphagia: Mouth, Vagus Root, Pharynx and Larynx

Method: Choose 3-5 points for a session. Puncture bilaterally with filiform needles and apply moderate stimulation. Treat daily or once every other day. The needles are left in place for 30-60 minutes.

2. Head acupuncture (suitable for the sequelae)

Points: Opposite Motor Area, Leg Motor and Sensory Area, Sensory Area, Speech Area

Method: Insert the needles horizontally in the scalp to a depth of 0.5-1 *cun*, and rotate frequently. Encourage the patient to exercise the affected side. Treat once every other day.

3. Hydro-acupuncture (suitable for limb paralysis)

Points: Jianyu (L.I. 15), Quchi (L.I. 11), Hegu (L.I. 4), Fengshi (G.B. 31), Yanglingquan (G.B. 34), Zusanli (St. 36)

Method: Inject a 0.1 mg Vitamin B_{12} or 100 mg Vitamin B_1 solution into the above-mentioned points. Treat once every other day.

4. Cutaneous acupuncture (suitable for hemiplegia)

Points: Ganshu (U.B. 18), Shenshu (U.B. 23), Baliao (U.B. 31-34), Jiaji points (Extra, the 5th-21th vertebrae), Quchi (L.I. 11), Taiyuan (Lu. 9), Yanglingquan (G.B. 34), Fengshi (G.B. 31), Xuanzhong (G.B. 39)

Method: Tap with cutaneous needles until the skin becomes congested. Treat once every other day.

5. Cupping (suitable for hemiplegia)

Points: Jianyu (L.I. 15), Quchi (L.I. 11), Yangchi (S.J. 4), Huantiao (G.B. 30), Yanglingquan (G.B. 34), Qiuxu (G.B. 40)

Method: Choose 1-2 points on upper limbs and lower limbs for cupping in a session. Place the cups for 5-10 minutes. Treat once every 2-3 days.

Remarks: Acupuncture and moxibustion therapies are effective on cerebrovascular accident, and quite effective in the treatment of its sequelae. For an acute, severe case, Chinese and Western methods should be combined to save the patient. If the patient has paralyzed limbs and slurred speech, physical and speech therapy is encouraged.

REFERENCES:

1. Clinical observations of 167 cases using eye acupuncture in the treatment of apoplexy

Points: Bilateral Upper Jiao, Lower Jiao

Method: Press the skin around the eyeball with a finger to tighten it. Insert a gauge 32, 0.5 *cun* long, stainless steel needle horizontally to a depth of 0.2 *cun* in the area around the orbital ridge. Without manipulating, retain the needle for 5-10 minutes. Treat daily. Ten treatments constitute one course.

Results: Of 167 cases treated, 40 cases (24 percent) recovered, 66 cases (39.5 percent) showed marked success, 56 cases (33.5 percent) showed some improvement, and 5 cases (3 percent) showed no effect. The total effective rate was 97 percent.

(*Source:* Chinese Acupuncture & Moxibustion, (6):23, 1987)

2. Observation of the therapeutic results of moxibustion in treating hemiplegia

Points: Tianchuang (S.I. 16), Baihui (Du 20)

Method: Burn moxa cones on each point for 15 minutes. Treat once or twice a day. Thirty treatments constitute one course. The interval between courses is 3-5 days.

Results: After treatment, 13 cases recovered, 13 cases showed marked improvement, 6 cases showed some level of improvement, and 1 case showed no effect. The total effective rate was 97 percent.

(*Source:* Shandong Journal of Traditional Chinese Medicine, (6):12, 1987)

3. The results of cutaneous acupuncture used to treat 106 cases of hemiplegia

Principal points: The opposite slanted line starting from the vertex to the temporal region, Upper 1/3, Middle 1/3, and Lower 1/3 (Motor Area)

Supplementary points:

Hypertension: Mid-line of the vertex

Slurred speech: Mid-line of the forehead

Method: Adopt the lift-thrust and rotate-twirl method to produce reinforcing or reducing. This method is repeated 3-5 times. Keep needles inserted for 2-24 hours. Treat daily or once every other day. Ten treatments constitute one course. Encourage the patient to do functional exercises.

Results: The treatment cured 18 cases and produced a marked effect in 63 cases; 23 cases showed some improvement, and 2 cases showed no effect. The total effective rate was 98.1 percent.

(*Source:* Journal of Zhejiang College of Traditional Chinese Medicine, 12(2):53, 1988)

4. A study on plum-blossom needling of Shegen (Extra, root of the tongue) in the treatment of aphasia in apoplexy

Principal points: Shegen (Extra), Zhimai (Extra), Zengyin (Extra)

Supplementary points:

Dysphagia: Yifeng (S.J. 17), Fengfu (Du 16)

Dysphonia: Biantaoti (Extra)

Method: Insert a round-sharp gauge 20 needle to a depth of 0.5 *cun*, lifting and thrusting several times until the needling sensation under the tongue extending to the throat is felt. When needling the supplementary points, insert a common filiform needle towards the root of the tongue to a depth of 1.5-2 *cun*. Puncture with a lifting-thrusting method and strong stimulation until the needling sensation reaches the bottom of the tongue. Once a needling sensation is obtained, remove the needles. Treat daily or once every other day. If bleeding occurs, rinse with cold water.

Results: The method cured 24 cases and produced a marked effect in 4 cases; 2 cases showed some improvement, and 1 case showed no effect after 15 treatments.

(*Source:* Hebei Journal of Traditional Chinese Medicine, (1):38, 1987)

5. Therapeutic results observed in the treatment of 144 cases of cerebral apoplexy, using head acupuncture

Points:

Paralysis of lower limbs: Upper 1/5 of the opposite anterior slanted line from the vertex to the temple, the first line parallels with mid-line of head

Paralysis of upper limbs: Middle 2/5 of the opposite anterior slanted line from the vertex to the temple

Facial paralysis, salivation, deviation of the tongue and aphemia: Lower 2/5 of the opposite anterior slanted line from the vertex to the temple

Cerebellar degeneration: The line lateral to and below the external occipital protuberance, parallel to mid-line of head

Motor impairment of the hand: Voluntary Movement Area

Method: Insert a gauge 28 filiform needle horizontally, to a depth of 1-5 *cun*. After the needling sensation is obtained, leave the needles in place for 30-40 minutes. Manipulate the needles for 5-8 minutes, 2-3 times, while still inserted. Encourage the patient to exercise the affected limbs during the manipulations. Treat daily. Fifteen treatments constitute one course. The interval between courses is 3-5 days.

Results: This treatment cured 44 cases, or 30.56 percent, and produced a marked effect in 62 cases, or 43.06 percent. Some improvement was seen in 37 cases, or 25.69 percent, and only 1 case, or 0.69 percent, showed no effect.

(*Source:* Henan Traditional Chinese Medicine, (4):21, 1987)

6. The observed results of the treatment of 35 cases of cerebrovascular disease (bulbar paralysis) by the use of body acupuncture and head acupuncture

Points: Stomach Area, Zusanli (St. 36), Renzhong (Du 26), Baihui (Du 20), Fengfu (Du 16), Fengchi (G.B. 20), Chengjiang (Ren 24), Hegu (L.I. 4), Lianquan (Ren 23), Tongli (H. 5), Yamen (Du 15), Dicang (St. 4), Xiaguan (St. 7), Jiache (St. 6), Zhaohai (K. 6), Neiting (St. 44), Sanyinjiao (Sp. 6), Fenglong (St. 40), Yinlingquan (Sp. 9)

Method: Connect needles to an electro-stimulator. Treat daily. Ten treatments constitute one course.

Results: Among 35 cases, 21 were cured, 12 showed marked effect, 1 case showed some improvement and only 1 case showed no effect.

(*Source:* Beijing Medicine, 2(6):379, 1980)

7. Observations of the effects of acupuncture in treating 20 cases of pseudobulbar paralysis

Points: Bilateral Fengchi (G.B. 20), Yamen (Du 15)

Method: Make a perpendicular insertion at Fengchi (G.B. 20) to a depth of 0.5-1 *cun*, keeping the tip of the needle pointing to the opposite orbital ridge. Swiftly rotate the needle with a wide range of motion for 2-3 minutes. Rotate, but do not lift and thrust, three times in a session. At Yamen (Du 15), slowly and straightly insert without lifting, thrusting or rotating. Withdraw the needle after the needling sensation is obtained. Treat daily, and 7-10 treatments constitute one course.

Results: This method cured 8 cases and produced a marked effect in 5 cases. Some improvement was seen in 6 cases, and only 1 case showed no effect.

(*Source*: Shaanxi Journal of Traditional Chinese Medicine, 7(2):75, 1986)

4. Sciatica

Principal points: Jiaji points (Extra, L2-L5), Zhibian (U.B. 54), Huantiao (G.B. 30), Yanglingquan (G.B. 34)

Method: When needling the Jiaji points (Extra), slant the tip of the needle towards the spine, to a depth of 1.5 *cun*. Gently lift and thrust the needle after insertion. It is best if an electric stroke-like sensation or burning sensation is caused. Jiaji points (Extra) on the healthy side can also be needled. Try to make the needling sensation of each point extend downward. The needles are left in place for 30 minutes with periodic manipulation.

Supplementary points:

Pain along the gall bladder meridian: Fengshi (G.B. 31), Xuanzhong (G.B. 39), Qiuxu (G.B. 40)

Pain along the urinary bladder meridian: Yinmen (U.B. 37), Weizhong (U.B. 40), Chengshan (U.B. 57), Kunlun (U.B. 60)

Blood stagnation: Geshu (U.B. 17), pricking Weizhong (U.B. 40) to cause bleeding

Frequent recurrent sciatica: Shenshu (U.B. 23), Zusanli (St. 36), combined with moxibustion

Other therapies:

1. Moxibustion

Points: Ashi points

Method: Use warm needle, or indirect moxibustion with ginger. Apply 5-7 moxa cones to each tender spot for indirect moxibustion. Treat daily.

2. Cupping

Points: Shenshu (U.B. 23), Zhibian (U.B. 54), Ashi points

Method: On the affected side, cup Shenshu (U.B. 23), Zhibian (U.B. 54) and 2-3 tender spots. The duration of cupping should be 5-10 minutes. Treat once every other day.

3. Ear acupuncture

Points: Sciatic Nerve, Buttocks, Lumbosacral Vertebrae

Method: Taking Pt. Sciatica Nerve as the main point, puncture with strong stimulation. The needles left inserted for 30-60 minutes. Treat daily or once every other day.

4. Pricking collaterals and cupping

Points: Lumbosacral region, Ashi points

Method: Tap with cutaneous needles until bleeding occurs, then apply cupping for 5-10 minutes. Treat once every 2-4 days.

5. Electro-acupuncture

Points:

Pain arising from the nerve root: Jiaji points (Extra, L4-L5), Yanglingquan (G.B. 34), or Weizhong (U.B. 40)

Pain arising from the nerve trunk: Zhibian (U.B. 54), or Huantiao (G.B. 30), Weizhong (U.B. 40), or Yanglingquan (G.B. 34)

Method: After insertion, connect the needles to an electro-stimulator with dense pulsation, or sparse-dense pulsation. Begin with moderate stimulation, progressing to strong stimulation. Treat daily. Each treatment should last 10-15 minutes. Ten treatments constitute one course.

Remarks: Acupuncture and moxibustion therapies are definitely effective in the treatment of primary sciatica. However, with secondary sciatica, the primary cause should be found and treated, acupuncture and moxibustion can be used as supplementary measures. When needling Huantiao (G.B. 30), Zhibian (U.B. 54) and Jiaji points (Extra) of the lumbar vertebrae, a radiating sensation may occur. At this point, no more manipulation should be applied, and the needle should be withdrawn a little bit, so as to avoid damaging the nerve.

REFERENCES:
   1. Results of acupuncture treatment in 140 cases of sciatica
   Point: Zhibian (U.B. 54)
   Method: Use a filiform needle, 4 *cun* in length; rotate and insert to a depth of 3-4 *cun*. Let the needling sensation extend to the diseased area. Retain the needle for 30 minutes. Treat daily. After 6-10 treatments, treat once every other day. Continue treatments until symptoms disappear.
   Results: This method cured 89 cases and produced a marked effect in 32 cases. Improvement was shown in 18 cases, with only 1 case which showed no effect.
   (*Source:* Chinese Acupuncture & Moxibustion, (2):38, 1987)
   2. Clinical observations on acupuncture in the treatment of 400 cases of sciatica
   Points: On affected side, Dachangshu (U.B. 25), Guanyuanshu (U.B. 26), Huantiao (G.B. 30), Tunzhong (Extra, middle point of the buttock)
   Method: Choose one point in each session. Treat daily or once every other day. When needling Dachangshu (U.B. 25) or Guanyuanshu (U.B. 26), insert the needle to a depth of 2.5 *cun*. Apply the sparrow-pricking method 3-10 times to cause the electric stroke-like needling sensation to reach the end of limbs. You may either leave the needle inserted for 20 minutes or not.
   Results: This treatment cured 352 cases and produced a marked effect in 41 cases. Improvement was seen in 3 cases and no effect was shown in 4 cases.
   (*Source:* Shanghai Journal of Acupuncture and Moxibustion, (2):18, 1986)
   3. Results of puncturing the experience point in the treatment of 200 cases of sciatica
   Principal point: Experience point (1 *cun* below and lateral to the spinous process of the second lumbar vertebra)
   Supplementary point: Yanglingquan (G.B. 34)
   Method: Insert a filiform needle 5 *cun* in length at a 90-degree angle to a depth of 3-4 *cun*, manipulating with a lifting, thrusting, twirling and rotating motion. Let the needling sensation pass through the posterior part of the thigh to the foot, then withdraw the needle from this point. Treat daily. Seven treatments constitute one course.
   Results: Needling the experience point cured 42 cases and showed

a marked effect in 97 cases. Some improvement was seen in 38 cases and 23 cases manifested no effect.

(*Source:* Liaoning Journal of Traditional Chinese Medicine, 8(8):26, 1984)

4. Clinical observations on acupuncture in the treatment of 80 cases of sciatica

Points and method:

1) Yaobangxue (Extra, 10 points located 1 *cun* lateral to and below the spinous process of the 1st-5th lumbar vertebrae)

Puncture to a depth of 2-3 *cun* with "sparrow-pricking" method of lifting and thrusting.

2) Jingbangxue (Extra, six points located 1 *cun* lateral to and below the spinous process of the 4th, 5th and 6th cervical vertebrae)

Puncture to a depth of 2 *cun* with the "sparrow-pricking" method.

3) Dazhui (Du 14)

Insert to a depth of 0.5-1 *cun* with the "sparrow-pricking" method.

4) Yaoyangguan (Du 3), Ciliao (U.B. 32), Huantiao (G.B. 30), Yinmen (U.B. 37), Yanglingquan (G.B. 34), Chengshan (U.B. 57), Kunlun (U.B. 60)

Needle and then apply cupping after withdrawal of the needles.

These four groups can be used separately or in combination.

Results: These 4 methods cured 41 cases and produced a marked effect in 25 cases. Improvement was seen in 10 cases, with no effect in 4 cases.

(*Source:* Henan Traditional Chinese Medicine, (3):42, 1981)

5. Trigeminal Neuralgia

Points:

Pain at the first branch: Zanzhu (U.B. 2), Taiyang (Extra), Yangbai (G.B. 14), Fengchi (G.B. 20), Yifeng (S.J. 17), Zhiyin (U.B. 67)

Pain at the second branch: Sibai (St. 2), Yingxiang (L.I. 20), Nose-Juliao (St. 3), Xiaguan (St. 7), Neiting (St. 44), Yifeng (S.J. 17)

Pain at the third branch: Jiache (St. 6), Chengjiang (Ren 24), Hegu (L.I. 4), Jiachengjiang (Extra), Yifeng (S.J. 17)

Method: Puncture Zanzhu (U.B. 2) with the tip of the needle pointing to the lateral and inferior. Let the needling sensation extend to the forehead. Puncture Sibai (St. 2) with the tip of the needle pointing to the lateral and superior. Let the needling sensation radiate to the upper lips. Puncture Jiachengjiang (Extra) with medial and inferior insertion. Let the needling sensation radiate to the lower lip. All points are needled with moderate stimulation. Keep the needles in place for 15-30 minutes with periodic manipulation.

Other therapies:

1. Ear acupuncture

Points: Cheek, Forehead, Shenmen

Method: Choose 2-3 points in a session. Puncture with strong stimulation. The needles are left inserted for 20-30 minutes with manipulation once every five minutes, or needle-embedding may be used.

2. Hydro-acupuncture

Point: Tender spots on the face

Method: Inject a Vitamin B_1, or Vitamin B_{12} solution into the tender spots. Choose 1-2 tender spots for injection in each session. Inject 0.5 ml of the solution into each spot. Treat once every 2-3 days.

3. Head acupuncture

Points: The opposite Sensory Area

Method: Use the routine procedure of head acupuncture.

Remarks: Acupuncture therapy is quite effective in relieving pain associated with primary trigeminal neuralgia, however, with secondary trigeminal neuralgia, its cause should be found and treated.

REFERENCES:

1. Results of the use of acupuncture in the treatment of 33 cases of trigeminal neuralgia

Points:

Pain at the first branch: Yangbai (G.B. 14), Taiyang (Extra), or Touwei (St. 8)

Pain at the second branch: Sibai (St. 2), Yingxiang (L.I. 20)

Pain at the third branch: Xiaguan (St. 7), Daying (St. 5), or add Renzhong (Du 26), Chengjiang (Ren 24), connected with an electro-stimulator

Invasion by exogenous wind: Hegu (L.I. 4), combined with Zusanli (St. 36)

Deficient *yin* and hyperactivity of *yang*: Taixi (K. 3), Taichong (Liv. 3)

Results: Among 33 cases, a short-term cure was obtained in 12 cases, a marked effect in 13 cases, improvement in 7 cases, and no effect in 1 case. Most cases showed some effect after 6 treatments.

(*Source:* Yunnan Journal of Traditional Chinese Medicine, 2(1): 38, 1981)

2. Results of puncturing Xiahexue (Extra) in the treatment of 15 cases of pain at the mandibular branch

Points: Xiahexue (Extra, in the depression, at the medial aspect of the mandibular notch, 1.5-2 cm away from the mandibular angle and on the inferior border of the mandibular), combined with Xiaguan (St. 7)

Method: Use strong stimulating needling, then connect the needle with a pulse current apparatus for 15-20 minutes. Retain the needle for 20-30 minutes with periodic manipulation once every ten minutes.

Results: This method cured 12 cases and produced a marked effect in 3 cases.

(*Source:* Journal of Traditional Chinese Medicine, 21(10):35, 1980)

3. Observed results of deeply inserting into Sancha 1, 2, 3 (Extra) in the treatment of trigeminal neuralgia

Points and method:

1) Sancha 1 (Extra, on supraorbital foramen)

Insert to a depth of 1-1.2 *cun*, at a 90-degree angle, until a needling sensation is obtained.

2) Sancha 2 (Extra, on infraorbital foramen)

Insert towards the mouth at a 45-degree angle, to a depth of 1.2-1.4 *cun*.

3) Sancha 3 (Extra, on mental foramen)

Insert towards Jiache (St. 6) at a 20-degree angle, to a depth of 1.2-1.4 *cun*.

Results: This method produced marked effects in the relief of pain.

(*Source:* Jiangsu Chinese Medical Journal, 1(6):45, 1980)

6. Hypochondriac Pain

Principal points: Zhigou (S.J. 6), Yanglingquan (G.B. 34), Qimen (Liv. 14)

Method: Use filiform needles with moderate stimulation. Leave the needles in place for 20-30 minutes with periodic manipulation. Insert a needle into Qimen (Liv. 14) slantly and shallowly. Treat daily.

Supplementary points:

Qi and blood stagnation: Taichong (Liv. 3), Qiuxu (G.B. 40), Geshu (U.B. 17), Ganshu (U.B. 18), Xuehai (Sp. 10)

Internal retention of phlegm: Fenglong (St. 40), Zusanli (St. 36)

Deficient blood of the liver, malnutrition of meridians and collaterals: Ganshu (U.B. 18), Sanyinjiao (Sp. 6), Taixi (K. 3)

Intercostal neuralgia: Corresponding Jiaji points (Extra), Ashi points

Other therapies:

1. Tapping and cupping

Points: Ashi points

Method: Tap tender spots on the hypochondriac region, using a plum-blossom needle, until the local skin becomes congested. Then apply cups for five minutes. This method is applicable in the treatment of intercostal pain due to traumatic injury.

2. Ear acupuncture

Points: Chest, Shenmen, Liver, Occiput

Method: Choose 2-3 points on the affected ear. Rotate and twirl the needles with moderate stimulation. Leave the needles in place for 10-20 minutes. During an attack of pain, the therapeutic result will be achieved when needling is done.

3. Hydro-acupuncture

Points: Corresponding Jiaji points (Extra) related to intercostal neuralgia

Method: A 2 ml of 2% procaine hydrochloride solution is injected into the above points. Treat once every 1-2 days.

Remarks: Acupuncture and moxibustion are quite effective in the treatment of hypochondriac pain.

REFERENCE:

Results of a primary study on the use of a warm needle in the treatment of 20 cases of costal chondritis

Principal points: Ashi points

Supplementary points: Shanzhong (Ren 17), Waiguan (S.J. 5)

Method: Insert a 0.5 *cun* filiform needle at an acute angle into the center of the affected area. Then apply 2-3 moxa cones on the needle at the main point, and 1-2 moxa cones at each of the supplementary points. Treat daily. Seven treatments constitute one course.

Results: Among 20 cases, 17 cases were cured and improvement was seen in 3 cases.

(*Source:* Chinese Acupuncture & Moxibustion, (1):16, 1983)

7. Diaphragm Spasms (Hiccups)

Principal points: Neiguan (P. 6), Zhongwan (Ren 12), Tiantu (Ren 22)

Method: Normally, Neiguan (P. 6) and Zhongwan (Ren 12) are needled first, with continuous manipulation for several minutes. If the spasm has not been relieved, needle Tiantu (Ren 22).

Supplementary points:

Retention of food: Juque (Ren 14), Lineiting (Extra)

Qi Stagnation in the liver: Shanzhong (Ren 17), Taichong (Liv. 3)

Coldness in the stomach: Moxi Shangwan (Ren 13), Liangmen (St. 21)

Qi deficiency: Moxi Qihai (Ren 6), Zusanli (St. 36)

Other therapies:

1. Ear acupuncture

Points: Middle of Ear, End of Inferior Helix Crus, Stomach, Shenmen

Method: Use filiform needles to puncture bilateral points with strong stimulation. Leave the needles inserted for 60 minutes. With a chronic case, needle-embedding can be used.

2. Cupping

Points: Geshu (U.B. 17), Geguan (U.B. 46), Ganshu (U.B. 18), Zhongwan (Ren 12), Rugen (St. 18)

Method: Use medium cups. Place the cups for 10-15 minutes.

3. Finger pressure

Points: Zanzhu (U.B. 2), bilateral

Method: Press Zanzhu (U.B. 2) bilaterally with the fingers of both two hands for 5-10 minutes.

4. Moxibustion

Points: Shanzhong (Ren 17), Zhongwan (Ren 12), Guanyuan (Ren 4)

Method: Apply 5-7 cones of moxa to each point. This method is suitable for severe cases.

5. Hydro-acupuncture

Points: Geshu (U.B. 17), Neiguan (P. 6)

Method: Inject 0.5 ml of Vitamin B$_1$ solution into each point. Treat once every other day. Ten treatments constitute one course.

Remarks: Acupuncture and moxibustion therapies are quite effective in the short-term treatment of diaphragm spasms.

REFERENCES:

1. Positive therapeutic result observed with the use of acupuncture on Yifeng (S.J. 17) in the treatment of hiccups

Point: Yifeng (S.J. 17)

Method: Press with fingers.

Results: There were 2 cases. Each was cured with 1 treatment.

(*Source:* New Journal of Traditional Chinese Medicine, (7):32, 1984)

2. Results of needling Anding (Extra) in the treatment of diaphragm spasms

Points: Anding (Extra, 0.5 *cun* directly above Suliao, Du 25, 0.3 *cun* lateral to the border of alae nasi)

Method: Use a filiform needle to rapidly needle the point with an upwardly slanted insertion to a depth of 0.3 *cun*. Rotate the needle gently for one minute or until the spasm is checked. Leave the needle in place for 15-20 minutes. Treat daily.

Results: Ten cases were treated. Only 1 case showed no effect.

(*Source:* Hubei Journal of Traditional Chinese Medicine, (3):13, 1981)

3. Results of ear acupuncture in the treatment of 47 cases of hiccups

Principal points: Middle of Ear, Stomach, Liver, Spleen, End of Inferior Helix Crus

Supplementary points: Shenmen, Brain, Lower Apex of Tragus

Method: Puncture with a filiform needle.

Results: All were cured within 1-2 treatments.

(*Source:* Chinese Acupuncture & Moxibustion, (2):46, 1987)

4. Results of needling Zhongkui (Extra) in the treatment of 50 cases of stubborn hiccups

Points: Zhongkui (Extra), bilateral

Method: Insert the needle at a 90-degree angle to a depth of 0.2 *cun*, applying strong stimulation. When needling, instruct the patient to breathe deeply through the nose and hold for a while. During manipulation, ask the patient to repeat this 3-5 times. When hiccups are checked, deep abdominal breathing is required. The needles are kept in place for 30 minutes. Manipulate the needle once every five minutes, or the needles may be connected with an electro-stimulator.

Results: This treatment cured 49 cases and had no effect in only 1 case.

(*Source:* New Journal of Traditional Chinese Medicine, 20(1):38, 1988)

5. Results of needling Shaoshang (Lu. 11) in the treatment of stubborn hiccups

Points: Shaoshang (Lu. 11), bilateral

Method: Use filiform needles, 0.5-1 *cun* in length, to puncture bilateral Shaoshang (Lu. 11) at a 90-degree angle. Apply moderate stimulation every 1-2 minutes. Withdraw the needles after three repeated manipulations. Treat daily.

Results: This treatment proved effective in 23 cases, but had no effect in 2 cases. A therapeutic result can usually be obtained within 2 treatments.

(*Source:* Hunan Journal of Traditional Chinese Medicine, 3(1):33, 1987)

8. Gastrocnemius Spasm

Principal points: Houxi (S.I. 3), Chengshan (U.B. 57)

Method: During the attack of the spasm, needle the opposite Houxi (S.I. 3), using strong stimulation and continuous manipulation. Or needle Chengshan (U.B. 57) on the affected side, using strong stimulation. The spasm will subside at once. With a chronic case, needle these two points, using moderate stimulation, even method. Leave the needles in place for 30-60 minutes. Treat daily.

Supplementary points:

Severe attack: Yanglingquan (G.B. 34), Chengjin (U.B. 56), or Zusanli (St. 36), Sanyinjiao (Sp. 6), with reinforcing method

Other therapies:

1. Moxibustion

Points: Chengshan (U.B. 57), Zusanli (St. 36)

Method: Apply moxibustion with a moxa stick to each point for 10 minutes. Treat daily. This method is successful, not only as a treatment, but also as a prevention.

2. Finger pressure

Points: Chengshan (U.B. 57), Zanzhu (U.B. 2)

Method: During the attack, use the pad of the thumb to massage Chengshan (U.B. 57) on the affected side or bilateral Zanzhu (U.B. 2) until the spasm is totally relieved.

3. Wrist-and-ankle acupuncture

Points: Lower 1, 6, bilateral

Method: Use the routine procedure in wrist-and-ankle acupuncture.

Remarks: Acupuncture is quite effective in the treatment of gastrocnemius spasm.

REFERENCE:

The results of acupuncture and moxibustion in the treatment of 56 cases of gastrocnemius spasm

Points and method: During the attack, needle the opposite Houxi (S.I. 3), applying strong stimulation. Or needle Chengshan (U.B. 57), Yanglingquan (G.B. 34), Chengjin (U.B. 56) on the affected side, using the reducing method. With frequent attacks, combine Zusanli (St. 36) and Sanyinjiao (Sp. 6). Keep the needles in place for 1-2 hours. Treat daily. Five treatments constitute one course. If attacks often occur during sport activities, preventive moxibustion can be applied to Chengshan (U.B. 57) and Chengjin (U.B. 56).

Results: Among 28 cases which suffered on attack, 26 cases were immediately relieved, and the symptoms of 2 cases were greatly reduced. There were 13 cases suffering from frequent attacks and 15 cases with occasional attacks. Acupuncture and moxibustion cured all within 2-5 treatments.

(*Source:* Journal of Traditional Chinese Medicine, 25(3):23, 1984)

9. Facial Spasm

Principal points: Sibai (St. 2), Xiaguan (St. 7), Jiache (St. 6), Dicang (St. 4), Taiyang (Extra), Hegu (L.I. 4), Taichong (Liv. 3)

Method: Apply mild stimulation and even method to the points. Leave the needles inserted for 30 minutes. Treat daily or once every other day. Ten treatments constitute one course.

Supplementary points and method:

Invasion by exogenous wind and cold: Waiguan (S.J. 5). Apply a warm needle or moxibustion with a moxa stick to the points on the face.

Deficiency of *qi* and blood: Zusanli (St. 36), Sanyinjiao (Sp. 6), Qihai (Ren 6). Needle with reinforcing method.

Yin deficiency of the liver and kidney: Taixi (K. 3), Fengchi (G.B. 20)

Excessive phlegm and fire: Zhongwan (Ren 12), Yanglingquan (G.B. 34), Fenglong (St. 40)

Other therapies:

1. Intradermal needle therapy

Points: Xiaguan (St. 7), Sibai (St. 2), Dicang (St. 4), Tongziliao (G.B. 1), Quanliao (S.I. 18), Jiache (St. 6), Ashi points

Method: Choose 2-3 points on the affected side for each session. Use intradermal needle to needle at a 90-degree angle until a needling sensation is obtained. Then withdraw the needle to the subcutaneous region for implantation, and fix with adhesive tape. Limit the duration of implantation to 1-3 days. During the second implantation, change points. 5-10 treatments constitute one course.

2. Hydro-acupuncture

Points: Xiaguan (St. 7), Jiache (St. 6), Taiyang (Extra), Fengchi (G.B. 20), Yifeng (S.J. 17), Hegu (L.I. 4), Fenglong (St. 40), Zhigou (S.J. 6), Xuanzhong (G.B. 39)

Method: Add 2 ml of 300 μg Vitamin B_{12} to 2 ml of 2% procaine hydrochloride solution. Inject 1 ml into each point. Choose 2-3 points on the affected face and combine each point with one on the opposite upper limb and lower limb. Manipulate according to the routine procedure of hydro-acupuncture. Treat daily. Ten treatments constitute one course. Begin another injection after a ten-day rest.

3. Laser acupuncture

Points: Sibai (St. 2), Dicang (St. 4), Jiache (St. 6), Chengqi (St. 1), Hegu (L.I. 4)

Method: Use a He-Ne laser machine to illuminate the points on the region of the facial spasm as well as Hegu (L.I. 4). Choose 2-5 points for a session. Stimulate each point for three minutes. Treat daily. Ten treatments constitute one course.

4. Ear acupuncture

Points: Mouth, Cheek, Occiput, Eye, Brain, Liver

Method: Choose 2-4 points for a session. Puncture with filiform needles and apply moderate stimulation. Keep the needles inserted for 30 minutes. Treat daily. Embedding needles can also be used.

Remarks: Acupuncture and moxibustion therapies are quite effective in the treatment of facial spasm.

REFERENCE:

Clinical summary on subcutaneous needling in the treatment of 30 cases of facial spasm

Points: Corresponding points on the frequent attack portion of facial spasm

Method: Use 15-30 filiform needles, gauge 30-32, 0.5-1.5 *cun* in length, to subcutaneously puncture the affected area of the facial spasm. Suspend and list the needles closely around the trigger point of the spasm. Maintain a 0.5-1 cm interspace between needles. Leave the needles in place for 20-30 minutes. Treat daily. Ten treatments constitute one course.

Results: Through 4 courses of treatments, 18 cases were cured, 5 cases showed marked effect, and improvement was seen in 7 cases. The cases effected within 3 courses of treatment were 24.

(*Source:* Journal of Traditional Chinese Medicine, 24(1):66, 1983)

10. Facial Paralysis

Principal points: Yangbai (G.B. 14), Sibai (St. 2), Dicang (St. 4), Jiache (St. 6), Hegu (L.I. 4), Xiaguan (St. 7), Quanliao (S.I. 18)

Method: A joining method can be adopted when needling points on the face. Such as: Dicang (St. 4) joins to Jiache (St. 6), Yangbai (G.B. 14) to Yuyao (Extra), and Sibai (St. 2) to Nose-Juliao (St. 3). During the initial stage, it is advisable to puncture shallowly with mild stimulation. However, needle the remote points with moderate stimulation. Keep the needles inserted for 10-20 minutes. After withdrawing the needles, apply moxibustion with a moxa stick to the facial points until congestion appears. Points on the affected side, except Hegu (L.I. 4), are often selected for treatment. Treat daily or once every other day.

Supplementary points:

Flat philtrum: Yingxiang (L.I. 20)
Deviation of the philtrum: Renzhong (Du 26)
Maxillary labial groove deviated: Chengjiang (Ren 24)
Pain at the mastoid region: Yifeng (S.J. 17)
Difficulty in frowning and raising the eyebrow: Zanzhu (U.B. 2)
Headache at occiput region: Fengchi (G.B. 20)
Numbness and taste impairment of the tongue: Lianquan (Ren 23)
Incomplete closing of the eye: Zanzhu (U.B. 2), Sizhukong (S.J. 23)
Tinnitus and deafness: Tinghui (G.B. 2)
Other therapies:
1. Cutaneous acupuncture
Points: Yangbai (G.B. 14), Sibai (St. 2), Dicang (St. 4), Jiache (St. 6), Hegu (L.I. 4)
Method: Tap points on the affected side, except Hegu (L.I. 4), using cutaneous needles, until the local skin becomes red in color. Treat daily or once every other day. Ten treatments constitute one course. This method should be applied during the recovery stage or the sequelae.
2. Moxibustion
Points: Taiyang (Extra), Jiache (St. 6), Dicang (St. 4), Nose-Juliao (St. 3), Xiaguan (St. 7)
Method: Apply moxibustion with moxa cones once every 3-5 days. 3-7 cones are needed for each point. This method should be applied in chronic cases.
3. Electro-acupuncture
Points: Dicang (St. 4), Jiache (St. 6), Yangbai (G.B. 14), Sibai (St. 2), Hegu (L.I. 4)
Method: Apply current which the patient can tolerate for 5-10 minutes, and which produces twitching of the facial muscle. If the teeth clench tightly, it means the needles have been inserted too deeply into the masseter muscle. Withdraw and reinsert the needles.
4. Cupping
Points: On affected side
Method: Consider as a supplementary treatment, apply small cups once every 3-5 days.
5. Hydro-acupuncture
Points: Qianzhen (Extra), Taiyang (Extra), Dicang (St. 4), Yifeng (S.J. 17), Yingxiang (L.I. 20)

Method: Insert and retain the needles for 5-10 minutes until a needling sensation is obtained. Inject 0.5-1 ml of 100 mg Vitamin B$_1$ solution in each point. Treat daily or once every other day. These points can be used in rotation.

6. Head acupuncture

Points: Facial Motor Area on either the affected or opposite side of the head

Method: Treat daily or once every other day, according to the routine procedure of head acupuncture. Ten treatments constitute one course.

Remarks: This condition should be distinguished as either peripheral or central nervous system facial paralysis. If it is related to the central nervous system, the treatment should proceed according to the method used in treating a cerebrovascular accident.

Acupuncture is relatively effective in the treatment of this illness. However, more rapid results will be obtained, if acupuncture is combined with massage, hot compress, or Chinese and Western oral medication.

REFERENCES:

1. Clinical report on electro-acupuncture in the treatment of 47 cases of deviated mouth and eye

Points: Fengchi (G.B. 20), Qianzhen (Extra), Yangbai (G.B. 14), Jiache (St. 6), Hegu (L.I. 4)

Supplementary points: Xiaguan (St. 7), Quanliao (S.I. 18), Chengjiang (Ren 24), Renzhong (Du 26), Taiyang (Extra), Zusanli (St. 36), Neiting (St. 44), Taichong (Liv. 3)

Method: Select a point on the affected side, except Hegu (L.I. 4). The joining method is often used on facial points. The remote points are usually combined with local points. After the needling sensation is obtained, connect the needles to an electro-stimulator with a sparse-dense or intermittent pulsation, using moderate stimulation for 10-20 minutes. For an acute case, treat daily, but for a chronic case, treat once every other day. Seven treatments constitute one course.

Results: Among 47 cases, 21 cases were cured, marked effect was shown in 14 cases, improvement was seen in 10 cases, and no effect appeared in 2 cases. The total effective rate reached 95.8 percent.

(*Source:* Fujian Journal of Traditional Chinese Medicine, (3):28, 1981)

2. Primary study on electro-acupuncture in the treatment of acute peripheral facial paralysis

Points: a) Xiaguan (St. 7), Taiyang (Extra); b) Xiaguan (St. 7), Sibai (St. 2); c) Xiaguan (St. 7), Quanliao (S.I. 18); d) Xiaguan (St. 7), Dicang (St. 4)

Method: After needling, use an electrostimulator with sparse-dense pulsation, and set to a frequency of 14-16 times per minute, with output around 0.8-1.2 v. Apply less than one minute of stimulation at the beginning. If improvement is seen after 10 days, the amount of stimulation can be increased to two minutes. After 15 treatments, rotate intermittent pulsation and sparse-dense pulsation. The amount of electric stimulation also depends on producing a slight contraction of the facial muscles, and on the tolerance of the patient. Treat daily. Ten treatments constitute one course. The patient should rest for one week following two courses. If no improvement is shown after two more courses, some other therapies should be used.

Results: Among 100 cases, 84 cases were cured and 16 cases showed improvement. The total effective rate reached 100 percent. The maximum number of treatments needed was 30, the minimum was 18, the average was 21.5.

(*Source:* Chinese Acupuncture & Moxibustion, (5):3, 1987)

3. Observed results of Vitamin B_{12} injections in the treatment of 200 cases of facial neuritis

Points: Tongziliao (G.B. 1), Xiaguan (St. 7), Jiache (St. 6), Dicang (St. 4) on affected side, Hegu (L.I. 4) on opposite side

Method: Using a gauge 5 hypodermic needle and syringe, inject 1 ml of 15 μg or 50 μg Vitamin B_{12} solution into the above five points. Gently lift and thrust the needle after insertion, the medicine can be injected when a needling sensation is felt. To avoid bleeding, press dry cotton balls on the points after withdrawing the needle. Insert needles at an acute angle into Dicang (St. 4) and Jiache (St. 6), and insert at a 90-degree angle into Xiaguan (St. 7) and Hegu (L.I. 4). Treat twice a week. Six treatments constitute one course.

Results: The total effective rate reached 99 percent.

(*Source:* Shanghai Journal of Acupuncture and Moxibustion, (3):11, 1984)

4. Clinical observations of the needling of the facial nerve trunk in the treatment of 220 cases of peripheral facial paralysis

Points: Head-Wangu (G.B. 12) and Yifeng (S.J. 17) on affected side, Erchuixia (Extra, 3 cm directly below the junction between rear lobe and buccal surface)

Method: Puncture the points with mild stimulation, using the "sparrow-pricking" method. Remove the needles after 20 minutes.

Results: This method cured 167 cases, or 75.91 percent; marked effect was seen in 38 cases, or 17.27 percent; improvement occurred in 13 cases, 5.91 percent, while no effect was seen in 2 cases, 0.91 percent. The total effective rate reached 99.09 percent.

(*Source:* Chinese Acupuncture & Moxibustion, (3):19, 1987)

5. Summary of the use of pricking combined with mustard paste in the treatment of 127 cases of simple facial paralysis

Points: The first point is located on the occlusal line of intrabuccal membranous part, level with the second molar teeth. The second and third points are located 0.5 cm anterior or posterior to the first point. Six other matching points are located on the parallel lines 0.5 cm above and below the occlusal line. There are a total of nine points (4-6 points can be chosen for child's treatment).

Method: First, instruct the patient to rinse off with a 1.3% saline solution. With a three-edged needle, use the sparrow-pricking method, pricking each point 15-20 times. (The amount of pricking is divided by two for children.) Prick to a depth of 1-2 mm, enabling the local skin to become congested. Then make a paste of mustard powder (10 grams) mixed with warm water and spread on a piece of gauze, 2-3 cm^2 in size and 0.5 cm thick. Place this over the affected cheek near Xiaguan (St. 7), Jiache (St. 6) and Dicang (St. 4), and fix with adhesive tape. With a severe case, some other points should be treated. For example, if the frontal wrinkle was disappeared, Yangbai (G.B. 14) is also treated. If the eye does not close completely, Taiyang (Extra) is treated. Application should last 12-24 hours. Swelling and blisters may appear. If so apply an ointment for burn injury, changing the dressing once in two days. Side effects, such as a hot sensation, pain or lacrimation, are considered normal when the medicine is applied. All the side effects should disappear after four hours. Ask the patient to exercise caution, and not to expose the treated area to wind and cold for the duration of recovery.

Results: This treatment cured 102 cases and showed improvement in 19 cases. No effect was seen in 6 cases. This method is adaptable for the treatment of acute facial paralysis which has lasted between 3 months and a half year.

(*Source:* New Journal of Traditional Chinese Medicine, 18(4):37, 1986)

6. Observed results of acupuncture in the treatment of 155 cases of facial paralysis

Points: Jiuzhengxue (Extra, on the ulnar side of the little finger, close to the end of transverse crease of the metacarpophalangeal joint, at the junction of the red and white skin) joining to Hegu (L.I. 4), Shousanli (L.I. 10)

Method: Inject a 5% Angelica sinensis liquid or Vitamin B_1 solution into Shousanli (L.I. 10), 2 ml in each point. Treat daily. Ten treatments constitute one course.

Results: Of the 155 cases, 125 were cured, 14 showed a marked effect, 11 showed some improvement while 5 showed no effect. The total effective rate was 96.7 percent.

(*Source:* Shaanxi Journal of Traditional Chinese Medicine, 9(5):216, 1988)

7. Observed effects of treating 57 cases of facial paralysis by applying a warm needle

Principal point: Xiaguan (St. 7)

Method: Insert a needle, a depth of 1.5 *cun*, into Xiaguan (St. 7) on the affected side. Once the needling sensation is obtained, leave the needle in place. Burn a clump of moxa, 1 *cun* in length, attached to the other end of the needle. Withdraw the needle when the moxa is completely burned. Treat daily. Seven treatments constitute one course.

Supplementary points:

Incomplete closing of the eye: Sibai (St. 2) joining to Yingxiang (L.I. 20), Taiyang (Extra) to Quanliao (S.I. 18)

Deviation of the mouth: Dicang (St. 4) joining to Jiache (St. 6), Nose-Juliao (St. 3) to Jiache (St. 6)

Severe paralysis: Hegu (L.I. 4)

Results: Of the 57 cases treated, all were cured.

(*Source:* Shandong Journal of Traditional Chinese Medicine, (6):346, 1982)

11. Periodic Paralysis

Principal points: Baihui (Du 20), Dazhui (Du 14), Quchi (L.I. 11), Yanglingquan (G.B. 34), Zusanli (St. 36), Sanyinjiao (Sp. 6)

Method: Use the even method with filiform needles to produce strong stimulation. Keep needles in place for 10-20 minutes and treat daily.

Supplementary points:

Paralysis of the upper limbs: Jianyu (L.I. 15), Shousanli (L.I. 10), Hegu (L.I. 4)

Paralysis of the lower limbs: Huantiao (G.B. 30), Fengshi (G.B. 31), Taichong (Liv. 3)

Other therapies:

1. Electro-acupuncture

Points: The same as above.

Method: Select 2-3 pairs of points during an attack. Connect the electro-acupuncture apparatus with the needles after the arrival of *qi*. The frequency should be 120-200 times per minute and the intensity of the current must be adjusted according to the patient's tolerance. Use electric stimulation for 10-20 minutes each time and treat daily.

2. Hydro-acupuncture

Points: Jianyu (L.I. 15), Quchi (L.I. 11), Yanglingquan (G.B. 34), Ganshu (U.B. 18), Shenshu (U.B. 23)

Method: Treat 2-4 points each time. Inject 1 ml of Vitamin B_1 (10 mg/ml) or Vitamin B_{12} (15 μg/ml) solution into each point. The injections are administered daily or once every other day.

Remarks: The above methods have produced fair effects in the treatment of periodic paralysis and effectiveness has been obtained quickly in most cases.

12. Parkinsonism

Principal points: Baihui (Du 20), Dazhui (Du 14), Fengchi (G.B. 20), Hegu (L.I. 4), Taichong (Liv. 3)

Method: Employ filiform needles to produce moderate stimulation and continuously rotate the needles after the insertion until the tremor is relieved. Keep the needles inserted for 20-30 minutes, during which intermittent manipulation of needles is given. Treat daily and 10 treatments constitute one course.

Supplementary points:

Tremor of the upper limbs: Quchi (L.I. 11), Waiguan (S.J. 5)

Tremor of the lower limbs: Yanglingquan (G.B. 34), Xuanzhong

(G.B. 9)

Appearance of "mask face" : Taiyang (Extra), Renzhong (Du 26), Jiache (St. 6), Dicang (St. 4) with shallow insertion and retention of needles

Hyperhidrosis: Yinxi (H. 6), Zusanli (St. 36)

Insomnia or dream-disturbed sleep: Shenmen (H. 7), Neiguan (P. 6), Sanyinjiao (Sp. 6)

Involuntary salivation: Dicang (St. 4), Lianquan (Ren 23)

Emotional depression: Renzhong (Du 26), Neiguan (P. 6), Xinshu (U.B. 15)

Other therapies:

1. Ear acupuncture

Points: Shenmen, Brain, Occiput, Heart, Liver, Brain Stem, Central Rim

Method: Utilize filiform needles to produce moderate stimulation and then retain the needles for 20-30 minutes. Treat daily. Embedding needles or acupressure with seeds can also be applied.

2. Head acupuncture

Points: Chorea and Tremor Control Area

Method: In a case of unilateral tremor, use points on the opposite side, but bilateral points should be employed when both sides are involved. Perform the routine operation of head acupuncture daily or once every other day. Ten treatments constitute one course.

Remarks: Acupuncture has certain therapeutic effects in the treatment of Parkinsonism.

13. Agraphia with Tremulous Hand

Principal points: Jianzhen (S.I. 9), Quchi (L.I. 11), Fengchi (G.B. 20), Shousanli (L.I. 10), Waiguan (S.J. 5), Hegu (L.I. 4)

Method: Use filiform needles to puncture with moderate stimulation, retaining the needles for 20 minutes with periodic manipulation once every 10 minutes. Treat daily. Moxibustion can also be used on Quchi (L.I. 11), Shousanli (L.I. 10), Waiguan (S.J. 5) and Hegu (L.I. 4) for 10-20 minutes.

Supplementary points:

For chronic cases: Baihui (Du 20), Yanglingquan (G.B. 34)

Other therapies:

1. Ear acupuncture

Points: Liver, Heart, Kidney, Spleen, Wrist, Finger, Brain

Method: Choose 2-3 points on one side, rotating each time. Embedding needles are used for 24 hours. Treat once every other day. Ten treatments constitute one course.

2. Electro-acupuncture

Points: a) Shousanli (L.I. 10), Hegu (L.I. 4); b) Jianzhen (S.I. 9), Quchi (L.I. 11)

Method: Use one group of points for each treatment, rotating between treatments. After the needling sensation is obtained, connect the needles to an electro-stimulator with sparse-dense pulsation, set the stimulating intensity to the tolerance of the patient. Treat once every other day. Duration of the electro-acupuncture will be 10-15 minutes. Ten treatments constitute one course.

Remarks: The above-mentioned methods are quite effective for agraphia with tremulous hand.

14. Multiple Neuritis

Principal points:

The upper limbs: Jianyu (L.I. 15), Quchi (L.I. 11), Waiguan (S.J. 5), Hegu (L.I. 4), Baxie (Extra)

The lower limbs: Huantiao (G.B. 30), Yanglingquan (G.B. 34), Sanyinjiao (Sp. 6), Xuanzhong (G.B. 39), Bafeng (Extra)

Method: Puncture with moderate stimulation. Leave the needles in place for 30 minutes. Treat daily. Joining method can also be used. For coldness of the limbs, warm needles or moxibustion with moxa sticks can be applied. If it is necessary, electro-acupuncture may also be applied to the points on the upper and lower limbs. 2-4 points are usually chosen in a session. Use intermittent pulsation for 15-20 minutes.

Supplementary points:

Chronic muscle atrophy: Ganshu (U.B. 18), Shenshu (U.B. 23), Taixi (K. 3), Zusanli (St. 36), Mingmen (Du 4); combined with moxibustion

Numbness and stabbing pain on the tips of the fingers and toes: Prick Shixuan (Extra) with a three-edged needle to cause a few drops of blood out; treat once every 3-5 days.

Paralysis: Mingmen (Du 4), Yaoyangguan (Du 3)

Wrist dropping: Yanglao (S.I. 6), Yangchi (S.J. 4)

Foot dropping: Jiexi (St. 41), Zusanli (St. 36), Qiuxu (G.B. 40), Shangqiu (Sp. 5)

Irritability, hot feeling, night sweating: Yinxi (H. 6), Fuliu (K. 7)

Other therapies:

1. Cutaneous acupuncture

Points: Points along the large intestine and stomach meridians are taken as the main points, combined with points on affected region. If the patient suffers paralysis, points along the Du meridian and the corresponding Jiaji points (Extra) should be added.

Method: Tap with moderate stimulation until the skin becomes congested or slight bleeding is produced. Treat once every other day.

2. Ear acupuncture

Points: Corresponding points, Shenmen, End of Inferior Helix Crus

Method: Puncture with moderate stimulation. The needles are left in place for 20-30 minutes. Treat daily.

3. Head acupuncture

Points: Motor Area, Sensory Area, Leg Motor and Sensory Area

Method: Retain the needles for 30-60 minutes with periodic rotating manipulation. Treat once every other day.

Remarks: This disease needs many courses.

REFERENCE:

Clinical observations of acupuncture in the treatment of 56 cases of multiple neuritis

Points:

The upper limbs: a) Quchi (L.I. 11), Waiguan (S.J. 5), Baxie (Extra); b) Shousanli (L.I. 10), Hegu (L.I. 4), Houxi (S.I. 3)

The lower limbs: Yanglingquan (G.B. 34), Sanyinjiao (Sp. 6), Taibai (Sp. 3)

Weakness of the spleen and stomach: Zhongwan (Ren 12), Weishu (U.B. 21), Pishu (U.B. 20)

Stagnation of *qi* and blood: Reinforcing Hegu (L.I. 4), reducing Sanyinjiao (Sp. 6) and Taichong (Liv. 3)

Dampness in the limbs: Yinlingquan (Sp. 9), Gongsun (Sp. 4)

Method: After the needling sensation is obtained, connect the needles with a Model 6805 electro-stimulator. Retain the needles for 20-30 minutes. Fifteen treatments constitute one course.

Results: This method cured 29 cases, and caused improvement in 11 cases. However, 16 cases showed no effect.

(*Source:* Hubei Journal of Traditional Chinese Medicine, (6):30, 1987)

15. Neuritis of Lateral Cutaneous Nerve of Thigh

Principal points: Biguan (St. 31), Femur-Futu (St. 32), Yinshi (St. 33), Fengshi (G.B. 31), Ashi points

Method: Puncture the points shallowly, with strong stimulation. Warm needles or moxibustion with a moxa stick may be used after needling. Select 3-5 Ashi points on the sensory impairment area of the thigh and puncture subcutaneously towards the center of the affected area. The needles are retained for 20-30 minutes. Treat daily or once every other day. Ten treatments constitute one course.

Supplementary points:

Chronic disease with blood stagnation: Xuehai (Sp. 10)

Other therapies:

1. Cutaneous acupuncture

Points: The local sensory impairment area

Method: Tap the local sensory impairment area from the outline to the center until the local area becomes congested. Treat once every other day.

2. Moxibustion

Points: Ashi points

Method: Select 5-7 Ashi points at the local sensory impairment area. Apply indirect moxibustion with ginger and 5-7 moxa cones to each point. Treat daily or once every other day.

3. Tapping and cupping

Points: Fengshi (G.B. 31), Biguan (St. 31), Femur-Futu (St. 32), Yinshi (St. 33)

Method: First, tap the points with cutaneous needles until the local skin becomes congested or until tapping produces slight bleeding, then apply cups for five minutes. Treat once every other day.

4. Electro-acupuncture

Points: Biguan (St. 31), Femur-Futu (St. 32), Yinshi (St. 33), Fengshi (G.B. 31), Femur-Zhongdu (G.B. 32), Yanglingquan (G.B. 34)

Method: Cutaneously joining method can be adopted at points on the local affected area. Puncture Yanglingquan (G.B. 34) at a 90-degree angle. After the needling sensation is obtained, connect the needles to an electro-stimulator with sparse-dense pulsation and adjust the intensity to the tolerance of the patient. Treat once every other day. Duration of the electro-acupuncture should be 10-15 minutes.

5. Hydro-acupuncture

Points: Biguan (St. 31), Femur-Futu (St. 32), Fengshi (G.B. 31)

Method: Use a mixed solution of 50 mg Vitamin B_1 and 100 μg Vitamin B_{12} and inject according to the routine procedures of hydro-acupuncture. Inject each point with 1 ml of solution. Treat once every other day.

Remarks: The above-mentioned methods are quite effective in the treatment of neuritis of the lateral cutaneous nerve of the thigh. Usually, 2-3 kinds of methods are used in combination for treatment.

REFERENCES:

1. Observation of the use of "quintuple puncture" in the treatment of 25 cases of neuritis of the lateral cutaneous nerve of the thigh

Points and method: Choose a filiform needle, 2.5 *cun* in length, and puncture to a depth of 2-4 cm in the center of the sensory impairment area (close to the point of Fengshi, G.B. 31). Then select 4 points, 2-3 fingers' width away, around the center point, and puncture at the center to a depth of 3-5 cm, at a 25-degree angle to the skin. Use an even method with rotation, but no lifting or thrusting. Leave the needles inserted for 20 minutes. Treat once every other day. Ten treatments constitute one course.

Results: Each case received 3-36 treatments, the average was 10.5 treatments. This treatment cured 13 cases, showed marked effect in 9 cases, and produced no effect in 3 cases.

(*Source:* Journal of Traditional Chinese Medicine, 25(1):27, 1984)

2. Observed results of the application of a plum-blossom needle, cupping and moxibustion in the treatment of 10 cases of neuritis of the lateral cutaneous nerve of the thigh

Points: Ashi points

Method: Use plum-blossom needles to tap gently and cause a few drops of blood to surface. Then, apply cups for 10-15 minutes, followed by moxibustion with moxa sticks for 10 minutes.

Results: All 10 cases were totally cured by 3-5 treatments.

(*Source:* Shanghai Journal of Acupuncture and Moxibustion, (3):20, 1985)

3. Observed results of the use of a plum-blossom needle and "walking cups" in the treatment of 31 cases of neuritis of the lateral cutaneous nerve of the thigh

Points and method: After sterilization on the dull sensory area is complete, use plum-blossom needles to tap evenly until the local skin becomes congested or slight bleeding is produced. Then apply the liquid paraffin to the skin surface. Place a small cup on the affected skin and slowly move up and down, left and right, until the local skin becomes congested. Treat once every other day. 2-5 treatments are needed.

Results: Of the 31 cases treated, 27 cases were cured, 2 cases showed marked effect, improvement was seen in 1 case and no effect was obtained in 1 case.

(*Source:* Henan Traditional Chinese Medicine, (4):28, 1987)

16. Peripheral Nerve Injury

I. Brachia plexus injury

Principal points: Jiaji points (Extra) from the fourth cervical vertebra to the first thoracic vertebra on the affected side, Jianyu (L.I. 15), Quchi (L.I. 11), Shousanli (L.I. 10), Hegu (L.I. 4)

Supplementary points: Dazhui (Du 14), Binao (L.I. 14), Jianliao (S.J. 14), Yuji (Lu. 10), Houxi (S.I. 3)

Method: Insert at an oblique angle in Jiaji points (Extra), incline the needle towards the dorsal mid-line, and apply strong stimulation to all points except Jiaji points (Extra) and Dazhui (Du 14), using repeated lifting, thrusting and rotating of needles. Stimulate 4-5 points each time, leaving the needles in place for 30 minutes. While the needles are retained, moxibustion is also acceptable. After needling, cupping is performed on the thick muscle. Treat daily or once every other day. Ten treatments constitute one course.

II. Radial nerve injury

Principal points: Jianyu (L.I. 15), Jianliao (S.J. 14), Quchi (L.I. 11), Waiguan (S.J. 5), Hegu (L.I. 4)

Supplementary points: Jianzhen (S.I. 9), Shousanli (L.I. 10), Lieque (Lu. 7), Hand-Zhongzhu (S.J. 3)

Method: Select 2-3 principal and supplementary points for each treatment. Apply strong stimulation with deep insertion and retain the needles for 30 minutes. While the needles are in place, mild moxibustion with a moxa stick, or warm-needle moxibustion can be applied. Use cupping on the thick muscle after acupuncture. Treat daily or once every other day. Ten treatments constitute one course.

III. Median nerve injury

Principal points: Dazhui (Du 14), Jianzhen (S.I. 9), Chize (Lu. 5), Neiguan (P. 6), Hegu (L.I. 4)

Supplementary points: Quze (P. 3), Ximen (P. 4), Daling (P. 7), Yuji (Lu. 10)

Method: Select 2-3 principal and supplementary points for each treatment. Apply strong stimulation on all except Dazhui (Du 14). Retain the needles in place for 30 minutes and manipulate intermittently. Mild moxibustion with a moxa stick, or warm-needle moxibustion, can also be applied. Cupping is performed at the points on the shoulder after acupuncture is completed. Treat daily or once every other day. Ten treatments constitute one course.

IV. Ulnar nerve injury

Principal points: Jianzhen (S.I. 9), Xiaohai (S.I. 8), Shenmen (H. 7), Houxi (S.I. 3)

Supplementary points: Shaohai (H. 3), Hand-Wangu (S.I. 4), Hand-Zhongzhu (S.J. 3), Shaoze (S.I. 1)

Method: Select 2-3 principal and supplementary points for each treatment and provide strong stimulation. Retain the needles for 30 minutes and manipulate intermittently. Meanwhile, mild moxibustion with a moxa stick, or warm-needle moxibustion, can be applied. Treat daily or once every other day. Ten treatments constitute one course.

V. Femoral nerve injury

Principal points: Mingmen (Du 4), Jiaji points (Extra) from the first to fourth lumbar vertebrae on the affected side, Femur-Futu (St. 32), Yinshi (St. 33), Zusanli (St. 36)

Supplementary points: Yaoyangguan (Du 3), Xuehai (Sp. 10), Liangqiu (St. 34)

Method: Select 2-3 principal and supplementary points for each treatment and provide strong stimulation on all except Mingmen (Du 4), Yaoyangguan (Du 3) and Jiaji points (Extra). Retain the needles in place for 30 minutes and manipulate intermittently. Mild moxibustion with a moxa stick, or warm-needle moxibustion, may be combined at the same time. Cupping is performed on the thick muscles in the lower back, the hip and the thigh after acupuncture is completed. Treat daily or once every other day. Ten treatments constitute one course.

VI. Injury of common peroneal nerve

Principal points: Huantiao (G.B. 30), Weizhong (U.B. 40), Yanglingquan (G.B. 34), Zusanli (St. 36), Jiexi (St. 41)

Supplementary points: Weiyang (U.B. 39), Xuanzhong (G.B. 39), Qiuxu (G.B. 40), Kunlun (U.B. 60)

Method: Select 2-3 principal and supplementary points for each treatment and provide strong stimulation. Retain the needles in place for 30 minutes but manipulate intermittently. Moxibustion with a moxa stick, or warm-needle moxibustion, may be combined at the same time. Treat daily or once every other day. Ten treatments constitute one course.

Other therapies:

1. Ear acupuncture

Points: Liver, Spleen, Kidney, Shoulder, Elbow, Wrist, Finger, Lumbosacral Vertebrae, Sciatic Nerve, Buttocks, Knee, Ankle, Toe, etc., corresponding to the affected part

Method: Select 4-5 points for each treatment, according to the injured region. Perform strong stimulation with filiform needles. Retain the needles in place for 10 to 20 minutes. Treat once every other day, or needles are embedded for one to three days.

2. Electro-acupuncture

Points: 2-3 pairs of the body points mentioned above are selected and can be alternated.

Method: After connecting needles to the electro-acupuncture apparatus, increase the current gradually to bring on muscular contraction or local numbness, but not beyond the patient's tolerance. Connect the needles with the electricity for 15 minutes. Treat once every other day.

3. Cutaneous acupuncture

Points: The cutaneous areas dominated by the injured nerves

Method: Use a cutaneous needle to produce strong stimulation with heavy tapping, until causing the skin to bleed slightly. Treat twice weekly.

Remarks: Acupuncture and moxibustion have shown fair effects in the treatment of peripheral nerve injuries. During the treatment, encourage and assist the patient to do functional exercise, either actively or passively, so as to prevent muscular atrophy and deformity of joints.

REFERENCES:

1. Observed results of five cases of radial nerve injury treated with head acupuncture

Points:

Motor impairment: Upper Limb Motor Area (middle two-fifths) on the opposite side

Dysesthesia: Upper Limb Sensory Area (middle two-fifths) on the opposite side

Method: Insert a gauge 28 filiform needle, 2 or 2.5 *cun* in length, swiftly into the skin and then rotate down to the selected area. Perform the rotation of the needle for 30 seconds. When a needling sensation appears in the corresponding limb, give continuous rotation for five minutes. After a short period, manipulate the needle again, and this procedure is repeated three times. Treat daily. Twelve treatments constitute one course, with a three-day interval between courses.

Results: Marked effect was obtained in all the patients with 12-60 days of treatment.

(*Source:* Shanxi Traditional Chinese Medicine, 2(5):19, 1986)

2. Observed results of 30 cases of common peroneal nerve injury treated with electro-acupuncture

Points: a) Huantiao (G.B. 30), Yanglingquan (G.B. 34), Xuanzhong (G.B. 39), Foot-Linqi (G.B. 41); b) Zusanli (St. 36), Fuxi (U.B. 38), Xiajuxu (St. 39), Jiexi (St. 41)

Method: Select either of the two groups for each treatment. Connect the negative pole with the first two points and the positive pole with the two points behind. The frequency is 20-30 times per minute and the electric current is increased gradually to the extent of the patient's tolerance. The duration of electric treatment should be 20-30 minutes. Treat once every other day. Ten treatments constitute one course, with an interval of five days between courses.

Results: Of the 30 cases treated, 19 were cured, 3 showed marked effect, 4 showed some improvement and 4 showed no effect. The total effective rate was 86.7 percent.

(*Source :* Shanghai Journal of Acupuncture and Moxibustion, (4):18, 1986)

3. Observed results of 35 cases of superior cluneal nerve injury treated with acupuncture

Points and method: Insert three gauge 28-30 filiform needles into the tender spot of the superior cluneal nerve. Beginning at the top and

97

progressing downward, insert the needles at a 10-degree angle, to a depth of 2.5 *cun*. An electro-acupuncture apparatus is connected to one needle at the top and one at the bottom. Determine the intensity according to the patient's tolerance. Leave the needles in place for one hour.

Results: Of the 35 cases treated, 25 were cured, 7 showed marked effect, 2 showed improvement, and 1 showed no results. Usually a cure can be obtained with 1-2 treatments.

(*Source:* Jiangsu Chinese Medical Journal, 8(5):7, 1987)

17. Neurasthenia

Principal points: Shenmen (H. 7), Sanyinjiao (Sp. 6), Neiguan (P. 6), Sishencong (Extra)

Method: Puncture with moderate stimulation. Leave the needles in place for 15-30 minutes.

Supplementary points:

Deficiency of the heart and spleen: Xinshu (U.B. 15), Pishu (U.B. 20), Jueyinshu (U.B. 14)

Disharmony between the heart and kidney: Xinshu (U.B. 15), Shenshu (U.B. 23), Taixi (K. 3)

Upward attacking of fire in the liver: Ganshu (U.B. 18), Taichong (Liv. 3), Jianshi (P. 5)

Qi deficiency of the heart and gall bladder: Pangguangshu (U.B. 28), Danshu (U.B. 19)

Headache and vertigo: Touwei (St. 8), Fengchi (G.B. 20), Taiyang (Extra), Baihui (Du 20)

Palpitation: Xinshu (U.B. 15), Tongli (H. 5)

Tinnitus: Ermen (S.J. 21), Yifeng (S.J. 17)

Poor appetite: Zhongwan (Ren 12), Zusanli (St. 36), Weishu (U.B. 21)

Irregular menstruation: Guanyuan (Ren 4), Shenshu (U.B. 23), Baliao (U.B. 31-34)

Impotence, seminal emission: Guanyuan (Ren 4), Qihai (Ren 6), Shenshu (U.B. 23), Mingmen (Du 4), Taixi (K. 3)

Other therapies:

1. Ear acupuncture

Points: Shenmen, Heart, Spleen, Kidney, Central Rim, Brain

Method: Choose 2-3 points for each session. Puncture with moderate stimulation and rotation. The needles are left inserted for 20 minutes. Either needle-embedding or seed-embedding method can be used. Ask the patient to press them 2-3 times a day, massaging and pressing for 1-3 minutes, or until the points have a slight, distention sensation.

2. Cutaneous acupuncture

Points: Bilateral Jiaji points (Extra), Sacral Area, Head and Temporal Area

Method: Tap gently and cause the local area to become reddish in color. Treat once every other day.

3. Head acupuncture

Points: Motor Area, Sensory Area, Vertigo and Hearing Area, Leg Motor and Sensory Area

Method: Slowly insert the needle and rotate. Continue to rotate a little bit after a needling sensation is obtained. Retain the needles for 30 minutes.

4. Hydro-acupuncture

Points: Xinshu (U.B. 15), Pishu (U.B. 20), Neiguan (P. 6), Zusanli (St. 36)

Method: Select two points for each session. Inject a 100 mg Vitamin B_1 or 100 μg Vitamin B_{12} solution into the two points. Treat once every other day. Ten treatments constitute one course.

Remarks: Acupuncture and moxibustion are quite effective in the treatment of this illness. The best time for treatment is in the afternoon or just before the bedtime.

REFERENCES:

1. Effects of acupuncture in the treatment of 30 cases of insomnia
Points:

Disharmony between the heart and kidney: Shenshu (U.B. 23), Sanyinjiao (Sp. 6), Shenmen (H. 7)

Deficiency of the heart and spleen: Pishu (U.B. 20), Zusanli (St. 36), Sanyinjiao (Sp. 6), Shenmen (H. 7)

Excessive fire in the liver and gall bladder: Shenshu (U.B. 23), Shenmen (H. 7)

Method: Apply reinforcing method or even method in case of disharmony between the heart and kidney. Apply reducing method to treat excessive fire in the liver and gall bladder.

Results: Of the 30 cases treated, 5 cases were cured, 5 cases showed marked effect, 16 cases experienced some improvement, while 4 cases showed no effect.

(*Source:* Shanghai Journal of Traditional Chinese Medicine, (8):18, 1964)

2. Primary analysis on the use of needle-embedding method, applied to the ear, in the treatment of 100 cases of insomnia

Points: Heart, Shenmen, Kidney, Brain, Stomach

Method: Apply needle-embedding for 1-2 weeks. There is no obvious difference in the therapeutic results produced, due to the selection of unilateral points or bilateral points.

Results: With an established cure of 7-8 hours of sleep, 17 cases were cured. Improvement was evident in 65 cases, while 18 cases showed no effect. The total effective rate reached 82 percent.

(*Source:* New Journal of Traditional Chinese Medicine, (6):28, 1982)

3. Primary analysis on heel acupuncture in the treatment of neurasthenia

Point: The point is located at the center of heel where two lines cross, the transverse line on the sole, from the line drawing a vertical line starting from the mid-point of the external malleolus, and the middle line of the sole.

Method: Rotate the needle gently and insert rapidly to a depth of 0.1-0.2 *cun*. Retain the needle for 1-2 minutes. Treat daily. Six treatments constitute one course.

Results: There were 77 cases in the group. Marked effect was seen in 60 cases after 1-4 courses' treatment. In the control group of 21 cases, marked effect was seen in only 6 cases.

(*Source:* Journal of Traditional Chinese Medicine, (8):16, 1964)

4. Observed results of acupuncture in treating excessive sleep

Point and method: First, puncture bilateral Xinshu (U.B. 15) with the tip of the needle at an oblique angle to the root of the spinal process, and insert to a depth of 1 *cun*. Continue rotating, twirling, lifting and thrusting until the needling sensation extends to the chest. Puncture bilateral Zusanli (St. 36) and Sanyinjiao (Sp. 6) with a deep insertion. Continue rotating, twirling, lifting and thrusting until the needling sensation extends to the feet. Needle Baihui (Du 20) subcutaneously at a forward angle until the needling sensation is obtained. Apply the even method to all points. Retain the needles for 15-20 minutes, with periodic manipulation. Ten treatments constitute one course.

Results: Among 26 cases, 20 cases were cured, improvement was seen in 5 cases, while no effect was seen in only 1 case.

(*Source:* New Journal of Traditional Chinese Medicine, (11):33, 1986)

18. Hysteria

Principal points: Renzhong (Du 26), Neiguan (P. 6), Shenmen (H. 7)

Method: First, puncture bilateral Neiguan (P. 6) and Shenmen (H. 7). Then puncture Renzhong (Du 26) at an upward angle. Apply moderate stimulation to each point. Leave the needles in place for 20 minutes, with periodic manipulation.

Supplementary points:

Obstructed by wind and phlegm: Hegu (L.I. 4), Taichong (Liv. 3), Fenglong (St. 40)

Qi stagnation of the liver: Shanzhong (Ren 17), Taichong (Liv. 3), Tiantu (Ren 22)

Blood failing to nourish the heart: Sanyinjiao (Sp. 6)

Stupor: Baihui (Du 20), Daling (P. 7), Yongquan (K. 1)

Convulsion of the limbs: Houxi (S.I. 3), Yanglingquan (G.B. 34)

Paralysis of the limbs: Quchi (L.I. 11), Huantiao (G.B. 30), Yanglingquan (G.B. 34)

Restlessness: Dazhui (Du 14), Taichong (Liv. 3)

Hysterical aphasia: Lianquan (Ren 23), Tongli (H. 5)

Hysterical blindness: Fengchi (G.B. 20), Sizhukong (S.J. 23), Jingming (U.B. 1)

Constricted throat: Tiantu (Ren 22), Taichong (Liv. 3)

Deafness: Yifeng (S.J. 17), Tinghui (G.B. 2)

Sudden laughing or crying: Daling (P. 7), Sanyinjiao (Sp. 6), Shaoshang (Lu. 11)

Lack of appetite: Zusanli (St. 36), Gongsun (Sp. 4)

Vomiting: Zhongwan (Ren 12)

Hiccups: Shangwan (Ren 13), Geshu (U.B. 17)

Diarrhea: Shangjuxu (St. 37), Tianshu (St. 25)

Frequent urination: Guanyuan (Ren 4), Sanyinjiao (Sp. 6)

Other therapies:

1. Ear acupuncture

Points: Heart, Kidney, Brain Stem, Occiput, Shenmen, corresponding ear points related to the affected area

Method: Choose 3-4 points, according to symptoms. Puncture bilaterally with filiform needles and strong stimulation. Leave the needles in place for 20 minutes. Treat once every other day. Mild stimulation should be applied during recovery stage.

2. Electro-acupuncture

Points: Renzhong (Du 26), Neiguan (P. 6), Hegu (L.I. 4), Taichong (Liv. 3), corresponding points related to the affected area

Method: Ask the patient to assume a prone position. After the needling sensation is obtained, connect the needles with an electro-stimulator. Use dense pulsations. During hysterical seizure, adjust the electric power to 60-70 v. and stimulate for 10 seconds. If the symptoms are not checked, begin a second stimulation at the same voltage. When symptoms are relieved, change the output power to 8-12 v. and stimulate mildly for 15 minutes. Treat daily or once every other day.

Remarks: Acupuncture and moxibustion therapies can obtain a relatively good therapeutic result in the treatment of this illness. The therapeutic result can be strengthened by a combination of oral medication and the suggestive therapy.

REFERENCES:

1. Summary on acupuncture in the treatment of 1,316 cases of hysterical paralysis

Points and method: Rapidly insert Yongquan (K. 1), applying a combination of lifting, thrusting and rotating. First, enable the patient to restore feeling, then instruct the patient to exercise the affected limbs. The suggestive therapy is carried on at the same time. If the desired effect is not obtained, Quchi (L.I. 11), Waiguan (S.J. 5), Zusanli (St. 36) and Xuanzhong (G.B. 39) are also treated. Leave the needles in place for 3-10 minutes. If desired effect is still not obtained, the needles can be connected with an electro-stimulator, using intermittent or continuous pulsations to the tolerance of the patient, or the appearance of muscle twitching in the affected limbs.

Results: Of the 1,316 cases treated, 1,287 were cured, 16 showed improvement and only 13 cases showed no effect.

(*Source:* Journal of Traditional Chinese Medicine, 27(8):43, 1986)

2. Report on the effects of acupuncture in the treatment of 100 cases of hysteria

Points and method:

Flaring-up of the heart fire attacking the lung: Puncture Hegu (L.I. 4), Shenmen (H. 7), with reducing method

Deficient *qi* and blood in the heart: Puncture Neiguan (P. 6), Shenmen (H. 7), with reinforcing method

Palpitation, stifling sensation, deep and rapid pulse: Puncture Shenmen (H. 7), Neiguan (P. 6), Hegu (L.I. 4), with even method

Results: The hysterical seizure was immediately checked after the treatment in 83 cases, symptoms were reduced in 10 cases, and no effect was seen in 7 cases.

(*Source:* Jiangxi Journal of Traditional Chinese Medicine, (3):65, 1980)

3. Observed effects of acupuncture in the treatment of 105 cases of manic mental disorders

Principal points: Shenmen (H. 7), Taichong (Liv. 3)

Supplementary points: Shanzhong (Ren 17), Qimen (Liv. 14)

Method: Puncture with reducing method. Treat daily. Twenty treatments constitute one course.

Results: Through 1-6 courses' treatment, 95 cases were cured, marked effect was shown in 7 cases, and improvement was seen in 3 cases.

(*Source:* Academic Journal of Chinese Medicine and Medica Materia, (2):36, 1987)

4. Observed effects of head acupuncture in the treatment of 296 cases of hallucination

Principal points: Houding (Du 19) joining to Baihui (Du 20)

Supplementary points:

Visual hallucination: Head-Qiaoyin (G.B. 11) joining to Tianzhu (U.B. 10)

Olfactory hallucination: Fengfu (Du 16) joining to Fengchi (G.B. 20)

Viscero-hallucination: Head-Qiaoyin (G.B. 11) joining to Luxi (S.J. 19)

Method: Insert transversely at a 15 degree angle to the scalp, joining one point to another. Puncture with twirling and rotating, applying a vibrating method, for 1-3 minutes. Retain the needles for 1-3 hours after a needling sensation is obtained. Treat daily. Ten treatments constitute one course.

Results: Of the 296 cases treated, 209 were cured, marked effect was seen in 56 cases, improvement in 19 cases and no effect in 12 cases. The total effective rate reached 95.9 percent.

(*Source:* Journal of Traditional Chinese Medicine, 28(6):52, 1987)

19. Menopausal Syndrome

Principal points: Baihui (Du 20), Dazhui (Du 14), Shenmen (H. 7), Sanyinjiao (Sp. 6), Guanyuan (Ren 4), Zusanli (St. 36)

Method: Utilize filiform needles with even method to produce a mild stimulation, and retain the needles for 20-30 minutes. Treat daily or once every other day. Ten treatments constitute one course.

Supplementary points:

Tidal fever with nocturnal sweating: Taixi (K. 3), Yinxi (H. 6)

Palpitation with insomnia: Neiguan (P. 6)

Restlessness: Jianshi (P. 5), Ligou (Liv. 5)

Depression with fullness in the chest: Neiguan (P. 6), Shanzhong (Ren 17), Jianli (Ren 11)

Irregular menstruation: Zhongji (Ren 3), Qihai (Ren 6)

Hypertension: Quchi (L.I. 11), Taichong (Liv. 3)

Sore throat: Tiantu (Ren 22), Lianquan (Ren 23)

Other therapies:

1. Ear acupuncture

Points: End of Inferior Helix Crus, Shenmen, Intertragicus, Heart, Kidney, Occiput, Uterus, Ovary

Method: Select 2-4 points for each treatment. Needle with mild or moderate stimulation and retain the needles for 15 to 20 minutes. Treat daily or once every other day. Ten treatments constitute one course. The needle-embedding method is also applicable.

2. Hydro-acupuncture

Points: Xinshu (U.B. 15), Pishu (U.B. 20), Shenshu (U.B. 23), Sanyinjiao (Sp. 6), Zusanli (St. 36)

Method: Select 2-4 points for each treatment. Inject 0.5-1 ml of Vitamin B, solution into each point. The therapy is administered once every other day. Ten treatments constitute one course.

3. Wrist-and-ankle acupuncture

Points: Upper 1 and 2, bilateral

Method: Treat using the routine method of wrist-and-ankle

acupuncture.

Remarks: Acupuncture can obtain fair effect in treating menopausal syndrome.

20. Epilepsy

Principal points: Renzhong (Du 26), Baihui (Du 20), Shenmen (H. 7), Xinshu (U.B. 15), Pishu (U.B. 20), Jiuwei (Ren 15), Jianshi (P. 5)

Method: Apply moderate stimulation to each point.

Supplementary points:

Qi stagnation in the liver: Shanzhong (Ren 17), Taichong (Liv. 3)

Dizziness, headache: Fengchi (G.B. 20), Sishencong (Extra)

Other therapies:

1. Ear acupuncture

Points: Central Rim, Brain Stem, Brain, Heart, Liver, Kidney, Shenmen

Method: Choose 2-5 points for each session. Puncture with strong stimulation. Leave the needles in place for 20-30 minutes. Treat once every other day. Puncture two ears alternatively.

Remarks: Although acupuncture therapy has shown a certain effectiveness in the treatment of this illness, it should only be taken as a supplementary measure.

REFERENCES:

1. Observed therapeutic results of head acupuncture as the main method of treatment in 70 cases of epilepsy

Points: Thoracic Cavity Area, Motor Area, Vertigo and Hearing Area, Epilepsy Control Area (4 cm above Thoracic Cavity Area) Chorea and Tremor Control Area

Severe attack of seizures: Motor Area, Chorea and Tremor Control Area

Mild attack of seizures: Thoracic Cavity Area, Epilepsy Control Area

Psycholeptic episode: Vertigo and Hearing Area

Method: Adopt transversing and quick insertions. Keep the needles inserted for 30 minutes, with periodic manipulation. Rotate three times. The speed of rotation should be 200 times per minute. If it is necessary, needle-embedding may be inserted into the Thoracic Cavity Area and Motor Area, and left embedded for 3-5 days. Instruct the patient, or a relative, to press and massage the points for one minute, three times a day. Press and massage at any time the pre-signs of epilepsy occur.

For some patients, Shenmen (H. 7), Neiguan (P. 6), Zusanli (St. 36), and Sanyinjiao (Sp. 6) may be punctured. Also, Dazhui (Du 14), Taodao (Du 13), Xinshu (U.B. 15), Changqiang (Du 1), Shanzhong (Ren 17), and Guanyuan (Ren 4) may be bled with a three-edged needle. Treat once every other day. Ten treatments constitute one course.

Results: Marked results reached 46.88 percent; the effective rate was 67.71 percent.

(*Source:* Chinese Acupuncture & Moxibustion, (3):13, 1981)

2. Observed results of puncturing Dazhui (Du 14) in the treatment of 95 cases of epilepsy

Point: Dazhui (Du 14)

Method: Puncture with a 30-degree insertion, to a depth of 1.5 cun. Withdraw the needle and do not repeat the lifting and thrusting if an electro-stroke sensation extends to the limbs. Treat once every other day. Ten treatments constitute one course.

Results: Marked effect was seen in 25.2 percent, improvement was seen in 47.4 percent, while no effect developed in 27.4 percent of the cases.

(*Source:* Chinese Acupuncture & Moxibustion, (2):4, 1982)

21. Paraplegia

Principal points: Bilateral Jiaji points (Extra) or the Back-Shu points which are distributed from 1-2 vertebrae above and 1-2 vertebrae below the damaged surface

Supplementary points:

Paralysis on the upper limbs: Dazhui (Du 14), Jianyu (L.I. 15), Quchi (L.I. 11), Waiguan (S.J. 5), Hegu (L.I. 4), Houxi (S.I. 3), Baxie (Extra)

Paralysis on the lower limbs: Ciliao (U.B. 32), Zhibian (U.B. 54), Chengfu (U.B. 36), Yinmen (U.B. 37), Femur-Futu (St. 32), Biguan (St. 31), Zusanli (St. 36), Jiexi (St. 41), Fengshi (G.B. 31), Yanglingquan (G.B. 34), Xuanzhong (G.B. 39), Weizhong (U.B. 40),

Kunlun (U.B. 60), Chengshan (U.B. 57), Xuehai (Sp. 10), Sanyinjiao (Sp. 6), Taixi (K. 3), divided into several groups for use in turn

Retention of urine or incontinence of urine: Shenshu (U.B. 23), Pangguangshu (U.B. 28), Zhongji (Ren 3), Sanyinjiao (Sp. 6), Ciliao (U.B. 32)

Constipation or uncontrolled bowel movements: Dachangshu (U.B. 25), Tianshu (St. 25), Zhigou (S.J. 6)

Yin deficiency of the liver and kidney, malnutrition of the tendon and bone: Ganshu (U.B. 18), Shenshu (U.B. 23), Taixi (K. 3), Sanyinjiao (Sp. 6)

Blood stasis obstructed in the meridians: Xuehai (Sp. 10), Geshu (U.B. 17), Sanyinjiao (Sp. 6)

Remarks: In the treatment of paraplegia, the primary cause should be dealt with first. Acupuncture and moxibustion therapies are usually applied during the recovery stage. With flaccid paralysis, strong stimulation and repeated manipulation are needed. However, with spastic paralysis, puncture gently, so as to avoid causing a spasm on the affected limbs, which could cause a broken needle or bent needle. Leave the needles in place for 30 minutes, applying periodic manipulation. During the treatments, moxibustion with a moxa stick can be applied around the acupuncture points, or, after withdrawing the needles, apply cupping on the back and thick muscles of the lower limbs. Due to sensory impairment associated with this illness, needling may fail to produce a needling sensation. Deep insertion and repeated manipulation are needed. The more obvious the needling sensation, the quicker recovery will be. For the treatment of urination and defecation disorders, use strong stimulation and repeated manipulation. Keep the needles in place for 30 minutes. If it is necessary, moxibustion can be applied. For retention of urine, shallow insertion at an acute angle should be applied at points on the lower abdominal region, so as to avoid injuring the bladder.

Other therapies:

1. Electro-acupuncture

Points: Selecting points according to above prescriptions

Method: Choose 2-3 pairs of points for each session. After a needling sensation is obtained, connect the needles to the electro-stimulator for 20-30 minutes. Set the current at a level which produces a slight muscle twitching at the local region around the acupuncture points of the affected limb. Treat daily or once every other day. This method is suitable for the treatment of flaccid paralysis.

2. Cutaneous acupuncture

Points: Jiaji points (Extra) and the Back-Shu points, meridians of the large intestine, stomach, lung, spleen, urinary bladder, small intestine, *sanjiao*, and gall bladder of the affected limb

Method: Select and tap the corresponding Jiaji points and Back-Shu points. Another 1-2 meridian pathways should also be tapped, up to down, until congestion appears. Treat once every 2-3 days.

3. Hydro-acupuncture

Points: Corresponding Jiaji points (Extra), Back-Shu points, Jianyu (L.I. 15), Quchi (L.I. 11), Waiguan (S.J. 5), Biguan (St. 31), Zusanli (St. 36), Yanglingquan (G.B. 34), Xuanzhong (G.B. 39)

Method: Choose 3-5 points for each session. Inject 0.5-1.0 ml of 100 mg Vitamin B_1 or 100 μg Vitamin B_{12} solution into each point. Treat once every other day. Ten treatments constitute one course.

Remarks: To enhance the therapeutic result, herbal medicine, drugs, physiotherapy, or massage can be combined. During the treatments, functional exercise is, of course, necessary.

REFERENCE:

Therapeutic result observations of acupuncture in the treatment of 124 cases of paraplegia

1) Body acupuncture

Points: One middle point (Extra, in the distance of one spinal process above the damaged portion and the spinal process of L5) and eight corresponding Jiaji points (Extra)

To regulate urination and defecation: Baliao (U.B. 31, 32, 33, 34), Tianshu (St. 25), Qihai (Ren 6), Zhongji (Ren 3), 0.5 *cun* lateral to Zhongji (Ren 3), Sanyinjiao (Sp. 6), and points according to symptoms

Method: When needling points on the back, the needling sensation is required to extend to the lower part of the lesion of paralysis. Puncture Tianshu (St. 25) until the needling sensation extends to the inguinal groove. Puncture the points on the Ren meridian to cause the needling sensation to extend to the genitalium. Apply mild stimulation and the reinforcing method to a spinal cord lesion, however, apply moderate stimulation and the even method to a cauda equina lesion.

2) Hydro-acupuncture

Points: Xuehai (Sp. 10), Zusanli (St. 36), Chengshan (U.B. 57), Shenshu (U.B. 23), Sanyinjiao (Sp. 6)

Method: Inject a solution of Safflower, Red Sage Root or Vitamin B$_{12}$ into the points in turn. Each point requires 0.5-0.6 ml. Treat once every other day.

Results: Of the 124 cases treated, 10 cases were cured, 102 showed some improvement and 12 displayed no effect. The normal bowel movement rate was increased from 9.7 percent (before treatment) to 81.5 percent (after treatment), and the normal urination rate from 8.1 percent to 76.61 percent. The flaccid paraplegia cases showed some improvement.

(*Source:* Journal of Traditional Chinese Medicine, 26(12):34, 1985)

22. Acute Soft Tissue Injury of the Waist

Principal points: Renzhong (Du 26), Yinmen (U.B. 37), Shenshu (U.B. 23), Zhishi (U.B. 52), Yaoyangguan (Du 3), Huantiao (G.B. 30)

Method: Puncture Renzhong (Du 26) or Huantiao (G.B. 30) first, with strong stimulation. To needle Renzhong (Du 26), instruct the patient to exercise the lumbar region for 3-5 minutes. At this time, thrust Huantiao (G.B. 30), until the needling sensation is conducted down to the foot. After removing the needle, puncture the remaining points with moderate stimulation. Leave the needles in place for 30 minutes, during which, mild moxibustion can be performed with a moxa stick. After withdrawing the needles, cupping can be provided on the tender spot. Treat mild cases daily, but severe cases can be treated twice daily.

Supplementary points:

Local swelling: Xuehai (Sp. 10), Geshu (U.B. 17)

Other therapies:

1. Bleeding with cupping

Points: Ashi points

Method: Use a cutaneous needle to tap the skin until it causes bleeding. Then perform cupping for five minutes to suck out a small amount of blood.

Remarks: This method is beneficial to reducing local swelling of a fresh case and long-standing blood stagnation of a chronic case.

2. Hydro-acupuncture

Points: Ashi points

Method: Inject 10 ml of 10% glucose solution, or combine this with 2 ml of 2% novocain solution, into the tender muscle bundle. Provide the injection once every 2-5 days, and 2-3 treatments constitute one course.

3. Ear acupuncture

Points: Lumbosacral Vertebrae, Shenmen

Method: Use strong stimulation. Leave the needles in place for 30 minutes, manipulating once a minute. Instruct the patient to exercise the lumbar region while the needles are left in place. One more treatment can be given the next day, if one treatment proves insufficient.

4. Electro-acupuncture

Points: Weizhong (U.B. 40), Houxi (S.I. 3), Shenshu (U.B. 23), Zhishi (U.B. 52)

Method: First use a dense wave for five minutes and then change to a sparse-dense wave. Slowly increase the output of the current and adjust according to the patient's tolerance. Connect for 10-30 minutes each time and treat once or twice daily.

5. Acu-pressure with fingers

Points: Feiyang (U.B. 58), Ashi points

Method: Using a thumb, press and knead the tender spot in the lumbar region first, then press bilateral Feiyang (U.B. 58). Massage each point for 5-10 minutes.

6. Wrist-and-ankle acupuncture

Points: Lower 5 and 6, bilateral

Method: As described above.

Remarks: Acupuncture produces good effects in the treatment of acute lumbar sprains, and combined with different methods can obtain even better effects. Instruct the patient with a case of acute injury to limit his movement of the lumbar region and bed-rest is essential.

23. Soft Tissue Injury of Knee

Principal points: Xiyan (Extra), Ashi points, Weizhong (U.B. 40), Xiyangguan (G.B. 33)

Method: Ashi points are prescribed for an injury to the medial and lateral accessory ligaments. Puncture Xiyan (Extra) and Weizhong (U.B. 40) for a lesion of the infrapatellar fat pad and cruciate ligament, and treat Xiyangguan (G.B. 33) for all injuries to the soft tissues of the knee. Perform moderate stimulation on all the points, leaving needles in place for 20-30 minutes. Manipulate every 5-10 minutes. Treat daily or once every other day.

Supplementary points:
Painful swelling of the knee: Liangqiu (St. 34), Dubi (St. 35)
Other therapies:
1. Moxibustion
Points: Ashi points
Method: Apply mild moxibustion with a moxa stick for 10-15 minutes, or indirect moxibustion with ginger for 5-7 moxa cones, once daily.
2. Ear acupuncture
Points: Knee, Shenmen, Brain
Method: Apply moderate or strong stimulation with filiform needles, leaving the needles in place for 10-30 minutes. Treat daily.
Remarks: This treatment has notable analgesic effects.
3. Bleeding with cupping
Points: Ashi points
Method: Tap the tender spots of the knee with a skin needle to cause bleeding, and then perform cupping for 3-5 minutes.
4. Wrist-and-ankle acupuncture
Points: Lower 3, 4, and 5 (affected side)
Method: The routine operation is performed.
Remarks: Acupuncture and moxibustion therapies have satisfactory effect on analgesia and in reducing the swelling of the soft tissue of the knee.

24. Soft Tissue Injury of the Ankle

Principal points: Ashi points, Xuanzhong (G.B. 39), Jiexi (St. 41)
Method: Use the tender spot as the primary point and apply moderate stimulation, while combining Xuanzhong (G.B. 39) and Jiexi (St. 41) with strong stimulation. Leave the needles in place for 10-30 minutes and manipulate intermittently every 5-10 minutes. Treat daily.
Supplementary points: Kunlun (U.B. 60), Qiuxu (G.B. 40), Sanyinjiao (Sp. 6)

111

Other therapies:

1. Moxibustion

Points: Ashi points

Method: At the tender spot of the ankle, apply mild moxibustion with a moxa stick for 10-20 minutes, or indirect moxibustion with ginger, for 5-7 moxa cones, until the skin in the local region is flush. Treat once or twice daily.

2. Ear acupuncture

Points: Ankle, Shenmen, Brain

Method: Rotate filiform needles to produce moderate or strong stimulation, and then retain the needles for 10-30 minutes. Treat daily.

3. Bleeding with cupping

Points: Ashi points

Method: Tap the point with a cutaneous needle to cause bleeding, then provide cupping for 3-5 minutes.

Remarks: Acupuncture and moxibustion produce positive effects in treating analgesia and resolving swelling in the soft tissue of the ankle, but they are more helpful as treatments for sprains and contusions. If there is a rupture of a ligament, surgical treatment is recommended.

REFERENCES:

1. Observed results of 2,000 cases of acute soft tissue injury treated with contralateral needling

Points and method: Mark the tender spot in the injured area and provide the contralateral needling to the counterpart spot on the opposite side with swift insertion. Lift, thrust and rotate the needle. After a needling sensation of soreness, numbness and distention is obtained, the needle is left inserted for 20-30 minutes. During this time, gently massage the affected side to produce a hot sensation. When the pain disappears a few minutes later, fix the injured region with adhesive plaster, opposite to that causing the injury.

Results: Of the 2,000 cases treated, 1,980 cases were cured with only 1 treatment, making up 99 percent. The remaining 1 percent, or 20 cases, were cured with 2-3 treatments.

(*Source:* Chinese Acupuncture & Moxibustion, (4):17, 1987)

2. Observed results of 100 cases of acute joint sprain treated by needling the corresponding points

Points:

1) The hip joint corresponds to the shoulder; the anterior superior

iliac spine to the acromion;

2) The knee joint corresponds to the elbow; the patella to the olecranon; the patellar ligament to the tendon of the brachial triceps; the medial condyle of the femur to the lateral epicondyle of the humerus; and the lateral condyle of the femur to the medial epicondyle of the humerus;

3) The ankle joint corresponds to the wrist; the medial malleolus to the styloid process of the radius and the external malleolus to the styloid process of the ulna;

4) The toes correspond to the fingers;

5) The corresponding point of the lumbar sprain is located at the mid-point of the connection between both nipples (equal to the location of Shanzhong, Ren 17);

6) The corresponding points of the limbs are selected according to the proportion of the length of limbs.

Method: After the arrival of *qi*, produce strong stimulation and exercise the injured region, while the needles remain inserted for 20-30 minutes.

Results: The total effective rate was 99.4 percent and the cure rate was 89.1 percent.

(*Source:* Chinese Acupuncture & Moxibustion, (4):8, 1984)

3. Treatment of acute ankle sprain with ankle acupuncture

Points: Lower 1, 2, and 3

Method: Needle at a horizontal angle to skin, to a depth of 1.5 *cun*. Inferior 3 is supplemented if the pain appears when the heel touches the ground.

Results: Usually cure can be obtained within 2-4 treatments.

(*Source:* Journal of Henan College of Traditional Chinese Medicine, (1):50, 1978)

4. Treatment of ankle sprain with acupuncture

Points: Bafeng (Extra) as primary point; combined with Zusanli (St. 36) and Chongyang (St. 42)

Method: Select 1-2 loci of Bafeng (Extra) on the affected side and supplement Chongyang (St. 42) in cases of remarkable swelling. Employ gauge 23 filiform needles and insert to a depth determined by the arrival of *qi*. Leave the needles in place for 30 minutes, after the pain disappears. Treat daily.

Results: Of the 89 cases treated, all were cured. The minimum number of treatments was 1 and the maximum was 7. The cure rate was 100 percent.

(*Source:* Chinese Acupuncture & Moxibustion, (2):55, 1987)

5. Observed results of the treatment of 400 cases of acute lumbar sprain with acupuncture at Shangdu (Extra)

Point: Shangdu (Extra)

Method: Insert the needle towards the center of the sole to a depth of 1-1.5 *cun*, and leave the needle inserted for 20 minutes.

Results: The rate of cure was 89 percent.

(*Source:* Chinese Acupuncture & Moxibustion, (2):24, 1986)

6. Observed results of 56 cases of acute lumbar sprain treated with acupuncture in tender spots

Points and method: Require the patient to bend and stretch his lower back and to bend laterally as well. After finding the tender spot, insert a 1.5 *cun* needle to a depth of 1-1.2 *cun*. After the arrival of *qi*, lift the needle 0.3-0.5 *cun* subcutaneously and rotate clockwise. Wrap the needle under the skin and allow the patient to exercise the lumbar region. Simultaneously hold the handle of the needle, applying the sparrow-pricking method for 2-3 minutes. Rotate the needle counterclockwise, insert again to a depth of 1-1.2 *cun* to obtain the arrival of *qi*, and then withdraw. After withdrawal, allow the patient to move freely, and the pain should disappear.

Results: Of the 56 cases treated, most were cured with 1-2 treatments.

(*Source:* Academic Journal of Chinese Medicine and Medica Materia, (2):31, 1981)

7. Observed results of 150 cases of acute lumbar sprain treated by needling Yintang (Extra)

Point: Yintang (Extra)

Method: Thrusting downward, apply strong stimulation and leave the needles in place for 10-15 minutes.

Results: Of the 150 cases treated, 126 cases were cured, 11 showed improvement, and 13 showed no effect.

(*Source:* Chinese Acupuncture & Moxibustion, (2):26, 1984)

8. Observed results of the treatment of 81 cases of acute lumbar sprain by acupuncture at three back points

Points: Chengjin (U.B. 56), Yaoyangguan (Du 3), Yaoyan (Extra)

Method: First puncture Chengjin (U.B. 56) with the tip of the needle slanted upward. After the arrival of *qi*, with the thumb of the assisting hand, press Chengshan (U.B. 57) and rotate the needle to conduct the propagation of the needling sensation up to the lumbar region. Then needle Yaoyangguan (Du 3) and Yaoyan (Extra) and the sensation is also directed to the focus of the pain. Leave the needles inserted for five minutes.

Results: Of the 81 cases treated, 76 cases were cured with only 1 treatment and 5 were cured with 2 treatments.

(*Source:* Chinese Acupuncture & Moxibustion, (4):21, 1987)

9. Observed results of 30 cases of acute lumbar sprain treated with needling at Houxi (S.I. 3)

Point: Houxi (S.I. 3)

Method: Needle the point applying strong stimulation and instruct the patient to exercise the lower back at the same time.

Results: 15 cases were cured with 1 treatment, 8 were cured with 2 treatments and 7 with 3-4 treatments.

(*Source:* Hubei Journal of Traditional Chinese Medicine, (1):25, 1984)

10. Clinical observation of the treatment of 1,000 cases of acute lumbar sprain by needling Renzhong (Du 26) and Jingming (U.B. 1)

Points and method:

1) If the sprain takes place at the mid-line of the lumbar spine, 1 cm lateral from both sides of Renzhong (Du 26), insert the needle from the left side and penetrate to the right to produce strong stimulation for 5-10 seconds. The operator holds the patient at the junction of the lumbar region and the abdomen to assist the exercise of the lower back. The force should increase gradually and the movement should alternate between clockwise and counterclockwise, 20 times for each.

2) If the sprain is of the soft tissues, needle Jingming (U.B. 1) on the affected side and the same exercise is performed.

3) After the above treatment, the symptoms will be considerably alleviated. Dachangshu (U.B. 25) can be punctured. Cupping is done at Ashi point in the lumbar region and Weizhong (U.B. 40) can be also combined. Contralateral needling is also applicable.

Results: The cure rate was 77.2 percent, marked effective rate was 19.9 percent and rate of failure was 2.9 percent, so the total effective rate was 97.1 percent.

(*Source:* Yunnan Journal of Traditional Chinese Medicine, 3(1):34, 1982)

11. Clinical observation of 100 cases of acute lumbar sprain

treated by acupuncture to Yaoning (Extra)

Points: Place the palm of the affected side on the chest, with the tip of the thumb resting at Tiantu (Ren 22), and raise the elbow. In the depression on the anterior border superior to the elbow joint, among Quchi (L.I. 11), Hand-Wuli (L.I. 13) and Xiabai (Lu. 4), you will find a tender spot when you press with moderate force. That is the point Yaoning (Extra).

Method: Apply slow and perpendicular insertion to a depth of 0.5-1.5 *cun* and after the arrival of *qi*, apply strong stimulation for 10-20 seconds. Retain the needle for 15-30 minutes, during which, manipulate the needle 3-5 times, 5-10 seconds each time. Meanwhile require the patient to exercise his lower back. Remove the needle when the pain disappears or is markedly relieved.

Results: There were 98 cases cured, 1 case showed marked effect and 1 case displayed no results.

(*Source:* Journal of Integrated Traditional and Western Medicines, 6(7), 1986)

12. Preliminary observation of 358 cases of lumbago treated with abdomen acupuncture

Point: Corresponding point of the lower backache on the abdomen

Method: Apply standard needling techniques.

Results: There were 303 cases cured, 29 showed marked effects, 7 showed improvement and 19 showed no results.

(*Source:* Chinese Acupuncture & Moxibustion, (1):24, 1982)

25. Cervical Spondylosis

Principal points: Jiaji points (Extra, parallel to the affected vertebrae), Yanglao (S.I. 6), Dazhui (Du 14), Jianjing (G.B. 21)

Method: To puncture Jiaji points (Extra), angle the tip of the needle obliquely towards the spine. Puncture Dazhui (Du 14) with the needle deviating slightly to the affected side to obtain the propagation of the needling sensation down to the shoulder and arm. Strong stimulation is necessary in Yanglao (S.I. 6), while moderate stimulation is necessary in Jianjing (G.B. 21). The needles are retained for 20-30 minutes and warm-needle moxibustion or suspending moxibustion with a moxa stick over the point can be applied. Treat daily and 10 treatments

116

constitute one course.

Supplementary points:

Painful shoulder and arm: Jianyu (L.I. 15), Quchi (L.I. 11)

Numbness of fingers: Waiguan (S.J. 5), Baxie (Extra)

The pain localized in subscapular fossa: Tianzong (S.I. 11)

Localized pain in anterior aspect of the shoulder: Jianneiling (Extra)

Headache and dizziness: Fengchi (G.B. 20)

Other therapies:

1. Ear acupuncture

Points: Neck, Cervical Vertebrae, Shoulder, End of Inferior Helix Crus

Method: Apply strong stimulation with filiform needles and then retain the needles for 20-30 minutes. Treat daily or once every other day

2. Electro-acupuncture

Points: Jiaji points (Extra, parallel to the affected vertebrae), Dazhui (Du 14), Dazhu (U.B. 11), Tianzong (S.I. 11), Jianzhongshu (S.I. 15)

Method: Select 2-3 pairs of points for each treatment. After the arrival of *qi*, connect the electro-acupuncture apparatus with the needles to give stimulation with an impulsed current for 20-30 minutes. Treat daily or once every other day.

3. Bleeding combined with cupping

Points: Dazhui (Du 14), Dazhu (U.B. 11), Jianzhongshu (S.I. 15), Jianwaishu (S.I. 14)

Method: Tap the points with a cutaneous needle until the skin becomes flushed with a few bleeding spots in the local area, on which cupping is then applied.

4. Hydro-acupuncture

Points: Dazhu (U.B. 11), Jianzhongshu (S.I. 15), Jianwaishu (S.I. 14), Tianzong (S.I. 11)

Method: Select 2-3 points for each treatment. Inject 0.5-1.0 ml of 1% procaine solution into each point, once every other day.

Remarks: Acupuncture is fairly effective in relieving the symptoms of this disease. If traction, massage, and dirigation can be incorporated, the effectiveness will increase.

REFERENCE:

Observed results of 22 cases of cervical spondylosis treated with warm-needle acupuncture at Jiaji points (Extra)

Points: Jiaji points (Extra) parallel to the affected vertebrae

Pain in the nape of the neck and occipitus, and sensory disturbance: Jiaji points (Extra) 1.5 cm lateral to the interspace between the spinous processes of the third and fourth cervical vertebrae

Pain in the nape of the neck and the radiating pain and numbness from the shoulder down to the lateral aspect of the upper arm, the radial side of the forearm and the wrist: Jiaji points (Extra) 1.5 cm lateral to the interspace between the spinous processes of the fourth and fifth vertebrae

Pain and numbness going down to the thumb and the index finger: Jiaji points (Extra) 1.5 cm lateral to the interspace between the spinous processes of the fifth and sixth vertebrae

Pain and numbness radiating to the index finger and the middle finger: Jiaji points (Extra) 1.5 cm lateral to the interspace between the spinous processes of the sixth and seventh vertebrae

Numbness and pain radiating down to the medial aspect of the upper arm, the ulnar side of the forearm, the ring finger and the little finger: Jiaji points (Extra) 1.5 cm lateral to the interspace between the spinous processes of the seventh cervical vertebra and the first thoracic vertebra

Method: Apply warm-needle acupuncture once every other day. Ten treatments constitute one course.

Results: Of 22 cases treated, 7 were cured, 12 showed marked effect and 3 failed.

(*Source:* Shanghai Journal of Acupuncture and Moxibustion, (2):18, 1984)

26. Stiff Neck

Principal points: Laozhenxue (Extra), Xuanzhong (G.B. 39), Houxi (S.I. 3), Ashi points, Yanglao (S.I. 6)

Method: All the points are punctured on the affected side. Usually, Laozhenxue (Extra), Xuanzhong (G.B. 39), or Yanglao (S.I. 6) is needled at first with moderate or strong stimulation. When you rotate the needle, require the patient to move his neck around. Puncture

Houxi (S.I. 3) and tender spot in the local region when the pain is alleviated. Retain the needles for 15-30 minutes and manipulate once or twice during that period. Moxibustion can also be applied at the same time, and after removing the needles, cupping can be performed on shoulder and scapular region, and at the tender spot as well. Treat daily.

Supplementary points:

Headache: Fengchi (G.B. 20), Waiguan (S.J. 5)

Painful shoulder and back: Quyuan (S.I. 13), Dazhu (U.B. 11), Jianwaishu (S.I. 14)

Inability to raise or lower the head: Lieque (Lu. 7), or Dazhu (U.B. 11) and Jinggu (U.B. 64)

Inability to look backward: Zhizheng (S.I. 7), Jianwaishu (S.I. 14)

Other therapies:

1. Cutaneous acupuncture

Point: Ashi point

Method: Perform tapping with a cutaneous needle, first on the painful and rigid area of the nape of the neck until the skin becomes flushed and then on the tender spot of the shoulder and back.

2. Ear acupuncture

Points: Neck, Cervical Vertebrae, and tender spot

Method: Produce strong stimulation with filiform needles. While rotating the needle, require the patient to turn his head slowly for a couple of minutes. Retain the needles for 30 minutes. Treat daily.

3. Bleeding with cupping

Points: Tender spots on the neck

Method: Tap the tender spots with a cutaneous needle to cause bleeding, and then provide cupping.

Remarks: Acupuncture is very good in the treatment of a stiff neck. Such a case can be cured with 1-3 treatments. The effect will be more satisfactory if hot compress and massage follow the needling.

REFERENCES:

1. Observations of treatment of 215 cases of stiff neck by needling Houxi (S.I. 3)

Point: Houxi (S.I. 3)

Method: Insert the point to a depth of 0.3-0.5 *cun.* Produce strong stimulation and connect an electro-acupuncture apparatus with the frequency of 40-50 times per minute. Retain the needles for 15-20 minutes.

Results: Of 215 cases treated, 163 cases were cured with 1 treatment, 38 were cured with 2 treatments and 14 were improved after three sessions.

(*Source:* Chinese Acupuncture & Moxibustion, (5):22, 1984)

2. Observed results of the treatment of eight cases of stiff neck by needling Xuanzhong (G.B. 39)

Point: Xuanzhong (G.B. 39)

Method: Insert a filiform needle 2 *cun* in length into the point, and retain the needle for 30 minutes. During this time, manipulate the needle and require the patient to turn his head.

Results: All the cases were cured with 1 treatment.

(*Source:* Hunan Journal of Medicine and Medica Materia, (4):4, 1984)

3. Observed results of joint needling from Yemen (S.J. 2) to Hand-Zhongzhu (S.J. 3) in the treatment of spasms of the tendon of the neck

Points: Yemen (S.J. 2), Hand-Zhongzhu (S.J. 3)

Method: The palm of the hand of the affected side should face downward and be slightly clenched. Insert the needle at Yemen (S.J. 2) and thrust further towards Hand-Zhongzhu (S.J. 3) through the subcutaneous soft tissues. The depth of insertion is 1 *cun*. After the patient begins to feel such needling sensations as soreness, distention, numbness and heaviness, lift the needle and thrust and rotate as much as possible without exceeding the patient's tolerance. While manipulating the needle, require the patient to exercise his neck. Manipulate the needle for 20-60 seconds. Leave the needle in place for 15 minutes and manipulate as mentioned every five minutes.

Results: The treatment was effective in all cases involving injury of the soft tissue of the neck. Fifty-six cases were cured with 1 treatment, 17 were cured with 2 treatments and 5 were cured with 3 treatments.

(*Source:* Chinese Acupuncture & Moxibustion, (1):30, 1987)

27. Periarthritis of Shoulder Joint

Principal points: Tiaokou (St. 38), Jianyu (L.I. 15), Jianliao (S.J. 14), Binao (L.I. 14), Quchi (L.I. 11), Waiguan (S.J. 5), Ashi points

Method: Instruct the patient to take a sitting position with legs bent in a right angle at the knees. Insert a needle 3 *cun* in length at Tiaokou (St. 38) but thrust further towards Chengshan (U.B. 57), and rotate continuously. After the arrival of *qi*, require the patient to move the affected arm by raising it, touching the upper and the lower back, and feeling the opposite shoulder. The action should be gentle at the beginning and gradually speeds up, so as to avoid sharp pain. Manipulate the needle for 3-5 minutes, and after the pain is alleviated, puncture other points with moderate or strong stimulation. Retain the needles for 20-30 minutes, but manipulate every 5-10 minutes, and apply mild moxibustion with a moxa stick or warm-needle moxibustion at the same time. Treat daily or once every other day. Jianyu (L.I. 15) and Jianliao (S.J. 14) can be punctured with penetrating method from various directions.

Supplementary points:

Pain in the medial aspect of the shoulder: Chize (Lu. 5), Taiyuan (Lu. 9)

Pain in the lateral aspect of the shoulder: Houxi (S.I. 3), Xiaohai (S.I. 8)

Pain in the front of the shoulder: Hegu (L.I. 4), Lieque (Lu. 7)

Other therapies:

1. Ear acupuncture

Points: Shoulder, Shoulder Joint, Clavicle, Lower Apex of Tragus, Ashi point

Method: Select 2-3 points each time. Produce strong stimulation by continuous rotation of the needles and require the patient to properly exercise the affected arm. Retain the needles for 10-20 minutes and treat once every other day.

2. Electro-acupuncture

Points: Jianyu (L.I. 15), Jianliao (S.J. 14), Jianzhen (S.I. 9), Binao (L.I. 14)

Method: Select 1-2 pairs of points for each treatment. After the arrival of *qi*, connect the electro-acupuncture apparatus to the needles for 15 minutes. Adjust the intensity according to the patient's tolerance. Treat daily. Ten treatments constitute one course.

3. Moxibustion

Point: Ashi point

Method: Perform suspending moxibustion with a moxa stick over the tender spot in the local region, once or twice daily, 10-20 minutes

121

each time. Ten treatments constitute one course.

4. Bleeding with cupping

Point: Ashi point

Method: By means of the routine operation of cutaneous acupuncture, heavily tap the tender spot in the local region to cause bleeding, and then perform cupping on it for 5-10 minutes to suck out a small amount of blood. Treat once every third or fourth day. Cupping may be used alone.

5. Hydro-acupuncture

Point: Ashi point

Method: Use a solution of 2 ml of 200 μg Vitamin B_{12}, 2 ml of 2% novocain and 1 ml of water. After the arrival of *qi*, inject the liquid into the tender spot by means of routine operation of hydro-acupuncture. Inject once every second or third day. Ten treatments constitute one course.

Remarks : Acupuncture and moxibustion are fairly effective in treating periarthritis of the shoulder joint. The pain can be relieved or even eradicated after treatment, and the motoring function of the affected arm can return to normal or at least become improved after only a few treatments. The combination of body acupuncture, electro-acupuncture and ear acupuncture can heighten the therapeutic effect. In cases involving the motor impairment of the joint, combine massage and functional exercise to obtain a better effect.

REFERENCES:

1. Observed result of 51 cases of periarthritis of the shoulder joint treated by needling Jiaji points (Extra)

Points: Jiaji points (Extra) on both sides of the fifth cervical vertebra

Method: After penetrating the skin, thrust the needle horizontally to obtain the arrival of *qi* and then connect with electro-acupuncture apparatus for 15-30 minutes. The frequency is 1,000-1,500 times per minute.

Results: There were 31 cases cured, 10 showed marked effectiveness, 6 showed improvement and 4 failed.

(*Source:* Chinese Acupuncture & Moxibustion, (2):31, 1983)

2. Observed results of 246 cases of periarthritis of the shoulder joint treated with acupuncture

Point: Jianyu (L.I. 15)

Method: After the insertion, thrust the needle to the ventral, the medial and the lateral aspects of the shoulder to a depth of 5 cm and flick the handle of the needle three times. The direction of the insertion is parallel to the humerus.

Results: The cure rate was 85.8 percent with 1-4 treatments and with 5-9 treatments was 14.2 percent.

(*Source:* Shanghai Journal of Acupuncture and Moxibustion, (3):24, 1987)

3. Observed results of 122 cases of periarthritis of the shoulder joint treated with head acupuncture

Points and method: Insert the needle to a depth of 1 *cun* in the middle one-third of the anterior oblique parietotemporal line, the line connecting Qianding (Du 21) and Xuanli (G.B. 6), if one shoulder is affected. If both sides are affected, the point on the opposite side is used as well. If the pain is located on the anterior aspect of the shoulder, thrust the tip of the needle in the ventral direction. If the pain is on the posterior aspect of the shoulder, insert the tip towards the back. Manipulate the needle with the air-pumping method. The transient disappearance or relieving of the pain in the affected area is considered as the arrival of *qi* and then retain the needle for more than one hour, and manipulate every 10-30 minutes. Meanwhile, require the patient to exercise the affected shoulder, like lifting, stretching backward, adduction, intorsion, and abduction. Increase the amplitude and the intensity slowly. Treat once every second day and 10 treatments constitute one course.

Results: Of 122 cases treated, 77 cases were cured, 23 showed marked effect, 21 were improved, and 1 failed. The total effective rate was 99.2 percent.

(*Source:* Zhejiang Journal of Traditional Chinese Medicine, 22(3):116, 1987)

4. Observations of 40 cases of periarthritis of the shoulder joint treated with electro-acupuncture

Principal points: Three shoulder points (Jianyu, L.I. 15; the locus 1 *cun* above the anterior end of the axillary fold; and 1 *cun* above the posterior end of the axillary fold), Quchi (L.I. 11), Tiaokou (St. 38)

Supplementary points: Jianliao (S.J. 14), Bingfeng (S.I. 12), Ashi point

Method: Connect with the electricity 20 minutes daily. One course of treatment consists of 10 times and there is a 5-7 day interval between two courses.

Results: With 1-3 courses, 24 cases were cured, 5 showed marked effect and 11 were improved.

(*Source:* Jiangxi Journal of Traditional Chinese Medicine, (3):37, 1987)

5. Observed results of 343 cases of omarthritis treated with the contralateral or opposite needling method

Points:

Pain in the middle of the acromion: Biguan (St. 31) on the opposite side

Pain posterior to the acromion: Huantiao (G.B. 30) on the opposite side

Pain anterior to the acromion: the corresponding point in the medial side of the opposite thigh

Method: Treat deficiency and cold with burning-mountain-fire technique. Treat excess and heat with penetrating-sky-coolness technique. Treat indistinguishable deficiency or excess with even method.

Results: Of 343 cases treated, 222 cases were cured (64.7 percent). The total effective rate was 98.1 percent.

(*Source:* Shaanxi Journal of Traditional Chinese Medicine, (6):40, 1982)

6. Observed results of the treatment of 92 cases of shoulder pain with acupuncture

Point: Xiajuxu (St. 39)

Method: Insert a needle to a depth of 1.5 *cun* and retain the needle for 10-15 minutes. At the same time, require the patient to exercise the shoulder. Treat once every other day. Five treatments constitute one course.

Results: The total effective rate was 96.7 percent.

(*Source:* Chinese Acupuncture & Moxibustion, (4):19, 1986)

7. Observed results of the treatment of shoulder and arm pain with wrist-and-ankle acupuncture

Points: Upper 5, bilateral

Method: Needle horizontally and subcutaneously to a depth of 1-1.5 *cun*, and retain the needle for 30 minutes. Treat daily.

Results: Cure was obtained with 3-5 treatments.

(*Source:* Guangxi Journal of Bare-footed Doctors, (10):17 1978)

8. Observed results of 103 cases of periarthritis of the shoulder joint treated with acupuncture and acupoint injection

Points and method: Perform penetrating method from Tiaokou (St. 38) to Chengshan (U.B. 57) in the leg of the healthy side if one shoulder is affected, but bilaterally if both shoulders get the disease. Retain the needles for 15-20 minutes. Simultaneously, inject 1 ml of 5% Danggui solution into each of the following points: 1 *cun* medial and superior to Tianzong (S.I. 11), 1 *cun* lateral and superior to Naoshu (S.I. 10), 1 *cun* lateral and anterior to Jianyu (L.I. 15), 0.5 *cun* below Jugu (L.I. 16) and the point of the acromioclavicular joint.

Results: Of 103 cases treated, 78 cases were cured, 21 showed marked effect, 3 were improved, and 1 failed. The total effective rate was 99.03 percent.

(*Source:* Shaanxi Journal of Traditional Chinese Medicine, 5(4):28, 1984)

28. External Humeral Epicondylitis

Principal points: Ashi point at the elbow, Zhouliao (L.I. 12), Quchi (L.I. 11), Shousanli (L.I. 10)

Method: Apply moderate or strong stimulation to all points and puncture the tender spot with joint needling from various directions. Retain the needles for 20-30 minutes and manipulate every 5-10 minutes. Moxibustion can be combined or even used alone. Treat daily or once every other day, and ten treatments constitute one course.

Supplementary points:

Pain radiating down to the forearm: Waiguan (S.J. 5)

Pain radiating up to the shoulder: Jianyu (L.I. 15), Binao (L.I. 14)

Other therapies:

1. Bleeding with cupping

Point: Ashi point

Method: Tap with a cutaneous needle to bring about oozing of blood in the local region, and cup with cups of small diameter for 5-10 minutes. Treat once every three or four days.

2. Electro-acupuncture

Points: Ashi point, Quchi (L.I. 11)

Method: After the arrival of *qi*, connect the needles with an electro-acupuncture apparatus, and gradually strengthen the stimulation according to the patient's tolerance. The connection should last 10 minutes.

Treat daily or once every other day.

3. Ear acupuncture

Points: Elbow, Wrist, Brain, End of Inferior Helix Crus

Method: Produce moderate or strong stimulation with filiform needles which are retained for 15-20 minutes. Treat daily or once every other day, and 10 treatments constitute one course.

4. Wrist-and-ankle acupuncture

Points: Upper 3, 4 (affected side)

Method: Perform the routine operation of this therapy.

5. Hydro-acupuncture

Point: Ashi point

Method: Inject a solution of 0.5-1 mg of dexamethasone plus 2 ml of 1% procaine into the tender spot at the elbow by means of routine operating method of hydro-acupuncture. If the pain remains 7-10 days after the injection, the treatment can be repeated for once.

Remarks: Acupuncture therapy has fair effect in treating this disease but attention should be paid to resting the affected arm during the course of treatment.

REFERENCES:

1. Observation on the therapeutic effect of 100 cases of tennis elbow treated by needling the local points

Points: 1) Depression at the anterior border of the external epicondyle of humerus; 2) Depression at the posterior border of the external epicondyle of humerus

Impaired pronation of the forearm: Shousanli (L.I. 10) is added

Impaired supination of the forearm: Chize (Lu. 5) is added

Method: Perpendicularly puncture the depression at the anterior border of the external epicondyle of humerus and thrust a needle into the depression at the posterior border of the epicondyle in an angle of 45 degree towards the dorsum of the wrist from the middle of the epicondyle. Apply moderated stimulation and connect electricity with impulsed current for 20 minutes.

Results: Of the 100 cases treated, 62 cases were cured, 21 showed marked effect, and 17 showed some effect.

(*Source:* Journal of Traditional Chinese Medicine, 23(5):49, 1982)

2. Observed therapeutic results of the treatment of 20 cases of tennis elbow with plum-blossom needling in combination with moxibustion

Points: Ashi point, and one or two points above and below it, like Shousanli (L.I. 10) and Quchi (L.I. 11)

Method: Perform tapping with the plum-blossom needle. Begin gently in the local region. When there appears the sensation of soreness and distention, the performance is intensified until drawing blood. After cleaning the area, provide moxibustion for 15 minutes. Treat daily. Six treatments constitute one course and a 3-day interval is necessary between two courses.

Results: Of 20 cases treated, 12 cases were cured, 4 showed marked effect, 3 displayed some improvement, and 1 failed. The treatment can be repeated to those with recurrence and effectiveness can also be obtained.

(*Source:* Yunnan Journal of Traditional Chinese Medicine, 5(3):41, 1984)

3. Observed results of 20 cases of external humerus epicondylitis and tenosynovitis stenosans treated by electro-acupuncture incorporated with indirect moxibustion of ginger

Principal points: Ashi point, Zhouliao (L.I. 12), Quchi (L.I. 11), Lieque (Lu. 7), Jingqu (Lu. 8), Yangxi (L.I. 5)

Supplementary points: Shousanli (L.I. 10), Shanglian (L.I. 9), Waiguan (S.J. 5), Hegu (L.I. 4), Taiyuan (Lu. 9)

Method: Select 2-3 points daily, mainly the principal points. After the arrival of the sensation of soreness, numbness, distention and heaviness produced by needling, connect the electro-acupuncture apparatus to the needles, positive pole with the principal points and negative pole with the supplemented points. Begin by employing a continuous wave with the frequency of 120 times per minute, and change to intermittent wave after 15-20 minutes, with the frequency of 40 times per minute. Remove needles 15-20 minutes later. Adjust the intensity of the current to the level the patient can tolerate and is still comfortable. Provide indirect moxibustion with ginger on the tender spot after withdrawing the needles.

Results: Of 20 cases treated, 8 cases were cured, 10 were improved and 2 failed.

(*Source:* Chinese Acupuncture & Moxibustion, (1):6, 1987)

4. Observation on the therapeutic effect of 33 cases of external humerus epicondylitis treated with acupuncture

Points and method: Needle at Quchi (L.I. 11) and Waiguan (S.J. 5), and apply moxibustion at Ashi point. Needle gently but provide heavy moxibustion. Treat daily. Retain the needles for 15-30 minutes.

127

Seven treatments constitute one course.

Results: Of 33 cases treated, 27 were cured, 3 showed some effect and 3 failed.

(*Source:* Shanghai Journal of Acupuncture and Moxibustion, (3):18, 1984)

29. Tenosynovitis

Principal point: Ashi point

Method: Use filiform needles to puncture 3-4 points around the swollen area. Retain the needles for 15-30 minutes. Treat daily or once every other day. Moxibustion may also be combined.

Supplementary points:

Tenosynovitis on the radial styloid process: Yangxi (L.I. 5), Lieque (Lu. 7)

Tenosynovitis on the flexor digitorum muscle: Daling (P. 7), Waiguan (S.J. 5), with the tips of needles pointing to the carpal tunnel

Pain at the first metacarpophalangeal joint: Lieque (Lu. 7)

Pain at the second and third metacarpophalangeal joints: Daling (P. 7)

Pain at the fourth and fifth metacarpophalangeal joints: Shenmen (H. 7)

Other therapies:

1. Cutaneous acupuncture

Point: Ashi point (tenderness on the swollen area)

Method: Use cutaneous needles to tap the local area until the skin becomes congested or bleeds slightly. Treat daily or once every other day.

2. Moxibustion

Point: Ashi point (tenderness on the swollen area)

Method: Apply direct moxibustion with moxa cones, 3-5 in number. Take caution not to burn the skin. Treat once every other day.

3. Hydro-acupuncture

Points: Ashi point (tenderness on the swollen area), Quchi (L.I. 11) on the affected side

Method: Using 1-3 ml of 0.25-0.5% procaine hydrochloride solution, inject the tender spot and Quchi (L.I. 11) on the affected side. With chronic tenosynovitis, a 0.5-1 mg of dexamethasone should be added to the procaine hydrochloride solution for injection. Treat once every 2-3 days.

Remarks: The above-mentioned therapies are quite effective in the treatment of this condition. During treatment, movement of the affected wrist should be limited and reduced.

30. Ganglion

Principal point: Ashi point (the focus of the cyst)

Method: Insert four needles around the cyst and after the insertion, lift and thrust the needles to penetrate the wall of the cyst. Then thrust a thicker needle from the top of the cyst to penetrate the wall and reach the bottom. Retain the needles for 10-15 minutes and after withdrawing, squeeze the focus. Jelly-like mucus should flow out of the hole of the needle. Perform moxibustion with a moxa stick over the focus after needling. Treat daily or once every other day. With 3-5 treatments, the cyst will be gradually resolved. Or, use a three-edged needle to thrust the cyst in 3-4 foci which are then squeezed to press out the fluid. Bind the cyst tightly for a couple of days. If the cyst recurs, the same procedure can be repeated. Moxibustion is also applicable.

Remarks: Strict sterile technique is essential during the treatment in order to prevent an infection.

REFERENCES:

1. Observed results of the treatment of 38 cases of ganglion with deep insertion of quintuple punctures

Point: Cyst

Method: Antisepsis is essential in the treatment. Using the left hand, fix the cyst while thrusting needles 1-1.5 *cun* in length at the top and from the four sides to reach the inside of the cyst, then lift and thrust repeatedly to produce the sensation of soreness, numbness and distention. Retain the needles for 30 minutes and manipulate every five minutes.

Results: All the cases were cured within 3 treatments.

(*Source:* Shandong Medical Journal, (7):36, 1964)

2. Observed therapeutic results of red-hot needling in the treatment of 160 cases of thecal cyst

Point: Cyst

Method: Heat a three-edged needle to red-hot and swiftly thrust into the cyst. The mucus is then squeezed out.

Results: Of 160 cases treated, 152 cases were cured with 1 treatment, 7 were cured with 2 treatments and 1 with 3 treatments. No recurrence took place and no infection was caused.

(*Source:* Chinese Acupuncture & Moxibustion, (1):16, 1986)

31. *Bi* Syndromes (Painful Joints)

Principal points:

Pain in the shoulder joint: Ashi point, Jianyu (L.I. 15), Naoshu (S.I. 10), Quchi (L.I. 11), Yanglingquan (G.B. 34), on the affected side

Pain in the elbow: Ashi point, Quchi (L.I. 11), Hegu (L.I. 4), Waiguan (S.J. 5), Yanglingquan (G.B. 34), on the affected side

Pain in the wrist: Ashi point, Yangchi (S.J. 4), Waiguan (S.J. 5), Yangxi (L.I. 5), Hand-Wangu (S.I. 4), Qiuxu (G.B. 40), on the affected side

Pain in the metacarpal joint: Ashi point, Baxie (Extra), Hegu (L.I. 4), Houxi (S.I. 3), on the affected side

Pain in the finger joints: Ashi point, Sifeng (Extra), Hegu (L.I. 4), on the affected side

Pain in the hip joint: Ashi point, Huantiao (G.B. 30), Femur-Juliao (G.B. 29), Xuanzhong (G.B. 39), on the affected side

Pain in the knee joint: Ashi point, Xiyan (Extra), Liangqiu (St. 34), Yanglingquan (G.B. 34), Xiyangguan (G.B. 33), Weizhong (U.B. 40), Quchi (L.I. 11), on the affected side

Pain in the ankle joint: Ashi point, Shenmai (U.B. 62), Zhaohai (K. 6), Jiexi (St. 41), Kunlun (U.B. 60), Qiuxu (G.B. 40), Yangchi (S.J. 4), on the affected side

Pain in the toe joints: Ashi point, Bafeng (Extra), Neiting (St. 44), Taichong (Liv. 3), on the affected side

Pain in the spine: Dazhui (Du 14), Shenzhu (Du 12), Yaoyangguan (Du 3), Jiaji points (Extra), Ashi point

Supplementary points:

Heat *bi* syndrome: Dazhui (Du 14), Quchi (L.I. 11)

Wind *bi* syndrome: Fengmen (U.B. 12), Geshu (U.B. 17), Xuehai (Sp. 10)

130

Cold *bi* syndrome: Shenshu (U.B. 23), Guanyuan (Ren 4)

Damp *bi* syndrome: Yinlingquan (Sp. 9), Pishu (U.B. 20), Zusanli (St. 36)

Method: Use principal local points and supplementary points in combination according to symptoms. Choose 4-6 points for each session. The above points can be used in rotation. Puncture with moderate stimulation. Retain the needles for 20-30 minutes with periodic manipulation. Treat daily. Ten treatments constitute one course. If it is a cold or damp pattern, acupuncture and moxibustion should be used in combination. Suspended moxibustion with a moxa stick or cupping may be applied on the affected area.

Other therapies:

1. Ear acupuncture

Points: Tender spot at the corresponding area, End of Inferior Helix Crus, Shenmen

Method: Puncture with strong stimulation. Retain the needles for 10 minutes. Treat daily or once every other day. Ten treatments constitute one course. This method is applicable in arthritis with severe pain as the main manifestation.

2. Cutaneous acupuncture

Points: Corresponding Jiaji points (Extra), Ashi points on the swollen area

Method: Use cutaneous needles to tap forcefully and cause a few drops of blood. Then apply cupping. Tap once every three days. Five treatments constitute one course. This method is applicable in swelling and painful joint.

3. Hydro-acupuncture

Points: Local points on the affected area, Ashi points

Method: According to the routine procedure of hydro-acupuncture, inject into each point 0.5-1 ml of 100 mg Vitamin B_1 or 5-10% glucose solution. Treat once every 1-3 days. Ten treatments constitute one course.

4. Electro-acupuncture

Points: Local points on the affected area

Method: Select 4-6 points in a session. After the needling sensation is obtained, connect the needles to a low frequent pulse stimulator for 10-20 minutes. Treat once every other day. Ten treatments constitute one course.

Remarks: Acupuncture and moxibustion can obtain good therapeutic results in the treatment of *bi* syndrome (painful joint).

REFERENCES:

1. Observations of clinical therapeutic results of moxibustion in the treatment of rheumatic arthritis with increasing erythrocyte sedimentation

Points: Moxi Dazhui (Du 14), Yanglingquan (G.B. 34)

Method: Each point needs 30 minutes for moxibustion. Treat daily. Ten treatments constitute one course. If it is necessary, begin another course after three days' rest.

Results: Among 52 cases in the group, through 12-50 treatments, 26 cases (50 percent) showed marked effect (symptoms disappeared, erythrocyte sedimentation became normal), 22 cases (42.3 percent) showed improvement (symptoms reduced, erythrocyte sedimentation lowered), and 4 cases showed no effect. The total effective rate reached 92.3 percent.

(*Source:* Fujian Journal of Traditional Chinese Medicine, 17(6):25, 1986)

2. Observed results of plum-blossom needle, plus cupping and moxibustion, in treating 90 cases of painful joint

Points: Ashi points, 1-2 points above and below the Ashi point along the meridian

Method: Tap with plum-blossom needles until the local skin becomes congested. Then apply cupping for 5-10 minutes. After cupping, use moxibustion for 3-7 minutes. Treat once every two days. Five treatments constitute one course.

Results: Of the 90 cases treated, 47.8 percent were cured, 38.9 percent showed marked effect, 12.2 percent showed some improvement, 1.1 percent showed no effect. The total effective rate reached 98.9 percent.

(*Source:* Chinese Acupuncture & Moxibustion, (1):11, 1983)

32. Lower Back Pain

Principal points: Weizhong (U.B. 40), Shenshu (U.B. 23), Huantiao (G.B. 30), Ashi points

Method: Use filiform needles with moderate stimulation. Retain the needles for 20-30 minutes. Treat daily or once every other day. With chronic lower back pain, moxibustion is combined. For acute and severe lower back pain, use a three-edged needle to prick Weizhong

(U.B. 40), and cause bleeding.

Supplementary points:

Acute lumbar sprain: Puncture Renzhong (Du 26) or Yanglao (S.I. 6) with moderate stimulation. Encourage the patient to exercise the lumbar region when needling. Withdraw the needle until the pain is relieved.

Lower back pain due to invasion by cold and damp: Yaoyangguan (Du 3), Fengfu (Du 16)

Lumbar muscle strain: Geshu (U.B. 17), Ciliao (U.B. 32)

Lower back pain due to deficiency of the kidney: Mingmen (Du 4), Zhishi (U.B. 52), Taixi (K. 3)

Other therapies:

1. Tapping

Points: Weizhong (U.B. 40), Ashi points

Method: Use the cutaneous needle to tap gently until causing bleeding, then apply cups. This method is applicable in the treatment of lower back pain due to invasion by cold and damp, as well as chronic lumbar muscle strain.

2. Cupping

Points: Ashi points

Method: Cupping in combination can be used on the local tender spots in treating various lower back pains.

3. Ear acupuncture

Points: Lumbosacral Vertebrae, Kidney, Shenmen

Method: Use filiform needles with strong stimulation at points on the affected side. After insertion, frequently rotate the needles, and at the same time ask the patient to exercise the lumbar region. Retain the needles for ten minutes in each session. Treat daily or once every other day.

4. Electro-acupuncture

Points: Shenshu (U.B. 23), Ashi points

Method: Select and puncture Shenshu (U.B. 23) and a local tender spot. After insertion, connect the needles to a high frequency electro-pulse stimulator with strong stimulation for 5-10 minutes. Treat daily or once every other day.

5. Head acupuncture

Points: Bilateral Lower Limb Sensory Area, Leg Motor and Sensory Area

Method: After insertion, rotate the needles for 3-4 minutes. Retain the needles for 5-10 minutes. Then continue rotating the needles for another 3-4 minutes before withdrawing the needles.

Remarks: Acupuncture and moxibustion are quite effective in the treatment of lower back pain. With chronic lower back pain, encourage the patient often to massage the lumbar region by himself, 5-10 minutes each time. This can help to reduce pain on the lumbar or to prevent an attack of lower back pain.

REFERENCES:

1. Observed results of treating 300 cases of lumbar muscle strain by needling Tianzhu (U.B. 10)

Point: Tianzhu (U.B. 10)

Method: The patient is in sitting position with the head slightly forward. Rapidly insert the needle to a depth of 0.5-0.8 *cun*, let the tip of the needle slant towards the intervertebral foramen, without going deeply into the medial and superior aspect. Retain the needle for 20-30 minutes. Ask the patient to exercise the lumbar region. Treat daily. Eight treatments constitute one course.

Results: Of 300 cases treated, 152 cases were cured, marked effect was seen in 47 cases, 73 cases showed improvement, no effect appeared in 28 cases.

(*Source:* Guangxi Journal of Traditional Chinese Medicine, 9(2):30, 1986)

2. Observed results of treating back rigidity and pain in the spine by needling Jiaji points (Extra)

Point and method: Use the thumb to press downward from the Jiaji points (Extra, 0.5 *cun* lateral and below the spinal process of the first thoracic vertebra) to search for tender spot. Then use a filiform needle 1.5-2 *cun* in length to puncture at an angle towards the spine, until an electro-stroke sensation or numbness and distention sensation is obtained. At the same time insert another needle into the opposite point related to the tenderness with the above-mentioned method. Then apply two cups, with two needles in the points, for 20 minutes.

Results: Of 168 cases treated, 112 cases were cured, 54 cases showed improvement, 2 cases showed no effect.

(*Source:* Liaoning Journal of Traditional Chinese Medicine, 10(8):39, 1986)

33. Painful Heels

(Calcaneal spur, bursitis under the heel and fat pad inflammation are included.)

Principal points: Ashi points, Kunlun (U.B. 60), Taixi (K. 3)

Method: Tender spot should be found in the local area of the sole, and puncture Kunlun (U.B. 60) and Taixi (K. 3) of the affected foot. Produce moderate or strong stimulation with filiform needles and use an even method. Retain the needles for 15-20 minutes. Moxibustion with a moxa stick can be performed over the focus after the needles are taken out. Treat daily and 10 treatments constitute one course.

Supplementary points:

Kidney *yin* deficiency: Zhaohai (K. 6), Yongquan (K. 1)

Severe pain of the heel: Pushen (U.B. 61)

The pain referred to the lower leg: Yanglingquan (G.B. 34), Chengshan (U.B. 57);

Long-standing pain unable to be cured: Xiaguan (St. 7), after the arrival of *qi*, retaining the needle for 20-30 minutes during which require the patient to walk slowly

Other therapies:

1. Electro-acupuncture

Points: Ashi points, Kunlun (U.B. 60)

Method: After the arrival of *qi*, connect the electro-acupuncture apparatus with the needles for 15 minutes. Treat daily.

2. Red-hot needling

Points: Ashi points

Method: Select 3-5 points according to the area of tenderness and needle by means of routine operation of the red-hot needling. The treatment is once every other day and five treatments constitute one course.

3. Bleeding method

Points: Chengshan (U.B. 57), Ashi points

Method: Chengshan (U.B. 57) on the affected side, and 1-2 points in the tender area are prescribed. Bleed the points with the three-edged needle, and provide moxibustion with a moxa stick at Ashi points in the sole. Treat once every other day and five treatments constitute one course.

4. Ear acupuncture

Points: Heel, Shenmen

Method: Needle the points with moderate or strong stimulation. Retain the needles for 10-20 minutes. Treat daily. Needle-embedding method is also applicable.

Remarks: Acupuncture has fair effect in treating the painful heel, but attention should also be paid to moxibustion in the treatment.

REFERENCES:

1. Observed results of 115 cases of painful heels treated by indirect moxibustion with ginger

Point and method: Cut fresh ginger into a slice as thick as 0.3-0.5 cm. Thrust ginger with a needle to make several holes. Place the ginger slice on the affected heel and a moxa cone is put on the ginger and ignited. When the cone has burned out and the heel feels the burning pain, use the slice to rub the heel in the local area. Treat once or twice daily.

Results: Of the 115 cases treated, 102 cases were cured in a week, 8 were improved and the other 5 were treated with another method.

(*Source:* Hubei Journal of Traditional Chinese Medicine, (3):45, 1986)

2. Observed results of the treatment of 216 cases of painful heel by needling Fengchi (G.B. 20)

Point and method: If one heel is affected, puncture Fengchi (G.B. 20) perpendicularly to a depth of 0.5-1 *cun*, and after the arrival of *qi* rotate the needle 5-10 times, and retain the needle for 50 minutes. During this time, manipulate the needle every 10 minutes. When both heels are affected, employ the penetrating method. A point on either side can be punctured perpendicularly to a depth of 0.2-0.3 *cun* but the angle of insertion is changed, and the needle is thrust transversely towards the opposite point to a depth of 2-2.5 *cun*. (Skin on the opposite side should not be penetrated.) Then, lift and thrust the needle five times and rotate in large amplitude after that. Do not stimulate beyond the patient's tolerance. Retain the needle for 50 minutes.

Results: Of 216 cases treated, 134 cases were cured, 43 showed marked effect, 22 were improved and 17 remained unchanged. The total effective rate was 92.1 percent.

(*Source:* Journal of Traditional Chinese Medicine, 27(11):35, 1986)

34. Palpitation

Principal points: Xinshu (U.B. 15), Juque (Ren 14), Neiguan (P. 6), Shenmen (H. 7), Sanyinjiao (Sp. 6)

Method: Use filiform needles with moderate stimulation. Retain the needles for 20-30 minutes with periodic manipulation, once every 5-10 minutes. Treat daily or once every other day.

Supplementary points:

Tachycardia: Jianshi (P. 5)

Bradycardia: Suliao (Du 25), Tongli (H. 5)

Deficiency of the heart and kidney: Geshu (U.B. 17), Jueyinshu (U.B. 14), Shenshu (U.B. 23), Taixi (K. 3)

Disturbance of endogenous phlegm-fluid: Fenglong (St. 40), Chize (Lu. 5), Taichong (Liv. 3)

Stifling sensation in the chest: Shanzhong (Ren 17), Zhiyang (Du 9), Xuehai (Sp. 10)

Other therapies:

Ear acupuncture

Points: Heart, End of Inferior Helix Crus, Shenmen, Brain

Method: Choose 2-3 points in a session, puncture with moderate stimulation. Retain the needles for 20-30 minutes with periodic manipulation 2-3 times. Treat daily. Ten treatments constitute one course.

Remarks: Acupuncture and moxibustion are quite effective in the treatment of this illness.

REFERENCE:

Observed results of wrist-and-ankle acupuncture in the treatment of 30 cases of atrial fibrillation

Points: Neiguan (P. 6) on the left hand, Shenmen (H. 7)

Method: Use filiform needles 2-6 *cun* in length, and puncture a 30-degree angle against the skin. After rapidly penetrating the skin, adopt slow and horizontal insertion, so as not to cause any soreness, numbness, distention and pain sensation to the patient. If there is resistance of needling, insert the needle again. Treat daily or once every other day. Ten treatments constitute one course. Begin another course after 10-15 days' rest.

Results: Of the 30 cases treated, 19 showed marked effect (the symptoms disappeared, atrial fibrillation turned into sinus rhythm showing on E.C.G.), improvement (the symptoms obviously reduced, the fast atrial fibrillation rate lowered to the normal showing on E.C.G.) was shown in 2 cases, no effect was seen in 9 cases.

Remarks: With myocarditis complicated by atrial fibrillation, an excellent therapeutic result could be obtained by acupuncture, but for rheumatic heart disease, the results are not satisfactory

(*Source:* Liaoning Journal of Traditional Chinese Medicine, 10(5):38, 1986)

35. Hypertension

Principal points: Fengchi (G.B. 20), Quchi (L.I. 11), Hegu (L.I. 4)

Method: Insert a needle at Fengchi (G.B. 20) to a depth of 0.5-1 *cun*, with the tip of the needle pointing to the nose. Try to let the needling sensation extend to the vertex. Puncture this point with gentle manipulation by rotating, but not by lifting and thrusting. Retain the needles for 30 minutes. Treat daily or once every other day.

Supplementary points:

Hyperactivity of *yang* in the liver: Taichong (Liv. 3), Xingjian (Liv. 2), Taiyang (Extra)

Upward disturbance of turbid phlegm: Fenglong (St. 40)

Deficient *yin* and hyperactivity of *yang*: Sanyinjiao (Sp. 6), Taichong (Liv. 3), Taixi (K. 3)

Deficient *yin* and *yang*: Shenshu (U.B. 23), Guanyuan (Ren 4), Sanyinjiao (Sp. 6)

Palpitation and insomnia: Shenmen (H. 7)

Nausea and vomiting: Neiguan (P. 6)

Edema on the lower limbs: Yinlingquan (Sp. 9)

Other therapies:

1. Ear acupuncture

Points: Brain, End of Inferior Helix Crus, Shenmen, Heart, Lowering Blood Pressure Groove, Liver, Kidney

Method: Choose 3-5 points in a session. Puncture with moderate stimulation. Retain the needles for 1-2 hours. Treat daily. Ten treatments constitute one course.

2. Cutaneous acupuncture

Points: Both sides of the spine, especially the lumbar-sacral region, combined with cervical vertebrae, forehead, occipital region, ends of the four limbs, palms of the hands, and soles of the feet

Method: Adopt a mild stimulation. Tap first along the spine. The tapping order is from the upper portion to the lower portion, from the medial aspect to the lateral aspect. Afterward, areas on the head and neck can be tapped.

3. Cupping

Points: Points on the back along the first line of the urinary bladder meridians as the main points, combined with Jianyu (L.I. 15), Quchi (L.I. 11), Hegu (L.I. 4), Chengfu (U.B. 36), Weizhong (U.B. 40), Chengjin (U.B. 56), Chengshan (U.B. 57), Zusanli (St. 36)

Method: Select points according to specific symptoms. Choose a cup of proper size to fit the area to be treated. Generally, about 10 cups should be applied during each treatment, retaining the cups for 10-15 minutes.

4. Blood-letting on the ear

Points: Ear Apex, Lowering Blood Pressure Groove

Method: Prick with a three-edged needle to cause bleeding.

Remarks: Before treatment, the patient should be instructed to relax and avoid emotional excitement, tension and fear. Needling should not make the blood pressure suddenly rise, so strong stimulation is not advisable.

REFERENCE:

Observation of therapeutic results of needling with application of the principle "reducing the south and reinforcing the north" in the treatment of 60 cases of hypertension

Points: Taichong (Liv. 3) joining to Xingjian (Liv. 2), and Daling (P. 7) to Neiguan (P. 6) with reducing method; Ququan (Liv. 8), Taixi (K. 3) joining to Kunlun (U.B. 60), Fuliu (K. 7) with reinforcing method; Quchi (L.I. 11) and Fenglong (St. 40) first with reinforcing method and then with reducing method

Method: Treat daily or once every other day. Twenty days' treatment constitutes one course. Begin another course after 5-7 days' rest, and 2-3 courses may be needed.

Results: Among 60 cases, marked effect (the symptoms disappeared, and the blood pressure became normal) was seen in 24 cases, effectiveness (the most symptoms dissappeared, and the diastolic pressure was 20-30 mm down on the mercury column) was seen in 16 cases, improvement in 19 cases, no effect in 1 case. The total effective rate reached 98 percent. The average number of treatments was 15.

(*Source:* Journal of Traditional Chinese Medicine, 24(5):50, 1983)

36. Angina Pectoris

Principal points: Neiguan (P. 6), Xinshu (U.B. 15), Shanzhong (Ren 17)

Method: Insert the needle at Xinshu (U.B. 15), angled towards the spine. Apply moderate or strong stimulation. Let the needling sensation extend to the back or chest. Insert again subcutaneously and transverseiy along the sternum at Shanzhong (Ren 17). The above two points can be applied with moxibustion. Puncture Neiguan (P. 6) with moderate stimulation. Retain the needles for 20-30 minutes. Treat once every other day. 10-15 treatments constitute one course. The interval between courses is 3-5 days.

Supplementary points:

Inability to stop angina pectoris: Ximen (P. 4) with strong stimulation

Obstruction of turbid phlegm: Fenglong (St. 40)

Blood stasis blocking the collaterals: Geshu (U.B. 17)

Deficient *yang* in the heart and kidney: Shenshu (U.B. 23), Guanyuan (Ren 4), Qihai (Ren 6)

Other therapies:

1. Ear acupuncture

Points: Heart, Kidney, End of Inferior Helix Crus, Intertragicus, Brain, Shenmen

Method: Choose 2-4 points in a session. Puncture with strong stimulation. Retain the needles for 30 minutes. Treat daily or once every other day.

2. Electro-acupuncture

Points: Neiguan (P. 6), Shanzhong (Ren 17), Xinshu (U.B. 15), Jueyinshu (U.B. 14), Dushu (U.B. 16)

Method: Use sparse-dense pulsation with moderate stimulation to the tolerance of the patient for 10-15 minutes. Treat daily or once every other day.

140

3. Head acupuncture

Points: Thoracic Cavity Area, Blood Vessel Dilation and Constriction Area

Method: The routine procedure of head acupuncture.

Remarks: Acupuncture and moxibustion therapies are quite effective in the treatment of angina pectoris. In the case of an acute attack of angina pectoris or acute myocardia infarction, modern medicines should be combined to save the patient.

REFERENCE:

Observed results of electro-acupuncture in the treatment of 30 cases of angina pectoris

Points: Jueyinshu (U.B. 14) joining to Xinshu (U.B. 15), Neiguan (P. 6)

Method: After the needling sensation is obtained, connect the needles with an electro-stimulator, with continued pulsation, frequency 150 Hz and wave velocity 300 ms, to the tolerance of the patient. Treat daily. Twenty minutes are needed in a session. Seven treatments constitute one course.

Results: Among 30 cases (there were 17 cases accompanied with hypertension), 15 cases (88 percent) showed systolic pressure was 20 mm down on the mercury column, and 12 cases (70.6 percent) showed diastolic pressure was 10 mm down on the mercury column.

(*Source:* Chinese Acupuncture & Moxibustion, (2):4, 1987)

37. Thromboangiitis

Principal points:

Disease on the upper limb: Quchi (L.I. 11), Waiguan (S.J. 5), Hegu (L.I. 4), Hand-Zhongzhu (S.J. 3)

Disease on the lower limb: Zusanli (St. 36), Yanglingquan (G.B. 34), Yinlingquan (Sp. 9), Xuanzhong (G.B. 39), Xingjian (Liv. 2), Sanyinjiao (Sp. 6)

Method: Puncture the points with strong stimulation. After insertion, first manipulate the needles for 2-3 minutes. Then retain the needles for 20-30 minutes with periodic manipulation, once every five minutes. Warm needles may also be used. Treat daily. Some points can be joined to each other, for example, Quchi (L.I. 11) to Shaohai (H.

3), Waiguan (S.J. 5) to Neiguan (P. 6), Xuanzhong (G.B. 39) to Sanyinjiao (Sp. 6)

Supplementary points:

Disease on the upper limb: Jiaji points (Extra, from C6-T2)

Disease on the lower limb: Jiaji points (Extra, from L1-L3)

Pain of toes and fingers: Bafeng (Extra), Baxie (Extra)

Fever: Dazhui (Du 14), Quchi (L.I. 11)

Other therapies:

1. Ear acupuncture

Points: End of Inferior Helix Crus, Brain, corresponding points related to the affected limb, Heart, Liver, Kidney

Method: Choose 2-3 pairs of points in a session. Puncture with moderate stimulation. Retain the needles for 30-60 minutes with periodic manipulation. Treat daily. Ten treatments constitute one course.

2. Moxibustion

Points: Area on the affected limb

Method: Apply moxibustion with a moxa stick to the affected area for 10-20 minutes. Treat once or twice a day.

Remarks: Acupuncture and moxibustion may obtain a good therapeutic result in the treatment of thromboangiitis during the early stages. However, with necrotizing vasculitis at the advanced stage, the therapeutic results of acupuncture and moxibustion would be poor. Instead, use a combination of medications.

REFERENCE:

Clinical summary on acupuncture in the treatment of 181 cases of thromboangiitis

Main points for the lower limb: Maigen (Extra, level with the second sacral foramen, 3 *cun* lateral to and 0.5 *cun* below the posterior middle line), Xuehai (Sp. 10), Yinbao (Liv. 9)

Secondary points along the meridians:

For the big toe: Yinlingquan (Sp. 9), Diji (Sp. 8)

For the second or third toe: Zusanli (St. 36), Fenglong (St. 40)

For the fourth toe or the lateral aspect of the lower leg: Yanglingquan (G.B. 34), Xuanzhong (G.B. 39)

For the fifth toe or the posterior aspect of the lower leg: Chengshan (U.B. 57), Kunlun (U.B. 60)

For the sole of the foot: Taixi (K. 3)

Main points for the upper limb: Quchi (L.I. 11), Ximen (P. 4),

142

Qingling (H. 2)
    Secondary points along the meridians:
    For the thumb or index finger: Shousanli (L.I. 10)
    For the middle finger: Neiguan (P. 6)
    For the ring finger: Waiguan (S.J. 5)
    For the little finger: Tongli (H. 5)
    For the forearm or palm: Daling (P. 7)
    Method: Puncture with the lift and thrust method and enable the
needling sensation to reach the affected area. Do not retain the needles.
Choose 1-5 points in a session. Treat daily or once every other day. Fifteen treatments constitute one course. Begin another course after 3-5
days' rest.
    Results: The marked effective rate was 80.66 percent, and the
total effective rate was 97.78 percent.
    (*Source:* Chinese Acupuncture & Moxibustion (3):10, 1981)

38. Pulseless Disease (Aorto arteritis)

    Principal points: Xinshu (U.B. 15), Neiguan (P. 6), Taiyuan (Lu.
9)
    Method: Gently stimulate Xinshu (U.B. 15) with a filiform needle
which is withdrawn after being rotated for 2-3 minutes. Moderately
stimulate Neiguan (P. 6) and Taiyuan (Lu. 9) by means of the even
method but the needles are retained less than 15 minutes. Provide the
patient with cold limbs with mild moxibustion by a moxa stick. Treat
daily or once every other day and 10 treatments constitute one course.
    Supplementary points:
    Hypertension associated: Fengchi (G.B. 20), Quchi (L.I. 11), re-
duced with moderate stimulation
    Absence of pulse in the upper limb: Chize (Lu. 5), Shenmen (H.
7) with moderate stimulation
    Absence of pulse in the lower limbs: Taichong (Liv. 3), Taixi (K.
3), Qichong (St. 30), Jimen (Sp. 11) with acupuncture and mild
moxibustion with a moxa stick
    Other therapies:
    1. Ear acupuncture
    Points: Heart, Lung, Liver, Spleen, End of Inferior Helix Crus,
Lower Apex of Tragus, Brain, Intertragicus

Method: Select 2-4 points each time and stimulate intensely with filiform needles. Retain the needles for 1-4 hours, manipulating once every 30 minutes. Treat daily and 10 treatments constitute one course. Needle-embedding method is also applicable.

2. Electro-acupuncture

Points:

Pulselessness of the upper limbs: Neiguan (P. 6), Taiyuan (Lu. 9), Chize (Lu. 5), Quchi (L.I. 11)

Pulselessness of the lower limbs: Taichong (Liv. 3), Taixi (K. 3), Sanyinjiao (Sp. 6), Zusanli (St. 36)

Method: After the arrival of *qi*, connect the needles with the electro-acupuncture apparatus for 10-15 minutes. Treat once every other day. The method is most effective in the patient with a strong constitution.

3. Head acupuncture

Points: Blood Vessel Dilation and Constriction Area, Motor Area

Method: Apply the routine operation of head acupuncture.

Remarks: Acupuncture has certain benefits in the treatment of pulseless syndrome and some patients can obtain fair effects from it.

39. Raynaud's Disease

Principal points:

In cases of fingers affected: Waiguan (S.J. 5), Baxie (Extra)

In cases of toes affected: Sanyinjiao (Sp. 6), Bafeng (Extra)

Method: Perform lifting, thrusting and rotating of needles at Waiguan (S.J. 5) and Sanyinjiao (Sp. 6), until the needling sensation is conducted downward. You may provide Baxie (Extra) and Bafeng (Extra) with warm needling, or mild moxibustion by a moxa stick after the needling. Retain the needles for 10-30 minutes with intermittent manipulation, once every 5-10 minutes. Treat once every other day.

Supplementary points:

Red, painful and hot swelling of fingers and toes: Quchi (L.I. 11), Hegu (L.I. 4), or Xuehai (Sp. 10), Xingjian (Liv. 2)

Other therapies:

1. Ear acupuncture

Points: Finger, Toe, Wrist, Ankle, Heart, Liver, End of Inferior Helix Crus, Lower Apex of Tragus

Method: Select 4-5 points according to the affected region and moderately stimulate with filiform needles which are then retained for 30 minutes. Treat alternate ears daily. Needle-embedding method can also be applied with the needles being changed every 3-5 days.

2. Electro-acupuncture

Points: Quchi (L.I. 11), Waiguan (S.J. 5), Hegu (L.I. 4), or Xuehai (Sp. 10), Sanyinjiao (Sp. 6), Xuanzhong (G.B. 39)

Method: Select 4-6 points each time and connect the needles with the electro-acupuncture apparatus for 30 minutes, after the arrival of *qi*. Set the frequency at 200 times per minute and adjust the stimulation according to the patient's tolerance. Treat daily, and 10 treatments constitute one course.

Remarks: Acupuncture therapy has fair effect in treating this disease. The affected limbs should be kept warm.

REFERENCE:

Observed results of the treatment of 31 cases of Raynaud's disease with acupuncture

Points:

The fingers affected: Quepen (St. 12) in combination with Shixuan (Extra)

The thumb and index finger seriously affected: Hand-Wuli (L.I. 13)

The middle finger affected: Neiguan (P. 6)

The ring finger and little finger affected: Xiaohai (S.I. 8)

The toes affected: Sanyinjiao (Sp. 6), Zhaohai (K. 6) in combination with Shixuan (Extra), Huantiao (G.B. 30) or Zhibian (U.B. 54)

Method: Puncture Quepen (St. 12) with sparrow-pricking method without retention of needles. Bleed Shixuan (Extra) and puncture the rest of the points with needles retained for 20 minutes. A strong electro-shock sensation propagating down to the fingers or toes is essential in the treatment. Treat daily, and 18 treatments constitute one course, with a 7-day interval between the courses.

Results: After 2-4 courses, 21 cases were cured and 10 cases were markedly effected (slight recurrence of symptoms in winter, like discoloration and pain of fingers).

(*Source:* Chinese Acupuncture & Moxibustion, 8(4):25, 1988)

40. Erythromelalgia

Principal points: Dazhui (Du 14), Quchi (L.I. 11), Xuehai (Sp. 10), Weizhong (U.B. 40)

Method: Bleed Weizhong (U.B. 40) with a three-edged needle, and reduce the remaining points with strong stimulation. Retain the needles for 10-20 minutes and treat daily.

Supplementary points:

The upper limb affected: Chize (Lu. 5), Hegu (L.I. 4), Shixuan (Extra) with bleeding method by means of a three-edged needle

The lower limb affected: Zusanli (St. 36), Taichong (Liv. 3), Ashi point (tip of the toes) with bleeding method

Irritability and insomnia: Shenmen (H. 7) with moderate stimulation and retention of needles for ten minutes

Other therapies:

1. Ear acupuncture

Points: End of Inferior Helix Crus, Shenmen, Finger, Toe, Brain, Heart

Method: Apply moderate stimulation, retain the needles for 30-60 minutes and manipulate every 5-10 minutes. Treat daily or once every other day. The needle-embedding method is also applicable.

2. Moxibustion

Points: Ashi points

Method: To treat the persistent relapse, perform suspending moxibustion with moxa sticks over the focus, or provide indirect moxibustion with ginger. Select 3-5 points each time, with 5-7 cones on each point. Treat daily or once every other day.

3. Hydro-acupuncture

Points:

For the upper limb: Quchi (L.I. 11), Waiguan (S.J. 5), Hegu (L.I. 4)

For the lower limb: Zusanli (St. 36), Taichong (Liv. 3)

Method: Inject 1 ml of 0.5% procaine into each point by means of routine hydro-acupuncture. Inject daily or once every other day.

Remarks: Acupuncture therapy has good analgesic effect in the treatment of erythromelalgia. The condition of the disease therefore can be gradually alleviated.

146

REFERENCE:
Observation on 16 cases of erythromelalgia treated with electro-acupuncture on ear points
Points:
Group 1: End of Inferior Helix Crus, Shenmen
Group 2: Heart, Brain
Group 3: Heart, Shenmen
Method: All the points are prescribed bilaterally. Needle the points and then connect with an electro-acupuncture apparatus to stimulate with the impulse current. Treat for 30-60 minutes each time, once or twice daily, possibly adding another treatment before sleep.
Results: Six cases were treated with Group 1 and Group 2 in alternation and 10 were treated with Group 3 alone. Of the 16 cases treated, 14 cases were cured with 6-24 treatments and 2 were cured with 56 and 106 treatments. Ten cases have been followed up for 2-10 years and no relapse has taken place.
(*Source:* Jiangsu Chinese Medicine and Medica Materia, (1):32, 1984)

41. Anemia

Principal points: Dazhui (Du 14), Zhongwan (Ren 12), Zusanli (St. 36), Sanyinjiao (Sp. 6), Quchi (L.I. 11)
Method: Apply reinforcing method to each point. Puncture with moderate stimulation. Retain the needles for 15-20 minutes. Moxibustion with moxa sticks can be combined. Treat daily. Ten treatments constitute one course.
Supplementary points:
Deficiency of the heart and spleen: Geshu (U.B. 17), Pishu (U.B. 20)
Deficiency of the liver and kidney: Ganshu (U.B. 18), Shenshu (U.B. 23), Taixi (K. 3); combined with moxibustion
Deficient *yang* of the spleen and kidney: Pishu (U.B. 20), Shenshu (U.B. 23), Mingmen (Du 4), Qihai (Ren 6); combined with moxibustion
Epistaxis: Geshu (U.B. 17)
Amenorrhea: Xuehai (Sp. 10)
Profuse night sweating: Yinxi (H. 6)

147

Palpitation, insomnia: Shenmen (H. 7)

Menorrhagia: Moxi Yinbai (Sp. 1)

Other therapies:

1. Ear acupuncture

Points: Heart, Liver, Spleen, Kidney, Intertragicus, Lower Apex of Tragus

Method: Choose 3-5 points in a session. Puncture with moderate stimulation. Retain the needles for 15-20 minutes. Treat once every other day, or use needle-embedding for 3-5 days.

2. Hydro-acupuncture

Points: Xinshu (U.B. 15), Pishu (U.B. 20), Ganshu (U.B. 18), Geshu (U.B. 17), Zusanli (St. 36)

Method: Choose 2-3 points in a session. Manipulate according to the routine procedure of hydro-acupuncture. Use 0.5-1.0 ml of Vitamin B_{12} solution to inject into each point. Treat once every other day. Ten treatments constitute one course.

Remarks: Acupuncture and moxibustion therapies can obtain a good therapeutic result in the treatment of chronic anemia. Application of moxibustion in treating this illness should draw our attention.

REFERENCE:

Observed results of electro-acupuncture in treating 11 cases of aplastic anemia

Points: a) Dazhui (Du 14), Shenshu (U.B. 23), Zusanli (St. 36); b) Dazhui (Du 14), Gaohuangshu (U.B. 43), Hegu (L.I. 4), Xuehai (Sp. 10)

Method: After insertion, connect the needles with an electro-stimulator. The continuous and intermittent pulsation can be used in rotation. Set the frequency at 60-200 times per minute with a duration of 30 minutes in each session. Treat daily. Fifteen treatments constitute one course. The interval between courses is 1-3 days.

Results: Of the 11 cases treated, 1 was nearly cured, marked effect was seen in 2 cases, improvement in 2 cases and no effect in 6 cases.

(Source: Journal of Integrated Traditional and Western Medicines, 8(5):265, 1988)

42. Thrombocytopenia

Principal points: Geshu (U.B. 17), Xuehai (Sp. 10), Sanyinjiao (Sp. 6), Pishu (U.B. 20)

Method: Puncture with filiform needles and apply mild stimulation. Retain the needles for 20-30 minutes. Manipulate periodically every 5-10 minutes. Treat daily. Ten treatments constitute one course.

Supplementary points:

Hemorrhage due to heat of blood: Quchi (L.I. 11), Weizhong (U.B. 40)

Excessive fire due to *yin* deficiency: Shenshu (U.B. 23), Taixi (K. 3), with reinforcing method

Deficient *qi* and weakness of the spleen: Zusanli (St. 36), Pishu (U.B. 20), Sanyinjiao (Sp. 6), with reinforcing method; combined with moxibustion

Epistaxis: Shangxing (Du 23) with reducing method is applied to the patient with heat blood pattern, and moxibustion with 3-5 cones is applied to the patient with *qi* deficiency pattern.

Hemourine: Zhongji (Ren 3)

Bloody stool: Chengshan (U.B. 57), Guanyuan (Ren 4), with reinforcing method; combined with moxibustion

Uterine bleeding: Yinbai (Sp. 1), moxibustion with small moxa cone is applied.

Other therapies:

1. Moxibustion

Points: Baliao (U.B. 31-34), Yaoyangguan (Du 3)

Method: Apply indirect moxibustion with ginger. Duration of moxibustion should be about 45 minutes in a session. Treat daily. Ten treatments constitute one course.

2. Ear acupuncture

Points: Middle of Ear, Liver, Spleen, Kidney, Intertragicus, Lower Apex of Tragus

Method: Choose 2-4 points in a session. Puncture with filiform needles and moderate stimulation. Retain the needles for 30 minutes. Treat daily. Needle-embedding may be used.

Remarks: Acupuncture and moxibustion are quite effective in the treatment of certain cases. However, in a case of thrombocytopenia with severe bleeding, emergency measures should be resorted to. With secondary thrombocytopenia, its primary cause should be treated.

REFERENCES:

1. Clinical observation on acupuncture in the treatment of 28 cases of thrombocytopenic purpura

Points: Geshu (U.B. 17), Pishu (U.B. 20), Xuehai (Sp. 10), Sanyinjiao (Sp. 6)

Method: First, puncture Geshu (U.B. 17) and Pishu (U.B. 20) with a rapid motion at a 45-degree slanted insertion, pointing the tip of the needle towards the spine. Follow by twirling, rotating, lifting and thrusting needles. Retain the needles for five minutes after the needling sensation is obtained. Then puncture Xuehai (Sp. 10) and Sanyinjiao (Sp. 6) perpendicularly to the skin. Retain the needles for 30 minutes after the needling sensation is obtained. Treat daily. Thirty treatments constitute one course.

Results: There were 16 cases, in which after 1 course of treatment, bleeding was checked, and the blood platelet level was raised to more than $100,000/mm^3$; Improvement was seen in 5 cases, and no effect was evident in 7 cases. Nine cases were followed up after half a year. The therapeutic results of 6 cases were consolidated.

(*Source:* Shaanxi Journal of Traditional Chinese Medicine, "Additional Publication of Acupuncture and Moxibustion," 6, 1983)

2. Observed therapeutic results of vaccaria seeds applied on ear points in the treatment of 30 cases of thrombocytopenic purpura

Principal points: Spleen, Liver, Stomach

Secondary points: Lung, Mouth, Brain, Sanjiao

Method: Apply vaccaria seeds, fixed with adhesive tapes, to the ear points. Instruct the patient to press them for one minute, 3-5 times a day. Treat once every other day. Points on ears can be chosen in turn. Fifteen treatments constitute one course. The interval between courses is three days. The manifestations of most cases will disappear within 2-3 courses' treatment, but 1-2 courses of treatments are still needed for consolidation.

Results: Among 30 cases, 20 were cured (bleeding checked, purpura disappeared, blood platelet count ascended to the normal), marked effect (90% purpura disappeared, bleeding in the mouth checked, blood platelet count ascended) was shown in 7 cases, improvement (most purpura disappeared, bleeding in the mouth reduced, symptoms relapsed when ceased to press the ear points) was seen in 3 cases.

(*Source:* Shanxi Traditional Chinese Medicine, 2(4):22, 1986)

43. Leukopenia

Principal points: Zusanli (St. 36), Sanyinjiao (Sp. 6), Dazhui (Du 14), Pishu (U.B. 20), Xuehai (Sp. 10), Geshu (U.B. 17)

Method: Use filiform needles with mild stimulation. Retain the needles for 10-20 minutes. After needling, apply moxibustion with moxa sticks for 20-30 minutes. Treat daily or once every other day. Ten treatments constitute one course.

Supplementary points:

Lower fever, night sweating: Taixi (K. 3), Yinxi (H. 6)

Deficiency of the liver and kidney: Ganshu (U.B. 18), Shenshu (U.B. 23)

Other therapies:

1. Ear acupuncture

Points: Heart, Liver, Kidney, Spleen, Stomach, Intertragicus

Method: Choose 2-3 points in a session. Use filiform needles with moderate stimulation. Retain the needles for 20-30 minutes. Treat daily. Ten treatments constitute one course.

2. Hydro-acupuncture

Points: The same points as the body acupuncture.

Method: Use 0.5 ml (15 μg/ml) of Vitamin B_{12} solution to inject each point according to the routine procedure. Treat once every other day. Ten treatments constitute one course.

Remarks: Acupuncture and moxibustion therapies have certain effect in treating leukopenia, however, with secondary leukopenia, its primary cause should be found and treated.

REFERENCE:

Observed results of acupuncture in the treatment of 25 cases of leukopenia due to radiotherapy and chemical therapy

Principal points: Zusanli (St. 36), Sanyinjiao (Sp. 6), Xuanzhong (G.B. 39), Xuehai (Sp. 10), Geshu (U.B. 17)

Supplementary points: Taichong (Liv. 3), Taixi (K. 3)

Method: Treat daily or once every other day. Six treatments constitute one course, with 1-3 courses needed for recovery.

Results: Of 25 cases treated, 13 cases were cured, marked effect was seen in 9 cases, improvement was shown in 2 cases and no effect developed in 1 case. After treatments, the average leukocyte level rose to 5,128/mm^3.

(*Source:* Shaanxi Journal of Traditional Chinese Medicine, "Additional Publication of Acupuncture and Moxibustion," 9, 1981)

44. Vomiting

Principal points: Zhongwan (Ren 12), Zusanli (St. 36), Neiguan (P. 6), Gongsun (Sp. 4)

Method: Use filiform needles with moderate stimulation. Retain the needles for 20-30 minutes. For vomiting due to invasion by cold, combine moxibustion. Treat once or twice a day.

Supplementary points:

Severe vomiting: Jinjin-Yuye (Extra), prick and cause bleeding

Vomiting due to food overtaking: Xiawan (Ren 10), Xuanji (Ren 21)

Phlegm-damp obstructing in the middle *jiao*: Fenglong (St. 40), Shanzhong (Ren 17)

Weakness of the spleen and stomach: Pishu (U.B. 20), Weishu (U.B. 21)

Fire of the liver attacking the stomach with manifestation of vomiting, and sour regurgitation: Taichong (Liv. 3), Yanglingquan (G.B. 34)

Fever: Hegu (L.I. 4), Quchi (L.I. 11)

Other therapies:

1. Ear acupuncture

Points: Stomach, Liver, Shenmen, Brain, End of Inferior Helix Crus

Method: Choose 2-3 points in a session. Puncture with moderate stimulation. Retain the needles for 20-30 minutes. Treat daily.

2. Hydro-acupuncture

Points: Zusanli (St. 36), Zhiyang (Du 9), Lingtai (Du 10)

Method: Choose 2 points in each session. Use the points in rotation. Inject 2 ml of normal saline into each point. Treat daily.

3. Wrist-and-ankle acupuncture

Points: Upper 1, bilateral

Method: Puncture according to the routine procedure of wrist-

and-ankle acupuncture.

Remarks: Acupuncture has an excellent effect in the treatment of vomiting. These methods can also be used for the treatment of morning sickness or vomiting due to drug allergy.

REFERENCES:

1. Introduction of one acupuncture point in the treatment of vomiting

Point: 0.5 *cun* directly below Daling (P. 7)

Method: Use a filiform needle 1-1.5 *cun* in length, and insert at a 15-30-degree angle. Let the tip of the needle point to the middle finger. Puncture with strong stimulation. Retain the needle for about 10 minutes. With children, no retention is allowed. Needle the unilateral point for mild vomiting, but the bilateral points for severe vomiting.

Results: Among 26 cases, 21 were cured by 1 treatment, and 5 were cured by 2 treatments.

(*Source:* Liaoning Journal of Traditional Chinese Medicine, (1):31, 1979)

2. Observed results of electro-acupuncture in the treatment of 26 cases of neurotic vomiting

Points: Juque (Ren 14) joining to Xiawan (Ren 10), Burong (St. 19) to Taiyi (St. 23)

Method: Using a needle 5-6 *cun* in length, form a 25-degree angle against the skin and penetrate downward. Then connect the needle to an electro-stimulator for 20-30 minutes with a frequency of 14-16 times per second. 10-15 treatments constitute one course.

Results: Of 26 cases treated, 13 cases were cured, 9 cases showed marked effect and 4 cases improved. The total effective rate reached 100 percent.

(*Source:* Chinese Acupuncture & Moxibustion, (4):11, 1983)

45. Abdominal Pain

Principal points: Zhongwan (Ren 12), Zusanli (St. 36), Hegu (L.I. 4)

Method: First, puncture Zusanli (St. 36) and Hegu (L.I. 4), then needle Zhongwan (Ren 12). Apply moderate stimulation to the points. For abdominal pain due to deficiency and cold, add moxibustion to the above points. Retain the needles for 10-20 minutes.

    Supplementary points:

    Pain above the umbilicus: Liangmen (St. 21), Neiguan (P. 6)

    Pain below the umbilicus: Guanyuan (Ren 4), Zhongji (Ren 3), Sanyinjiao (Sp. 6), Dachangshu (U.B. 25)

    Pain around the umbilicus: Tianshu (St. 25), Qihai (Ren 6)

    Pain at the lateral abdomen: Yanglingquan (G.B. 34)

    Abdominal pain due to accumulation of cold: Indirect moxibustion with salt, or a moxa stick is applied at Shenque (Ren 8)

    Abdominal pain due to retention of food: Lineiting (Extra)

    Abdominal pain due to deficient *yang*: Shenshu (U.B. 23), Pishu (U.B. 20), combined with moxibustion

Other therapies:

1. Cupping

Points: Zhongwan (Ren 12), Tianshu (St. 25), Qihai (Ren 6), Guanyuan (Ren 4), Pishu (U.B. 20), Weishu (U.B. 21), Shenshu (U.B. 23)

Method: Choose 2-3 points in a session. Treat once or twice a day, using large size cups. This method is suitable in the treatment of abdominal pain due to food retention and cold accumulation.

2. Ear acupuncture

Points: Large Intestine, Small Intestine, Spleen, Stomach, Shenmen, End of Inferior Helix Crus

Method: Choose 2-3 points in a session. Puncture with moderate stimulation. Retain the needles for 10-20 minutes. Treat daily or once every other day.

Remarks: Acupuncture and moxibustion therapies are quite effective in relieving the symptoms of abdominal pain. However, for acute abdominal disorders, where therapeutic result is not desired, other therapeutic measures should be taken.

REFERENCES:

    1. Observed results of electro-acupuncture in the treatment of 164 cases of abdominal disorders

    Points:

    Biliary colic: Riyue (G.B. 24), Burong (St. 19), Juque (Ren 14), Dannangxue (Extra), Zusanli (St. 36), all on the right side; *qi* stagnation in the liver: Qimen (Liv. 14), bilateral Taichong (Liv. 3) are added; damp-heat in the liver and gall-bladder: bilateral Quchi (L.I.

11) are added.

Gastric spasm: Zhongwan (Ren 12), Zusanli (St. 36); cold in the stomach: Liangmen (St. 21), moxibustion with moxa sticks is combined; heat in the stomach: Neiting (St. 44) is combined; *qi* of the liver attacking the stomach: Taichong (Liv. 3) is combined.

Nephroureteral calculus: Shenshu (U.B. 23), Jingmen (G.B. 25), Fujie (Sp. 14), Sanyinjiao (Sp. 6), all on the affected side, bilateral Yinlingquan (Sp. 9)

Acute appendicitis: Maishidian (Extra), Tianshu (St. 25) on the right side, bilateral Lanweixue (Extra); fever: Quchi (L.I. 11) is added.

Dysmenorrhea: Guanyuan (Ren 4), Guilai (St. 29), Sanyinjiao (Sp. 6)

Method: With the exception of an angular insertion at Qimen (Liv. 14), Riyue (G.B. 24), and Burong (St. 19), the abdominal points are perpendicularly punctured first. After the needling sensation is obtained, continue the reducing method and let the needling sensation extend to the affected area. Then connect the needles to an electrostimulator with a sparse-dense pulsation frequency of 18 times per minute. Connect the line from the positive pole to the points around tenderness. Set the current intensity to the tolerance of the patient, with a duration of 30-60 minutes.

Results: Of 164 cases treated, those cured by 1 treatment made up 56.7 percent, those showing marked effect were 32.3 percent and improvements were seen in 7.3 percent. The total effective rate reached 96.3 percent.

(*Source:* Shanghai Journal of Acupuncture and Moxibustion, (3):15, 1987)

2. Observed results of needling Liangqiu (St. 34) in the treatment of 40 cases of acute abdominal pain

Point: Liangqiu (St. 34)

Method: Puncture according to normal acupuncture procedures.

Results: The short-term therapeutic effective rate was 100 percent. All pain disappeared, there was no relapse after two days' follow-up.

(*Source:* Chinese Acupuncture & Moxibustion, (3):10, 1987)

3. Observed results of needling Laogong (P. 8) in the treatment of 30 cases of gastric spasm

Point: Laogong (P. 8)

Method: Needle the point to a depth of 0.5-1 *cun* with even method. Retain the needle for 40 minutes with periodic manipulation, once every ten minutes.

Results: All were cured by 1 treatment.

(*Source:* Xinjiang Chinese Medicine and Medica Materia, (1):53, 1987)

4. Observed results of needling Zusanli (St. 36) and Liangqiu (St. 34) in the treatment of 20 cases of gastric spasm

Points: Zusanli (St. 36), Liangqiu (St. 34)

Method: Puncture Liangqiu (St. 34) and let the needling sensation extend upward. Needle Zusanli (St. 36) and cause the needling sensation to extend downward. Retain the needles for 5-10 minutes.

Results: The effective rate was 100 percent.

(*Source:* Chinese Acupuncture & Moxibustion, (5):13, 1984)

46. Diarrhea

I. Acute diarrhea

Principal points: Zhongwan (Ren 12), Tianshu (St. 25), Zusanli (St. 36), Yinlingquan (Sp. 9)

Method: Use filiform needles with strong stimulation. Retain the needles for 30 minutes. Treat once or twice a day. When the symptoms are reduced, treat daily until the symptoms disappear. With a case of acute diarrhea due to deficiency and cold, moxibustion should be applied to the points.

Supplementary points:

Abdominal pain: Hegu (L.I. 4), Sanyinjiao (Sp. 6)

Vomiting and diarrhea: Quze (P. 3), Weizhong (U.B. 40) for bloodletting

Nausea and vomiting: Neiguan (P. 6)

Fever: Quchi (L.I. 11)

II. Chronic diarrhea

Principal points: Pishu (U.B. 20), Zhangmen (Liv. 13), Tianshu (St. 25), Zhongwan (Ren 12), Zusanli (St. 36)

Method: Apply moderate stimulation. Retain the needles for 30 minutes. For diarrhea due to deficiency, moxibustion is added.

Supplementary points:

Morning diarrhea: Moxi Mingmen (Du 4), Taixi (K. 3), Shenshu (U.B. 23), Guanyuan (Ren 4)

Other therapies:

156

1. Ear acupuncture

Points: Large Intestine, Small Intestine, Spleen, Stomach, End of Inferior Helix Crus, Shenmen

Method: Choose 2-3 points in a session. Puncture with moderate stimulation. Retain the needles for 30 minutes. If acute diarrhea is present, treat once or twice a day. For chronic diarrhea, treat once every other day.

2. Cupping

Points: Tianshu (St. 25), Zusanli (St. 36), Guanyuan (Ren 4), Dachangshu (U.B. 25), Xiaochangshu (U.B. 27)

Method: The duration of cupping is five minutes. This method is applicable in the treatment of chronic diarrhea due to deficiency and cold.

Remarks: Acute diarrhea with dehydration should be treated and combined with modern medication.

REFERENCE:

Observed results of needling Zusanli (St. 36) and applying indirect moxibustion with ginger in the treatment of 60 cases of cold diarrhea.

Points: Zusanli (St. 36), Shenque (Ren 8)

Method: Needle Zusanli (St. 36), and apply indirect moxibustion with ginger at Shenque (Ren 8) for 15-20 minutes. Between 6 and 7 moxa cones are needed.

Results: Of 60 cases treated, 42 were cured (all symptoms relieved in 3 months, with 15-20 treatments), marked effect was seen in 15 cases and improvements were shown in 3 cases.

(*Source:* Inner-Mongolia Traditional Chinese Medicine, 5(4):32, 1986)

47. Dysentery

Principal points: Tianshu (St. 25), Shangjuxu (St. 37), Qihai (Ren 6)

Method: Puncture with strong stimulation. Retain the needles for 30 minutes with periodic manipulation, once every 5-10 minutes. For acute cases, give treatment 2-3 times a day. When the symptoms are relieved, change treatment to once a day. In cases of chronic dysentery, treat once every other day.

Supplementary points:

Fever, irritability and thirst: Quchi (L.I. 11), Dazhui (Du 14)

Fasting dysentery: Zhongwan (Ren 12), Neiguan (P. 6)

Nausea and vomiting: Neiguan (P. 6), Neiting (St. 44)

Tenesmus: Zhonglushu (U.B. 29), Yinlingquan (Sp. 9)

Chronic dysentery with prolapsed rectum: Changqiang (Du 1), moxi Baihui (Du 20)

Prolonged persistent dysentery or recurrent dysentery: Pishu (U.B. 20), Shenshu (U.B. 23); combined with moxibustion

Other therapies:

1. Moxibustion

Points: Shenque (Ren 8), Zhongwan (Ren 12), Tianshu (St. 25), Guanyuan (Ren 4), Pishu (U.B. 20), Shenshu (U.B. 23)

Method: Choose 3-4 points in a session. Apply indirect moxibustion with salt and 5-7 moxa cones at Shenque (Ren 8). Apply moxibustion with moxa sticks at the other points for 3-10 minutes each, or indirect moxibustion with ginger and 5-7 moxa cones can be used instead. Treat once every other day. Ten treatments constitute one course. This method is applicable to chronic dysentery.

2. Ear acupuncture

Points: Large Intestine, Small Intestine, Lower Portion of Rectum, Stomach, Shenmen, Spleen, Kidney

Method: Choose 3-5 points in a session. For acute bacillary dysentery, puncture with strong stimulation. Retain the needles for 20-30 minutes. Treat once or twice a day. For chronic bacillary dysentery, puncture with mild stimulation and retain the needles for 10-20 minutes. Treat once every other day.

Remarks: Acupuncture and moxibustion are quite effective in treating bacillary and amebic dysentery. They can not only control the symptoms, but also turn the bacteria culture into negative.

REFERENCES:

1. Observed results of acupuncture in the treatment of 192 cases of acute bacillary dysentery

Principal points: Zhongwan (Ren 12), Tianshu (St. 25), Zusanli (St. 36)

Supplementary points:

Fever: Hegu (L.I. 4), Quchi (L.I. 11)

At the recovery stage: Tianshu (St. 25), Zusanli (St. 36)

158

Method: Puncture with strong stimulation. Retain the needles for 30-120 minutes. Treat daily.

Results: All 192 cases were cured in an average of 3.3 days. The bacteria culture turned to negative in 66 cases, in an average of 2.7 days.

(*Source:* Chinese Acupuncture & Moxibustion, (4):6, 1982)

2. Observed results of acupuncture in the treatment of 30 cases of acute bacillary dysentery

Principal points: Shangjuxu (St. 37), Zusanli (St. 36), Tianshu (St. 25), Guanyuan (Ren 4), Zhixiexue (Extra, 0.5 *cun* above Guanyuan, Ren 4)

Supplementary points: Zhongwan (Ren 12), Quchi (L.I. 11), Neiguan (P. 6), Qihai (Ren 6), Hegu (L.I. 4), Zhigou (S.J. 6), Taichong (Liv. 3), Dachangshu (U.B. 25), Dazhui (Du 14)

Method: Puncture with moderate stimulation. Retain the needles for 10 minutes with periodic manipulation once every three minutes. Seven days' treatment constitutes one course. Treat twice daily during the first three days, and once a day during the later four days.

Results: Those cured (the routine examination of stool was normal for three times and the stool culture was shown negative for three times) in 1-3 days numbered 20 cases, in 4-6 days were 6 cases, in 7-8 days were 4 cases.

(*Source:* Fujian Journal of Traditional Chinese Medicine, 15(4):23, 1984)

48. Gastro-duodenal Ulcer

Principal points: Zhongwan (Ren 12), Zusanli (St. 36), Neiguan (P. 6), Pishu (U.B. 20), Ganshu (U.B. 18)

Method: Needle Zhongwan (Ren 12) with moderate stimulation, and puncture the other points with strong stimulation. Needling order starts with Neiguan (P. 6) and Zusanli (St. 36), and then goes to Zhongwan (Ren 12). If the stomach pain is not relieved, combine Ganshu (U.B. 18) and Pishu (U.B. 20). Retain the needles for 30 minutes. Treat 1-3 times a day, or every other day.

Supplementary points:

Qi of the liver transversely attacking the stomach: Taichong (Liv. 3), Yanglingquan (G.B. 34), Qimen (Liv. 14)

Weakness and cold of the spleen and stomach: Pishu (U.B. 20), Weishu (U.B. 21), Zhangmen (Liv. 13), Guanyuan (Ren 4); combined with moxibustion

Retention of food: Jianli (Ren 11), Lineiting (Extra)

Blood stagnation: Geshu (U.B. 17), Sanyinjiao (Sp. 6), Gongsun (Sp. 4)

Bloody stool: Xuehai (Sp. 10)

Vomiting with blood: Geshu (U.B. 17)

Other therapies:

1. Cupping

Points: Zhongwan (Ren 12), Liangmen (St. 21), Youmen (K. 21), Ganshu (U.B. 18), Pishu (U.B. 20), Weishu (U.B. 21) on the epigastric region and back

Method: Use large or medium cups. Duration of cupping is 10-15 minutes.

2. Ear acupuncture

Points: Stomach, Spleen, End of Inferior Helix Crus, Shenmen, Brain

Method: Choose 3-5 points. Retain the needles for 15-30 minutes.

3. Head acupuncture

Points: Stomach Area, bilateral

Method: Retain the needles for 20-30 minutes with periodic manipulation.

4. Hydro-acupuncture

Points: Weishu (U.B. 21), Pishu (U.B. 20), Zhongwan (Ren 12), Neiguan (P. 6), Zusanli (St. 36)

Method: Choose 1-3 points in a session. Inject 1-2 ml of 1% procaine solution into each point. Treat daily.

5. Wrist-and-ankle acupuncture

Points: Upper 1, Lower 1, bilateral

Method: The routine procedure for wrist-and-ankle acupuncture.

Remarks: Acupuncture and moxibustion are quite effective in relieving pain and promoting the healing of the ulcer for this illness.

REFERENCE:

Therapeutic result observation on acupuncture and moxibustion in the treatment of 50 cases of gastro-duodenal ulcer

Principal points: Neiguan (P. 6), Zusanli (St. 36), Gongsun (Sp. 4), or Zhongwan (Ren 12), Pishu (U.B. 20), Weishu (U.B. 21)

Supplementary points:

Stomach pain: Liangqiu (St. 34)

Abdominal distention: Tianshu (St. 25)

Sour regurgitation: Taichong (Liv. 3)

Constipation: Zhigou (S.J. 6)

Epigastric pain: Moxi Zhongwan (Ren 12)

Lassitude: Moxi Qihai (Ren 6)

Method: Puncture with even method. Retain the needles for les for 30 minutes. Treat once or twice a day. Ten treatments constitute one course. The interval between courses is three days.

Results: Of 50 cases treated, 14 cases were cured, marked effect was seen in 11 cases, improvement showed in 22 cases and no effect was seen in 3 cases.

(*Source:* Hubei Journal of Traditional Chinese Medicine, (2):50, 1984)

49. Acute Perforation of Gastro-duodenal Ulcer

Principal points: Zusanli (St. 36), Zhongwan (Ren 12), Tianshu (St. 25), Neiguan (P. 6)

Method: Puncture with strong stimulation. After the needling sensation is obtained, retain the needles for 30-60 minutes with periodic manipulation, once every 10-15 minutes. Treat once every 4-6 hours. Electro-acupuncture may also be used. Adopt continuous pulsation, high frequency, and power which can offer moderate or strong stimulation for 30-60 minutes in a session.

Other therapies:

Ear acupuncture

Points: Stomach, Abdomen, Shenmen, End of Inferior Helix Crus, Brain

Method: Choose 2-3 points in a session, puncture with strong stimulation and retain the needles for 20-30 minutes. Treat once every 4-6 hours.

Remarks: Acupuncture is applicable for a patient with a small perforation, but a good constitution. It has certain effectiveness in relieving pain. If, after 1-2 acupuncture treatments, there is no obvious improvement, surgery should be performed at once.

50. Gastroptosis

Principal points: Weishangxue (Extra), Zhongwan (Ren 12), Qihai (Ren 6), Guanyuan (Ren 4), Zusanli (St. 36), Baihui (Du 20)

Method: Insert a needle at an angle to a depth of 3-4 *cun* at Weishangxue (Extra). Puncture with twirling and rotating. The needle should not be retained. Apply strong stimulation to the other points. Retain the needles for 30 minutes. Apply moxibustion with moxa sticks to each point after the withdrawal of the needles. Treat once every other day. Ten treatments constitute one course.

Supplementary points:

Vomiting: Neiguan (P. 6)

Abdominal distention diarrhea: Tianshu (St. 25)

Splashing sound in the stomach: Yinlingquan (Sp. 9)

Constipation: Zhigou (S.J. 6), Shangjuxu (St. 37)

Other therapies:

Ear acupuncture

Points: Stomach, End of Inferior Helix Crus, Brain, Shenmen

Method: Use points on ears in rotation. Puncture with filiform needles and strong stimulation. Retain the needles for 20-30 minutes. Treat once every other day, or embed needles for 2-3 days.

REFERENCE:

Therapeutic result observation on acupuncture in the treatment of 24 cases of gastroptosis

Points and method: Place the patient in a supine position. Puncture bilateral Tianshu (St. 25) with 2 filiform needles, 4 *cun* in length. Form the tips of the needles in a 15-degree angle against the skin, and rotate towards Qihai (Ren 6). Needle bilateral Zusanli (St. 36). Ten treatments constitute one course. The interval between treatments is 2-3 days. For severe cases, combine Decoction for Reinforcing Middle *Jiao* and Replenishing *Qi,* or Decoction (Pill) of Cyperus and Amomum with Six Noble Ingredients or More.

Results: The recovery judged by barium fluoroscopy, in which the symptoms were markedly improved through 2-3 treating courses, was evident in 16 cases. There were 4 cases in which the stomach was elevated 2-3 cm. The symptoms were reduced in 3 cases, and no effect was seen in 1 case. The total effective rate reached 95.8 percent.

162

(*Source:* Xinjiang Chinese Medicine and Medica Materia, (1):49, 1986)

51. Acute Gastric Dilatation

Principal points: Zhongwan (Ren 12), Tianshu (St. 25), Zusanli (St. 36), Neiguan (P. 6), Lineiting (Extra)

Method: Thrust at Zhongwan (Ren 12) and Tianshu (St. 25) perpendicularly for about 2 *cun* and reduce with rotation of needles while the other points are reduced by means of lifting, thrusting and rotating the needles. Repeat the manipulation continuously until the bowel sound becomes normalized and the vomiting is relieved.

Supplementary points:

Shock: Renzhong (Du 26), Yongquan (K. 1)

Other therapies:

1. Ear acupuncture

Points: Stomach, End of Inferior Helix Crus, Shenmen, Brain, Spleen

Method: Employ filiform needles and give strong stimulation. Retain the needles for 30 minutes. Manipulate the needles every 10 minutes. Or needles are embedded in 2-3 points and changed every three days.

2. Wrist-and-ankle acupuncture

Points: Upper 1, Lower 1

Method: Select points bilaterally and retain the needles for 30 minutes.

Remarks: Acupuncture therapy can alleviate the symptoms of this disease but comprehensive measures must be taken to rescue the severe and critical cases.

52. Acute Appendicitis

Principal points: Lanweixue (Extra), Tianshu (St. 25), Zusanli (St. 36)

Method: Strong stimulation is necessary, and after the arrival of *qi*, rotate the needles for a few minutes, then retain for 30-60 minutes. Rotate the needles every 15 minutes during the retention. Treat 2-4 times daily until the symptoms are relieved or resolved.

Supplementary points:

Fever: Hegu (L.I. 4), Quchi (L.I. 11), Neiting (St. 44)

Nausea and vomiting: Neiguan (P. 6)

Abdominal pain and distention: Qihai (Ren 6)

Constipation: Dachangshu (U.B. 25), Zhigou (S.J. 6)

Other therapies:

1. Ear acupuncture

Points: Appendix, End of Inferior Helix Crus, Shenmen, Large Intestine

Method: Apply strong stimulation with filiform needles and retain the needles for 30-60 minutes. Treat once or twice daily. Alternate between two ears, until the symptoms are resolved.

2. Hydro-acupuncture

Points: Lanweixue (Extra), Zusanli (St. 36) on the right side

Method: Require the patient to lie supine with knees flexed or to sit straight with knees flexed. After locating the point, insert the needle swiftly for 3-4 cm, and after the arrival of *qi*, inject slowly 1-2 ml of injection water into each point, once or twice daily, until the symptoms are resolved.

3. Electro-acupuncture

Points: Lanweixue (Extra), Tianshu (St. 25, right side), Zusanli (St. 36, right side)

Method: Employ an electro-acupuncture apparatus with intensity set to the patient's tolerance. Connect the electricity for 30 minutes, 1-3 times daily.

Remarks: Acupuncture has fair therapeutic effect in treating simple acute appendicitis. In the treatment, patients are closely observed and timely surgical operation is recommended to those with unsatisfactory effect.

To treat chronic appendicitis, the same points as those for acute appendicitis can be prescribed. Treat daily or once every other day. The points in the lower abdomen can be provided with moxibustion with moxa sticks.

REFERENCES:

1. Observation on the short-term therapeutic effect on acute appendicitis with acupuncture as the sole treatment

Principal point: Zusanli (St. 36)

164

Supplementary points: Quchi (L.I. 11), Neiting (St. 44)

Method: After the arrival of *qi*, use reducing technique with strong stimulation. Retain the needles for one hour, and treat 2-3 times daily, decreasing to 1-2 times daily after the condition is improved. Surgery is necessary in failed cases.

Results: In 633 cases, 395 were cured for the short-term, 198 showed marked effect and 40 were unchanged. The total effective rate was 93.7 percent.

(*Source:* New Journal of Traditional Chinese Medicine, 13(8):402, 1983)

2. Observation on the therapeutic effect of abdominal distention after the operation of appendicitis treated with acupuncture in 24 cases

Points: Zusanli (St. 36), Hegu (L.I. 4), Neiguan (P. 6), all bilateral

Method: Swiftly insert filiform needles, 2 *cun* in length, into the points and towards the focus of the disease. After the arrival of *qi*, require the patient to breathe deeply a few times. Manipulate the needles every 2-3 minutes to bring on strong stimulation and withdraw swiftly after 15 minutes.

Results: Of the 24 cases treated, 10 cases were of quick effect (the distention disappears with only 1 treatment), 2 cases showed marked effect, in 11 cases the distention disappeared after 1 or 2 days, and in 1 case the distention disappeared after 3 days.

(*Source:* Jiangxi Journal of Traditional Chinese Medicine, (6):35, 1983)

3. Observation on 130 cases of postoperative abdominal distention treated with indirect moxibustion by scallion stalk and salt

Points: Tianshu (St. 25), Shangjuxu (St. 37)

Method: Smash together 90 grams of scallion stalk and 30 grams of salt, then place on the points 0.5-0.8 cm thick. Ignite 2 moxa sticks together to perform moxibustion on both points simultaneously, until the skin is flushed. Treat once or twice daily.

Results: Of 130 cases treated, 98 cases showed marked effect, 25 cases showed some effect and 7 cases failed.

(*Source:* New Journal of Traditional Chinese Medicine, 17(11):26, 1985)

53. Acute Intestinal Obstruction

Principal points: Tianshu (St. 25), Daheng (Sp. 15), Dachangshu (U.B. 25), Zusanli (St. 36), Neiguan (P. 6)

Method: Puncture with strong stimulation. Continue twirling and rotating for 2-3 minutes. Retain the needles for 30-60 minutes with periodic manipulation, once every 10 minutes. Treat once every 2-3 hours. When the symptoms are improved, treat 2-3 times a day until remission of symptoms. Electro-acupuncture can also be added, if it is necessary.

Supplementary points:

Abdominal distention: Ciliao (U.B. 32)

Retention of food: Zhongwan (Ren 12)

Accumulation of parasites: Sifeng (Extra), Xiawan (Ren 10), Gongsun (Sp. 4); prick and cause Sifeng (Extra) a few drops of white fluid.

Deficiency and cold: Reinforcing Guanyuan (Ren 4), Qihai (Ren 6); warm needle or moxibustion with moxa sticks is applied for 30-60 minutes.

Fever: Quchi (L.I. 11), Neiting (St. 44)

Other therapies:

1. Ear acupuncture

Points: Large Intestine, Small Intestine, Shenmen, Stomach, Abdomen

Method: Use filiform needles with strong stimulation. Retain the needles for 30-60 minutes. Treat once every 4-6 hours.

2. Hydro-acupuncture

Points: Zusanli (St. 36), bilateral

Method: Inject 0.25 mg of neostigmine into each point. This method is applicable in the treatment of paralytic intestinal obstruction.

Remarks: Acupuncture and moxibustion therapies can obtain a good therapeutic result in the treatment of intestinal obstruction in the early stage. If no desired effect is shown through 4-6 hours' treatment, operation should be taken into consideration.

54. Pancreatitis

Principal points: Zhongwan (Ren 12), Liangmen (St. 21), Neiguan

(P. 6), Zusanli (St. 36), Yanglingquan (G.B. 34)

Method: Intense stimulation is necessary. After insertion, rotate the needle for 2-3 minutes and retain for 30-60 minutes. Rotate every 5-10 minutes. During the acute stage, treat 3-4 times daily, and connect the electro-acupuncture apparatus with all the points for 30-60 minutes.

Supplementary points:

Fever: Quchi (L.I. 11), Hegu (L.I. 4)

Abdominal distention: Daheng (Sp. 15), Qihai (Ren 6)

Jaundice: Danshu (U.B. 19), Zhiyang (Du 9)

Chronic pancreatitis: Ganshu (U.B. 18), Pishu (U.B. 20), Qihai (Ren 6); combined with moxibustion

Other therapies:

Ear acupuncture

Points: Pancreas, Gall Bladder, End of Inferior Helix Crus, Shenmen

Method: Employ filiform needles to conduct strong stimulation and retain the needles for 30-60 minutes, or embed intradermal needles in the points for 2-3 days.

Remarks: To treat the severe cases, medication or even surgical operation might be incorporated. Acupuncture therapy has certain effect in alleviating the pain.

REFERENCE:

Observed results of the treatment of 13 cases of acute pancreatitis with acupuncture

Points: a) Shangwan (Ren 13), Pishu (U.B. 20), Zusanli (St. 36), Hegu (L.I. 4); b) Zhongwan (Ren 12), Weishu (U.B. 21), Xiajuxu (St. 39), Dazhui (Du 14); c) Danshu (U.B. 19), Neiguan (P. 6), Yanglingquan (G.B. 34), Daheng (Sp. 15)

Method: Needle each of the above three groups for 10-15 minutes and alternate every two hours. Provide strong stimulation and utilize an electric impulse of sparse-dense wave to intensify the stimulation.

Results: All the cases were treated with acupuncture alone except 1 case which was administered with intravenous dripping because of the persistent hyperpyrexia and vomiting. After the treatment with acupuncture for 5-7 days, the symptoms disappeared, thus a clinical cure was obtained.

(*Source:* Chinese Acupuncture & Moxibustion, (6):33, 1987)

55. Cholecystitis and Gallstone

Principal points: Zhangmen (Liv. 13), Qimen (Liv. 14), Danshu (U.B. 19), Dannangxue (Extra), Yanglingquan (G.B. 34), Quchi (L.I. 11)

Method: Moderate stimulation is necessary and after the insertion, lift, thrust and rotate the needles for 3-5 minutes, and then retain the needles for 30-60 minutes. During the retention, rotate the needles every 10 minutes. Treat daily. In case of an attack of colic, perform strong stimulation at Danshu (U.B. 19) and Yanglingquan (G.B. 34). Continuously rotate the needles until the pain is eased. Treat 2-3 times daily.

Supplementary points:
Nausea and vomiting: Neiguan (P. 6)
Hyperpyrexia: Dazhui (Du 14), Hegu (L.I. 4)
Constipation: Zhigou (S.J. 6)
Jaundice: Zhiyang (Du 9)
Other therapies:
1. Electro-acupuncture
Points: Riyue (G.B. 24, right side), Qimen (Liv. 14, right side), Dannangxue (Extra), Zusanli (St. 36)
Method: Employ a sparse-dense wave. Strong stimulation is essential, but not beyond the patient's tolerance. Treat daily, 30-60 minutes each time.
2. Hydro-acupuncture
Points: Qimen (Liv. 14, right side), Zusanli (St. 36, right side)
Method: Inject 2.5 ml of 0.5% novocain into each of the above points, once or twice daily.
3. Ear acupuncture
Points: Gall Bladder, Liver, Pancreas, Shenmen, Brain, End of Inferior Helix Crus
Method: Select 2-3 points above-mentioned each time, give strong stimulation, and retain the needles for 20-40 minutes. Electro-apparatus can also be connected with the needles. Treat once or twice daily.
4. Acu-pressure
Points: Danshu (U.B. 19), Ganshu (U.B. 18)
Method: Press the above points bilaterally with thumbs, 5-10 minutes for each point, once or twice daily.
Remarks: Acupuncture has good analgesic effect in treating simple

acute cholecystitis and gallstone.

REFERENCES:

1. Observed results of 150 cases of acute cholecystitis treated with acupuncture

Points: Xisixue (Extra, right side, located 4 *cun* above the lateral border of the patella with the knee flexed), Yanglingquan (G.B. 34), Qimen (Liv. 14)

Method: Insert perpendicularly and swiftly, and after the arrival of *qi*, rotate the needle counterclockwise. Insert at Yanglingquan (G.B. 34) in a 95-degree angle and rotate the needle counterclockwise to conduct the propagation upward along the thigh. Insert at Qimen (Liv. 14) at a 45-degree angle and rotate the needle clockwise after the arrival of *qi*. Retain the needles for 30 minutes, and rotate once every 10 minutes.

Results: Of 150 cases treated, 142 cases were cured and 8 failed.

(*Source:* Chinese Acupuncture & Moxibustion, 6(4):5, 1986)

2. Clinical observation on 63 cases of biliary colic treated with acupuncture

Points and method: According to the random sampling, 18 cases were punctured at Dannangxue (Extra), 18 were needled at Zusanli (St. 36), and 27 were also needled at Zusanli (St. 36), but connected with an electro-acupuncture apparatus for strong stimulation. All the cases were needled bilaterally. A 2.5 *cun* filiform needle was inserted perpendicularly at Zusanli (St. 36) and a 1.5 *cun* needle was thrust at Dannangxue (Extra, located at the site 5/12 on the medial side in the dorsal aspect of the second metacarpal bone). The needles were lifted and thrust for reduction, and after the needling sensation of numbness, distention, heaviness and soreness was acquired, the needles were retained for half an hour. At the same time, the medication of Major Bupleurum Decoction was administered orally.

Results: Of 63 cases treated, 6 cases showed marked clinical effect, 30 cases showed some effect, 21 cases improved and 6 cases failed.

(*Source:* Jiangxi Journal of Traditional Chinese Medicine, (4):34, 1988)

3. Observation on the therapeutical effect of 114 cases of gallstone treated with ear acupuncture

Points: Liver, Gall Bladder, Duodenum, Sanjiao

Method: Stick vaccaria seeds on the ear points with adhesive plaster, alternate two ears every second day. One course of treatment con-

169

sists of five weeks. Require the patient to press the points for 20 minutes after every meal and before sleep. Whenever abdominal pain appears, the points can be pressed immediately in order to ease the pain.

Results: Of 114 cases treated, 99 cases obtained the evacuation of stones, making up 86.8 percent; the minimal evacuation was more than 10 pieces of sand-like stones while the maximum was more than 100 pieces of stones 5-15 mm in diameter; 67 cases underwent Ultrasonic B examination after the treatment, and 6 cases of them evacuated all stones.

(*Source:* Chinese Acupuncture & Moxibustion, (5):23, 1987)

4. Clinical observation on 100 cases of gallstone treated with ear-acupoint pressure

Principal points: Gall Bladder, Liver, Spleen, Stomach, Lower Apex of Tragus

Supplementary points:

Constipation: Large Intestine

Insomnia: End of Inferior Helix Crus, Shenmen

Palpitation and stuffiness in the chest: Heart, Lung

Method: Put vaccaria seeds in the center of a plaster measuring 0.5 cm x 0.5 cm. Then stick on the ear points for pressure, alternate ears every second day. Thirty days constitute a course of treatment with a 10-day interval between two courses. Pressure is given once in the morning, afternoon, evening and before sleep, until a flush or burning sensation of the auricle is present, or even the propagation along the meridians and collaterals on the body. A fatty diet should be combined.

Results: Of 100 cases treated, 96 cases acquired the evacuation of stones and among them 3 cases had complete evacuation, 4 cases were unchanged. Usually the evacuation began after 1-15 treatments but those suffering from atrophic cholecystitis experienced evacuation after more than 16 treatments. When there was an acute attack of chronic cholecystitis, the evacuation of stones began after the inflammation was resolved. 1-4 courses were needed to evacuate all stones. The effect of evacuation was fair for the stones less than 8 mm in diameter, and the stones over 12 mm in diameter were seldom evacuated.

(*Source:* Shaanxi Journal of Traditional Chinese Medicine, 7(5):216, 1986)

170

56. Constipation

Principal points: Dachangshu (U.B. 25), Tianshu (St. 25), Zhigou (S.J. 6), Shangjuxu (St. 37)

Method: Produce moderately strong stimulation and provide continuous rotation of the needle at Tianshu (St. 25) for 5-10 minutes. Retain the needles for 10-20 minutes and treat daily.

Supplementary points:

Accumulated heat in stomach and intestines: Hegu (L.I. 4), Quchi (L.I. 11), Neiting (St. 44)

Constipation resulting from stagnation of *qi*: Zhongwan (Ren 12), Yanglingquan (G.B. 34), Xingjian (Liv. 2)

Deficiency of both *qi* and blood: Pishu (U.B. 20), Weishu (U.B. 21)

Stagnation of cold due to *yang* deficiency: Moxi Shenque (Ren 8), Qihai (Ren 6)

Other therapies:

1. Ear acupuncture

Points: Lower Portion of Rectum, Large Intestine, Brain

Method: Apply moderately strong stimulation, and intermittent manipulation of needles. Retain the needles for 10-20 minutes. Treat daily or once every other day.

2. Electro-acupuncture

Points: Daheng (Sp. 15), Xiajuxu (St. 39); or Zhigou (S.J. 6), Shimen (Ren 5)

Method: Connect the electro-apparatus with needles for 10-20 minutes with sparse-dense wave. Treat once every second day and alternate two groups of points.

Remarks: Acupuncture has good effect in treating this disease. The causative factors should be found out for those unchanged after a number of treatments.

REFERENCES:

1. Observed results of the treatment of 8 cases of habitual constipation by needling Chengshan (U.B. 57)

Point: Chengshan (U.B. 57)

Method: Apply acupuncture once daily.

Results: Of 8 cases treated, 7 cases were cured with 10 treatments, and 1 case was unchanged.

(*Source:* Journal of Traditional Chinese Medicine, 21(10):16, 1980)

2. Observed results of 53 cases of habitual constipation treated with ear acupressure

Principal points: Large Intestine, Lower Portion of Rectum, Abdomen, Middle of the Cymba

Supplementary points:

Constitutional debility after long-standing illness, senility, and postpartum: Spleen, Stomach, Intertragicus, Brain

Syndrome of excess: Lung, Sanjiao

Method: Press all points to find the tender spots. Then stick with vaccaria seeds for pressure. The seeds are changed every 5-7 days.

Results: Of 53 cases treated, 12 cases were basically cured, 24 showed marked effect, 12 were improved and 5 were unchanged.

(*Source:* Chinese Acupuncture & Moxibustion, (4):14, 1987)

57. Hemorrhoids

Principal points: Changqiang (Du 1), Baihuanshu (U.B. 30), Chengshan (U.B. 57), Erbai (Extra)

Method: Straightly insert Changqiang (Du 1) to cause the needling sensation extending to the anus. Needle Baihuanshu (U.B. 30) to the medial and inferior and let the needling sensation radiate to the anus. Puncture Chengshan (U.B. 57) slantly and upwardly to a depth of 2.5-3 *cun* with strong stimulation. Insert needle perpendicularly at Erbai (Extra) to a depth of 0.5-1 *cun*. Retain the needles for 30 minutes with periodic manipulation, once every 5-10 minutes. Treat daily.

Supplementary points:

Swelling and pain at the anus: Zhibian (U.B. 54)

Bleeding: Xuehai (Sp. 10), Qihaishu (U.B. 24)

Constipation: Dachangshu (U.B. 25), Tianshu (St. 25)

Other therapies:

1. Pricking therapy

Points: Select one or several round red rashes (the same size as the needle tip), from bilateral T7 to the lumbar sacral region, as the puncturing points.

Method: Use a thick needle to prick the points so as to cause bleeding. Treat once in seven days.

172

2. Ear acupuncture

Points: Lower Portion of Rectum, Shenmen, Brain

Method: Use filiform needles with moderate stimulation. Retain the needles for 20-30 minutes. Treat daily.

3. Electro-acupuncture

Points: Zhishu (Extra, 1 *cun* lateral to Mingmen, Du 4), Changqiang (Du 1), Chengshan (U.B. 57), Huiyang (U.B. 35)

Method: Choose 2-3 points in a session. After the needling sensations are obtained, connect the needles to an electro-stimulator for 5-10 minutes. Limit the amount of stimulation to the tolerance of the patient. Treat 2-3 times a week.

4. Blood-letting

Point: Mouth-Yinjiao (Du 28)

Method: Use a three-edged needle to prick the point and cause bleeding.

Remarks: Acupuncture and moxibustion are quite effective in relieving pain and swelling associated with hemorrhoids.

REFERENCE:

Observed results of puncturing Chengshan (U.B. 57) in treating 100 cases of pain associated with hemorrhoids

Points: Chengshan (U.B. 57), bilateral .

Method: Insert the needles to a depth of 1.5 *cun* with strong stimulation. Retain the needles for 30 minutes with periodic manipulation, once every five minutes.

Results: The effective rate for internal hemorrhoids reached 100 percent, external hemorrhoids 96 percent, and mixed hemorrhoids 96.7 percent.

(*Source:* Chinese Acupuncture & Moxibustion, (2):23, 1986)

58. Prolapse of Rectum

Principal points: Changqiang (Du 1), Baihui (Du 20), Chengshan (U.B. 57), Tigangxue (Extra, at the spot of three and nine o'clock around the anus, 0.5 *cun* lateral to the center of the anus)

Method: To puncture Changqiang (Du 1), insert the needle between the rectum and the coccyx 0.5-1 *cun* in depth, until the needling sensation has spread all around the anus. Provide moderately strong stimulation at Chengshan (U.B. 57). Needle Tigangxue (Extra) as deep as 1.5 *cun*, retain the needles for 10-20 minutes, and manipulate every four minutes. Offer mild moxibustion with a moxa stick over Baihui (Du 20) for 10-20 minutes, or moxi after the needling. Treat daily or once every other day. Ten times constitute one course.

Supplementary points:

Deficiency of *qi* and constitutional weakness: Qihai (Ren 6), Zusanli (St. 36), Pishu (U.B. 20)

Red, painful, feverish and swelling associated: Quchi (L.I. 11), Yinlingquan (Sp. 9)

Other therapies:

1. Pricking therapy

Points: Any locus 1.5 *cun* lateral to the posterior mid-line between the third lumbar vertebra and the second sacral vertebra

Method: Apply conventional sterile technique with iodine tincture and alcohol on the skin of the pricked locus. Hold the needle with the right hand and after thrusting the tip of the needle into the skin, with the index finger of the left hand push the skin of the loci gently towards the tip so as to penetrate the skin with the needle. Then raise the tip up and move slightly to prick out the subcutaneous fiber, or to cut several dozens of the white subcutaneous fibriform matters. After the operation, sterilize with iodine tincture and alcohol on the locus, which is then covered with the antiseptic gauze and fixed with plaster. Treat once a week or every 10 days, and prick one locus in each treatment.

2. Ear acupuncture

Points: Lower Portion of Rectum, Brain, Shenmen

Method: Select the above points on both ears and puncture with filiform needles to obtain moderate stimulation. Retain the needles for 30 minutes. Treat daily and 10 treatments constitute one course.

3. Cutaneous acupuncture

Points: Dachangshu (U.B. 25), Ciliao (U.B. 32), Jiaji points (Extra, from second to the tenth thoracic vertebra), Changqiang (Du 1), Baihuanshu (U.B. 30)

Method: Tap each point for 3-5 minutes, until the skin is flushed or caused slight bleeding. Treat once every other day.

4. Electro-acupuncture

Points: Changqiang (Du 1), Tigangxue (Extra), Chengshan (U.B. 57)

Method: Employ interrupted or sparse-dense wave. Set the frequen-

174

cy at 20 times per minute, and the intensity of stimulation to the extent of the patient's tolerance but with absence of pain. An intense contraction, numbness and distention of the perianal soft tissues will appear, after the currency is connected. One treatment lasts for 15-30 minutes. Treat once every other day. Ten treatments constitute one course and there should be 5-day interval between two courses.

Remarks: Acupuncture has fair effect in treating the prolapse of anus, but the effectiveness is only satisfactory for acute cases. Chronic cases will require further treatment.

REFERENCE:

Observed results of the treatment of 67 cases of pediatric prolapse of rectum in deficient syndrome with acupuncture

Points: Baihui (Du 20), Changqiang (Du 1), Huiyang (U.B. 35), Chengshan (U.B. 57)

Method: After the quick insertion of the needles, swiftly thrust and slowly lift each needle nine times and then retain the needles for 20 minutes. The depth in Changqiang (Du 1) is 1.5 *cun*, while the tip of the needle goes 1.5 *cun* deep interiorly and medially in Huiyang (U.B. 35). Treat daily, and six treatments constitute one course. Provide three courses consecutively.

Results: Of 67 cases treated, 63 cases were cured and 4 cases failed.

(*Source:* Chinese Acupuncture & Moxibustion, 5(6):7, 1985)

59. Ascariasis

I. Roundworm in the intestine

Principal points: Sifeng (Extra), Baichongwo (Extra), Tianshu (St. 25), Qihai (Ren 6), Daheng (Sp. 15)

Method: Prick Sifeng (Extra) with a thick filiform needle, and squeeze out the white fluid. Needle the other points with moderate stimulation and repeated manipulation. Retain the needles for 10-30 minutes. Treat daily.

Supplementary points:

Vomiting: Neiguan (P. 6), Zhongwan (Ren 12)

Abdominal distention: Ganshu (U.B. 18), Pishu (U.B. 20), with reinforcing method and moxibustion; Neiting (St. 44), with reducing method

II. Roundworm in the biliary tract

Principal points: Burong (St. 19), Juque (Ren 14), Yanglingquan (G.B. 34), Taichong (Liv. 3), Qimen (Liv. 14)

Method: Use filiform needles. Puncture shallowly with repeated manipulation. Withdraw the needles after pain is relieved. Treat 2-3 times a day.

Supplementary points:

Vomiting: Neiguan (P. 6), Zhongwan (Ren 12)

Severe pain: Sibai (St. 2) joining to Yingxiang (L.I. 20), Dannangxue (Extra)

Other therapies:

1. Ear acupuncture

Points: End of Inferior Helix Crus, Shenmen, Liver, Gall Bladder, Pancreas

Method: Use filiform needles with strong stimulation. Retain the needles for 30-60 minutes with periodic manipulation, or use an electrostimulator for 20 minutes. Treat once or twice a day. This method is applicable to roundworm in the biliary tract.

2. Electro-excited therapy

Points: Danshu (U.B. 19), Ashi points

Method: In acute biliary colic pain, put the cathode at Danshu (U.B. 19) on the right side, and place the anode at the Ashi point below the rib on the right side. Treat once for 3-5 minutes. If the desired results are not obtained, begin another treatment after 30 minutes.

Remarks: Acupuncture and moxibustion are quite effective in relieving pain and eliminating parasites in the treatment of ascariasis.

REFERENCES:

1. Observed results of the treatment of 34 cases of ascariasis with acupuncture

Principal points: Jiaji points (Extra, from T7) or Zhiyang (Du 9)

Supplementary points: Danshu (U.B. 19), Pishu (U.B. 20), Weicang (U.B. 50), on the right side

Method: Select bilateral T7 Jiaji points and insert at a perpendicular angle. Then, change the needles' direction to form a 65-degree angle against the skin to a depth of 1 *cun*. Try to let the tip of the needle reach the spinal periosteum. Apply reducing method with small amplitude until the patient feels the muscles relax in the chest and abdo-

176

men. Retain the needles for 20-30 minutes. As to the supplementary points, puncture according to the routine procedure.

Results: Of the 34 cases treated, 28 cases were cured (symptoms and signs disappeared after one treatment, no relapsing within 24 hours), marked effect (symptoms disappeared but some signs remained after one treatment) was seen in 4 cases, and improvement (after one treatment, symptoms disappeared and pain relapsed within 24 hours) in 2 cases.

(*Source:* Fujian Journal of Traditional Chinese Medicine, 16(6):57, 1985)

2. Clinical study on needling Danshu (U.B. 19) and Pishu (U.B. 20) in the treatment of 520 cases of ascariasis in the biliary tract

Points and method: Puncture Danshu (U.B. 19) and Pishu (U.B. 20).

Results: Those cured by 1-3 treatments numbered 309, by more than 4 treatments numbered 181, those with no effect numbered 30 cases.

(*Source:* Jiangxi Journal of Traditional Chinese Medicine, (4):27, 1981)

3. Observed results of ear acupuncture in the treatment of 18 cases of ascariasis in the biliary tract

Points: Pancreas, Duodenum, all on the right ear

Method: Insert the needles into the cartilage.

Results: Of 18 cases treated, 16 cases were cured, improvement was seen in 1 case and no effect was evident in 1 case.

(*Source:* Chinese Acupuncture & Moxibustion, (2):5, 1986)

4. Observation on acupuncture in relieving pain in the treatment of 70 cases of ascariasis in the biliary tract

Points: Juque (Ren 14), Jiuwei (Ren 15), Burong (St. 19), Shangwan (Ren 13), Zhongwan (Ren 12)

Method: Choose 1-2 points in a session. The patient is in supine position with the knees flexed. Insert the needle to 20-35 mm to get the needling sensation. Retain the needle for 10-30 minutes. If the desired effect is not seen, continue manipulation until the pain is completely relieved.

Results: Of the 70 cases treated, marked effect was seen in 48 cases, improvement in 21 cases, no effect in 1 case. The total effective rate reached 98.6 percent.

(*Source:* Chinese Acupuncture & Moxibustion, (5):13, 1987)

5. Therapeutic result observation on acupuncture in the treatment of 1,279 cases of ascariasis in the intestines of children

Points: Daheng (Sp. 15), Zusanli (St. 36)

Method: When needling Daheng (Sp. 15), the tip of the needle should point to the umbilicus and form 60-degree angle against the skin, and be inserted to a depth of 1.5-2.5 *cun.* Manipulate the needle with great amplitude 5-6 times. Do not retain the needle. Treat daily for 1-3 days.

Results: There were 472 cases in which the parasites were eliminated.

(*Source:* New Journal of Traditional Chinese Medicine, (4):37, 1980)

60. Infectious Hepatitis

Principal points: Zhiyang (Du 9), Danshu (U.B. 19), Yinlingquan (Sp. 9), Zusanli (St. 36)

Method: Puncture the above-mentioned points with filiform needles and apply moderate stimulation. Retain the needles for 20-30 minutes with periodic manipulation once every 5-10 minutes. Treat daily. Ten treatments constitute one course.

Supplementary points:

Damp-heat pattern: Dazhui (Du 14), Quchi (L.I. 11), Yanglingquan (G.B. 34), Taichong (Liv. 3), with reducing method

Cold-damp pattern: Pishu (U.B. 20), Yanggang (U.B. 48), Sanyinjiao (Sp. 6), with reinforcing method, and combined with moxibustion

Hypochondriac pain: Insert slantly at Qimen (Liv. 14), Zhigou (S.J. 6)

Stifling sensation in the chest, vomiting: Neiguan (P. 6), Gongsun (Sp. 4)

Poor appetite: Zhongwan (Ren 12)

Abdominal distention: Tianshu (St. 25), Qihai (Ren 6)

Diarrhea: Guanyuan (Ren 4), Tianshu (St. 25), with reinforcing method, and combined with moxibustion

Hard hepatomegaly: Ganshu (U.B. 18), Zhangmen (Liv. 13), Pigen (Extra)

Listlessness, chills: Mingmen (Du 4), Qihai (Ren 6)

Other therapies:

1. Ear acupuncture

Points: Liver, Gall Bladder, Spleen, Stomach, End of Inferior Helix Crus, Vagus Root

Method: Choose 4-6 points in a session. Puncture with filiform needles and moderate stimulation. Retain the needles for 30 minutes. Treat daily or once every other day. Ten treatments constitute one course.

2. Hydro-acupuncture

Points: Ganshu (U.B. 18), Pishu (U.B. 20), Foot-Zhongdu (Liv. 6)

Method: Choose 2-4 points in a session. Use 0.5-1 ml of Vitamin B_1 or B_{12} solution according to the routine procedure of hydro-acupuncture to inject each point. Treat once every other day. Ten treatments constitute one course.

3. Laser acupuncture

Points: Ganshu (U.B. 18), Zusanli (St. 36), groin or cervical lymph node

Method: The He-Ne laser machine is used to illuminate for 5 minutes each point applied with gentian violet. First, lead the laser light onto the lymph nodes, then Ganshu (U.B. 18), and then Zusanli (St. 36). Two lights on the two sides can be used in rotation. Treat daily. Twenty treatments constitute one course. If the symptoms and signs have nearly disappeared and the examination of the liver function shows it to be normal or close to the normal after one course, cease treatment and take ten days' rest for observation. If it is effective, another course can be continued. If it is of no effect or causes nausea, other therapies should be used.

Remarks: Acupuncture and moxibustion therapies are effective in the treatment of infectious hepatitis. As to severe, acute hepatitis, other combination therapies should be adopted to save the patient. During the treatment, strict sterilization of things, especially the needles, should be followed.

REFERENCES:

1. Observed results of acupuncture in the treatment of 121 cases of acute icterohepatitis

Points and method: Puncture Zusanli (St. 36) and Yanglingquan

179

(G.B. 34) to join to Yinlingquan (Sp. 9), and Taichong (Liv. 3) to Yongquan (K.1).Use the above bilateral points in rotation. Treat daily. If fever is present, add Quchi (L.I. 11), Hegu (L.I. 4) or Dazhui (Du 14); if vomiting is a symptom, combine Neiguan (P. 6) and Zhongwan (Ren 12). For abdominal distention, take into consideration Tianshu (St. 25) and Dachangshu (U.B. 25). Apply even method to mild cases. Use reducing method for cases with severe damp-heat pattern. After the needling sensation is obtained, connect the needles with an electro-stimulator.

Results: Of 121 cases treated, the cured numbered 115, improvement was seen in 5 cases and no effect was evident in 1 case.

(*Source:* Liaoning Journal of Traditional Chinese Medicine, (6):48, 1981)

2. Therapeutic result observation of acupuncture in the treatment of 29 cases of liver diseases

Principal points: Zusanli (St. 36), Ganyanxue (Extra, 2 *cun* below Sanyinjiao, Sp. 6), Zhongfeng (Liv. 4)

Supplementary points:

Abdominal distention and indigestion: Gongsun (Sp. 4), Zhongwan (Ren 12)

Nausea and vomiting: Zhigou (S.J. 6), Neiguan (P. 6)

Qi stagnation in the liver: Zhangmen (Liv. 13)

Jaundice: Hegu (L.I. 4), Houxi (S.I. 3)

Ascites: Shuifen (Ren 9), Qihai (Ren 6), Sanyinjiao (Sp. 6), Zhongji (Ren 3), or apply ear acupuncture

Method: Puncture with even method. Retain the needles for an hour. If using bilateral points, choose the points on one side in a session. Rotate the bilateral points. Fifteen treatments constitute one course. Begin another course after five days' rest.

Results: Among 11 cases of acute hepatitis, 10 were cured, improvement was seen in 1 case. Among 11 cases of chronic hepatitis, 10 were cured, improvement was seen in 1 case. Among the other 7 cases (3 cases had hepatocirrhosis at the early stage, 3 cases had ascites due to cirrhosis, 1 case had symptoms similar to liver disorders but no physical signs) except 1 case with hepatocirrhosis at the early stage, the other 6 cases were all improved. The number of treatments was from 23 to 155.

(*Source:* Shaanxi Journal of Traditional Chinese Medicine, "Additional Publication of Acupuncture and Moxibustion," 14, 1981)

61. Common Cold

Principal points: Fengchi (G.B. 20), Hegu (L.I. 4), Lieque (Lu. 7), Dazhui (Du 14)

Method: Apply moderate stimulation to all the points. Needle Fengchi (G.B. 20), and let the needling sensation extend to the nape and head.

Supplementary points:

Nasal obstruction: Yingxiang (L.I. 20)

Headache: Taiyang (Extra), Yintang (Extra)

Sore-throat: Shaoshang (Lu. 11), causing bleeding with a three-edged needle

Fever: Quchi (L.I. 11)

Soreness and pain on the back: Feishu (U.B. 13), applying cupping

Other therapies:

Ear acupuncture

Points: Lung, Internal Nose, Lower Apex of Tragus, Forehead

Method: Puncture with moderate stimulation and periodic manipulation for 2-3 minutes. Retain the needles for 20-30 minutes. If a sore-throat exists, add Tonsil (Extra). Treat daily.

Remarks: When the common cold is prevalent, puncture Zusanli (St. 36) and retain the needle for 10-15 minutes, or apply moxibustion with a moxa stick at Zusanli (St. 36) for 5-8 minutes. Treat daily for three days. This can prevent the disease.

REFERENCE:

Observed results of treating the common cold by needling one point

Point: Yemen (S.J. 2)

Method: Use a filiform needle to puncture at an angle towards the interspace of the metacarpal bones, rotating to the left and right several times. Generally, needle the point on one side for the treatment. If the desired effect is not produced, puncture the point on the opposite side. Retain the needle for 15-30 minutes.

Results: Of 394 cases treated, 247 cases, 63 percent, were cured with all symptoms disappearing, those with symptoms nearly disappearing numbered 82, 21 percent; marked effect was seen in 36 cases, 9 percent; improvement in 20 cases, 5 percent; no effect in 9 cases, 2

percent.

(*Source:* Henan Traditional Chinese Medicine, 8(4):19, 1988)

62. Acute Bronchitis

Principal Points: Feishu (U.B. 13), Chize (Lu. 5), Hegu (L.I. 4), Lieque (Lu. 7)

Method: Reduce all the above points by means of strong stimulation, and retain the needles for 10-20 minutes, manipulating them every five minutes. Treat once or twice daily according to the severity of the disease.

Supplementary points:

Chills and fever: Fengchi (G.B. 20), Fengmen (U.B. 12), performed with moxibustion after the needling

Hyperpyrexia: Dazhui (Du 14), Quchi (L.I. 11)

Severe cough: Tiantu (Ren 22)

Nasal obstruction with rhinorrhea: Yingxiang (L.I. 20)

Severe sore-throat: Shaoshang (Lu. 11), bleeded with a three-edged needle

Excessive sputum: Fenglong (St. 40)

Other therapies:

1. Ear acupuncture

Points: Lung, Trachea, Shenmen, End of Inferior Helix Crus, Lower Apex of Tragus

Method: Use filiform needles to produce moderate stimulation and then retain the needles for 20-30 minutes. Treat daily.

2. Hydro-acupuncture

Points: Feishu (U.B. 13), Dingchuan (Extra), Fengmen (U.B. 12), Dazhu (U.B. 11)

Method: Select two pairs of points for each treatment, prescribe one kind of antibiotic solution for intramuscular injection (carry out a dermal sensitivity test when necessary), and inject 0.5 ml of the medicinal liquid into each point by means of routine operation of hydro-acupuncture. Treat daily.

3. Cutaneous acupuncture

Points: Nape of the neck, urinary bladder meridian from first to seventh thoracic vertebrae, and stomach meridian on the anterior aspect of the neck

Method: Strongly tap with a cutaneous needle until the skin bleeds. Treat daily.

4. Cupping

Points: On the upper back, from Dazhu (U.B. 11) down to Geshu (U.B. 17), bilateral

Method: Apply movable cupping to cause the skin flushing. Treat daily.

Remarks: Acupuncture has fairly good effects in treating acute bronchitis.

63. Chronic Bronchitis

Principal points: Feishu (U.B. 13), Chize (Lu. 5), Dingchuan (Extra), Tiantu (Ren 22)

Method: Puncture the points with moderate stimulation and even method. Retain the needles for 20-30 minutes with periodic manipulation every 5-10 minutes. Or connect with an electro-stimulator for 15 minutes after the needling sensations are obtained. Treat daily or once every other day. Ten treatments constitute one course.

Supplementary points:

Asthma: Shanzhong (Ren 17)

Chest and hypochondriac pain: Shanzhong (Ren 17), Yanglingquan (G.B. 34), Zhigou (S.J. 6)

Excessive phlegm and dampness: Fenglong (St. 40), Pishu (U.B. 20)

Liver fire attacking the lung: Zhigou (S.J. 6), Xingjian (Liv. 2), with reducing method

Deficient *yin* of the lung and kidney: Shenshu (U.B. 23), Taixi (K. 3), Gaohuangshu (U.B. 43), with reinforcing method

Deficient *yang* of the spleen and kidney: Shenshu (U.B. 23), Pishu (U.B. 20), Qihai (Ren 6), Zusanli (St. 36), with reinforcing method, and combined with moxibustion

Other therapies:

1. Ear acupuncture

Points: Lung, Trachea, Lower Apex of Tragus, End of Inferior Helix Crus, Ear-asthma

Method: Choose 2-3 points in a session. Use filiform needles with moderate stimulation. Retain the needles for 30 minutes with periodic manipulation. Treat daily or once every other day. Ten treatments constitute one course. Or use needle-embedding for 1-2 days, treating once every other day. Five treatments constitute one course. Use the ear points in turn. Or vaccaria seeds can be applied at the ear points. Instruct the patient to press them 3-5 times a day. Remove and change the seeds every three days.

2. Embedding sutures in points

Points: Shanzhong (Ren 17), Feishu (U.B. 13), Dingchuan (Extra), Shenshu (U.B. 23)

Method: Operate according to the routine procedure of embedding sutures in points. Treat twice a month. Treatments of three months constitute one course.

3. Incision method

Points: Shanzhong (Ren 17), Feishu (U.B. 13)

Method: Operate according to the routine procedure of incision method. The method can be repeated after 2-3 weeks.

4. Hydro-acupuncture

Points: Feishu (U.B. 13), Dingchuan (Extra), Fengmen (U.B. 12), Quchi (L.I. 11), Chize (Lu. 5), Fenglong (St. 40)

Method: Choose 2-4 points in a session. Inject 0.5 ml of Vitamin B_1 solution (100 mg/ml) according to the routine procedure of hydro-acupuncture into each point. Treat once every other day. Ten treatments constitute one course.

5. Finger pressure

Points: The pair of points at inferior broads of the 1st-5th sternocostal joints, and tender spots as secondary points

Method: Choose 1-2 pairs of points in a session. Press and slip your fingers on the bone where the point is located. Maintain pressure on each point for 7-15 minutes. Treat twice a day. Ten treatments constitute one course.

Remarks: Combination of the above-mentioned methods can obtain a certain therapeutic result in the treatment of chronic bronchitis.

REFERENCE:

Observed results of ear acupuncture in the treatment of 100 cases of chronic bronchitis

Points: Trachea, Lower Apex of Tragus, Prostate

Excessive phlegm: Spleen

184

Method: Use mustard seeds, vaccaria seeds or intradermal needles for implantation on the ears. Change the seeds or needles after five days. Five treatments constitute one course.

Results: Of 100 cases treated, 47 cases were controlled, marked effect was seen in 43 cases, improvement in 6 cases, no effect was evident in 4 cases. The total effective rate in the short term reached 96 percent.

(*Source:* Shanghai Journal of Acupuncture and Moxibustion, (2): 12, 1987)

64. Bronchial Asthma

Principal points: Dingchuan (Extra), Feishu (U.B. 13), Shanzhong (Ren 17), Tiantu (Ren 22)

Method: Puncture Dingchuan (Extra), and Shanzhong (Ren 17) with viberating manipulation. Retain the needles for 20-30 minutes with periodic manipulation. Treat once or twice a day during the acute stage, but daily or once every other day during the remission stage.

Supplementary points:

Chronic bronchial asthma: Shenzhu (Du 12), Gaohuangshu (U.B. 43), applying indirect moxibustion with garlic

Weakness of the body: Zusanli (St. 36), Qihai (Ren 6), combined with moxibustion

Profuse phlegm: Fenglong (St. 40), Chize (Lu. 5)

Allergic bronchial asthma: Xuehai (Sp. 10)

Other therapies:

1. Cutaneous acupuncture (commonly used at the acute stage)
Points and method:

a) Use a cutaneous needle to tap gently the thenar eminences and the pathways of the lung meridians on the forearms for about 15 minutes. Then tap the bilateral muscle sternocleido-mastoideus for another 15 minutes. It has a relieving function.

b) Use a cutaneous needle to tap the upper back and nape of neck, particularly in the area between the left and right paths of the urinary bladder meridians. Continue tapping until the skin feels hot and the patient is breathing more freely.

Choose one of the above two methods for the treatment, or use the two methods in rotation.

2. Wrist-and-ankle acupuncture

Points: Upper 1 and 2, bilateral

Method: Apply the routine procedure of wrist-and-ankle acupuncture.

　3. Application method

Points: Bailao (Extra), Feishu (U.B. 13), Gaohuangshu (U.B. 43)

Method: Grind herbs of Brassica Alba, Euphorbia Kansui, Sarum Sieboldi and Corydalis Bulbosa, 15 grams each, into powders. During application, mix the powders with jinger juice to make six plasters. Spread a little bit of Flos Caryophylli and Cinnamon Twig powders on each plaster. Place the plasters on the above points for two hours. The patient will experience sensations of hotness, numbness or pain after application. The local skin may become congested and red in color, and sometimes blisters may arise. The method is applicable in children. Treat once every ten days during the 30 hottest days of the summer. The application may be continued for three years.

　4. Hydro-acupuncture

Points: Jiaji points (Extra, from T1-T6)

Method: Choose a pair of Jiaji points (Extra) in a session. After the needling sensation is obtained, inject 0.5-1 ml of placental tissue extract solution into each point. Begin with the upper points and progress downward. Change points daily for the treatment. This method is applicable to bronchial asthma during the remission stage.

　5. Ear acupuncture

Points: Ear-asthma, Lower Apex of Tragus, Trachea, Brain, End of Inferior Helix Crus

Method: Choose 2-3 points in a session. Puncture with strong stimulation. Retain the needles for 5-10 minutes. Treat daily. Ten treatments constitute one course.

　6. Head acupuncture

Points: Thoracic Cavity Area

Method: Perform the routine procedure of head acupuncture.

　7. Incision method

Point: Shanzhong (Ren 17)

Method: After the routine sterilization on the point, administer 2% novocaine as a local anesthetic. A transverse incision, 0.5 cm in length, is made at the point. Remove a little bit of fatty tissue, and stroke the wound with hemostatic forceps for half a minute. Then stitch the incision. Remove the thread after seven days.

186

8. Laser acupuncture

Points: Shanzhong (Ren 17), Tiantu (Ren 22), Dingchuan (Extra), Feishu (U.B. 13)

Method: Choose 2-4 points in a session. Illuminate each point for 5-10 minutes. Treat daily. Ten treatments constitute one course.

Remarks: For a severe attack of bronchial asthma or persistent bronchial asthma, other medication should be combined for the treatment. The points on the chest and back should be shallowly punctured to avoid injury of the internal organ. Moxibustion is suitable during the remission stage.

REFERENCES:

1. Observed results of puncturing Sifeng (Extra) in the treatment of 37 cases of infantile asthma

Point: Sifeng (Extra)

Method: Extend the patient's fingers with palm up. Use a three-edged needle to prick the point rapidly to a depth of 2-3 mm, drawing a small amount of yellow and white fluid. Treat once every two days.

Results: Of 37 cases treated, marked effect was seen in 13 cases, improvement in 21 cases, and no effect in 3 cases.

(*Source:* Liaoning Journal of Traditional Chinese Medicine, (2):14, 1981)

2. Clinical observation on electro-acupuncture in the treatment of 60 cases of bronchial asthma

Point: Kongzui (Lu. 6)

Method: Rapidly insert the needle to a depth of 0.3-0.5 *cun.* Apply reducing method after the needling sensation is obtained. Let the sensation extend upward to the chest, and downward to the thumb of the same side. Connect an electro-stimulator for 30-60 minutes.

Results: There were 60 cases under observation, of which 48 were completely or basically restored to the healthy conditions. The total effective rate was 100 percent.

(*Source:* Henan Traditional Chinese Medicine, (6):39, 1982)

65. Pneumonia

Principal points: Dazhui (Du 14), Feishu (U.B. 13), Hegu (L.I.

4), Chize (Lu. 5)

Method: Reduce all the points with strong stimulation and retain the needles for 30 minutes, manipulating intermittently. Treat once or twice daily.

Supplementary points:

Persistent fever: Weizhong (U.B. 40), twelve Jing-Well points (Lu. 11, L.I. 1, S.I. 1, S.J. 1, H. 9, P. 9) bleeded with a three-edged needle

Unconsciousness and delirium: Renzhong (Du 26), Yongquan (K. 1) intensely stimulated

Pain in chest and costal region: Zhigou (S.J. 6)

Excessive sputum: Fenglong (St. 40)

Blood-stained sputum: Geshu (U.B. 17)

Long-lasting cough consuming *qi* and *yin*: Taiyuan (Lu. 9), Gaohuangshu (U.B. 43), Sanyinjiao (Sp. 6), Zusanli (St. 36), all with even method

Unconsciousness with convulsion: Renzhong (Du 26), Neiguan (P. 6), Guanyuan (Ren 4), Qihai (Ren 6); Renzhong (Du 26) and Neiguan (P. 6) with strong stimulation by filiform needles, while Qihai (Ren 6) and Guanyuan (Ren 4) with moxibustion by big moxa cones.

Other therapies:

1. Ear acupuncture

Points: Lung, Trachea, End of Inferior Helix Crus, Lower Apex of Tragus

Method: Apply moderate stimulation with filiform needles which are retained for 30-60 minutes. Those cases with high fever can be bled at the first vein on the dorsum of the ear. Treat 2-3 times daily.

2. Hydro-acupuncture

Points: Feishu (U.B. 13), Quchi (L.I. 11)

Method: Inject 0.5 ml of intramuscular injectable antibiotics into each point by means of routine operation of hydro-acupuncture. Inject once or twice daily. Skin sensitivity test should be provided when it is necessary.

3. Cupping

Points: Fengmen (U.B. 12), Feishu (U.B. 13), Gaohuangshu (U.B. 43), Ashi point (where the wet rale can be heard on the back)

Method: The routine operation of cupping is performed once daily.

Remarks: Acupuncture has fair effect in treating pneumonia. Those with complications of heart failure, shock, and meningeal irritation symptoms should be rescued with Western and traditional Chinese medication in addition to acupuncture therapy.

66. Pulmonary Tuberculosis

Principal points: Chize (Lu. 5), Feishu (U.B. 13), Gaohuangshu (U.B. 43), Zusanli (St. 36), Jiehexue (Extra)

Method: Use filiform needles to give moderate stimulation. Retain the needles for 20-30 minutes with periodic manipulation. Apply moxibustion at Feishu (U.B. 13), and Gaohuangshu (U.B. 43). Treat daily, and 10-15 treatments constitute one course.

Supplementary points:

Coughing blood: Geshu (U.B. 17), Kongzui (Lu. 6)

Severe cough: Taiyuan (Lu. 9)

Afternoon fever, night sweating: Yinxi (H. 6), Taixi (K. 3)

Seminal emission: Zhishi (U.B. 52), Guanyuan (Ren 4), Sanyinjiao (Sp. 6)

Amenorrhea: Xuehai (Sp. 10)

Yang deficiency with cold limbs: Moxi Guanyuan (Ren 4)

Other therapies:

1. Ear acupuncture

Points: Lung, End of Inferior Helix Crus, Shenmen, Ear-asthma

Method: Use filiform needles with moderate stimulation. Retain the needles for 20 minutes with periodic manipulation, or connect an electro-stimulator. Treat daily or once every other day. Ten treatments constitute one course.

2. Hydro-acupuncture

Points: Jihexue (Extra), Feishu (U.B. 13), Gaohuangshu (U.B. 43), Quchi (L.I. 11)

Method: Choose 2-3 points in a session. Inject each point with 0.5 ml of 100 mg Vitamin B_1 solution according to the routine procedure of hydro-acupuncture. Treat daily. Ten treatments constitute one course.

3. Embedding sutures in points

Points: a) Gaohuangshu (U.B. 43); b) Jihexue (Extra), Jueyinshu (U.B. 14) joining to Geshu (U.B. 17), Zhongfu (Lu. 1) joining to Yunmen (Lu. 2)

Method: Choose one group in a session. Bury or embed small strands of surgical gut in the points, according to the routine procedure of embedding sutures. Use two groups of points in turn. The interval between two sessions is 20-30 days.

Remarks: Acupuncture and moxibustion are effective supplementary therapies in the treatment of pulmonary tuberculosis. They are especially applicable to the patient whose therapeutic result is not satisfactory after prolonged exposure to an anti-tuberculosis drug.

REFERENCE:

Observed results of acupuncture in the treatment of 132 cases of pulmonary tuberculosis

Points and method:

a) Deficient *yang*: Adopt the treating principle of promoting *qi* circulation and warming *yang*, while using moxibustion as the main measure.

Qi deficiency in the lung: Zhongfu (Lu. 1), Feishu (U.B. 13), Dazhui (Du 14), Gaohuangshu (U.B. 43)

Deficient *yang* of the lung and spleen: Weishu (U.B. 21), Zhangmen (Liv. 13), Zhongwan (Ren 12), Zusanli (St. 36)

Deficient *yang* of the lung and kidney: Guanyuan (Ren 4), Qihai (Ren 6), Mingmen (Du 4), Shenshu (U.B. 23)

b) Deficient *yin*: Acupuncture is taken as the main measure.

Yin deficiency of the lung: Reinforcing Taiyuan (Lu. 9), Feishu (U.B. 13), Pianli (L.I. 6)

Yin deficiency of the lung and spleen: Reducing Taibai (Sp. 3), and reinforcing Zusanli (St. 36), Tianshu (St. 25)

Yin deficiency of the lung and kidney: Reinforcing Fuliu (K. 7), Jingqu (Lu. 8), Shenshu (U.B. 23), Geshu (U.B. 17), Taixi (K. 3), and reducing Xingjian (Liv. 2), Laogong (P. 8)

Results: Among 132 cases, marked effect was evident in 16 cases, improvement in 39 cases, no effect in 74 cases, and 3 cases became worse.

(*Source:* Zhejiang Journal of Traditional Chinese Medicine, 16(1):22, 1981)

67. Retention of Urine, Incontinence of Urine

Principal points: Zhongji (Ren 3), Sanyinjiao (Sp. 6)
Method: Use filiform needles with strong stimulation. Retain the

needles for or 20-30 minutes with periodic manipulation. For retention of urine, pay attention to the condition of the urinary bladder and not to injure it. When needling Zhongji (Ren 3), insert the needle slantly with the tip pointing downward, and enable the needling sensation extend to the perineum. Treat several times a day until inducing urination. For incontinence of urine, treat daily or once every other day.

Supplementary points:

Deficient *yang* of the spleen and kidney: Shenshu (U.B. 23), Pishu (U.B. 20), Taixi (K. 3), Guanyuan (Ren 4), Mingmen (Du 4), combined with moxibustion

Qi stagnation in the liver: Ganshu (U.B. 18), Taichong (Liv. 3)

Accumulation of damp and heat: Yinlingquan (Sp. 9), Shuidao (St. 28)

Other therapies:

1. Ear acupuncture

Points: Urinary Bladder, Kidney, Urethra, End of Inferior Helix Crus, External Genitalia

Method: Choose 2-4 points in each session. Use filiform needles or connect with an electro-stimulator with moderate stimulation. Retain the needles for 15-20 minutes. Treat daily. Use the points on the ears in turn.

2. Electro-acupuncture

Point: Weidao (G.B. 28)

Method: Puncture bilateral Weidao (G.B. 28) with the tips of the two needles pointing to Qugu (Ren 2) to a depth of 2-3 *cun*. Then connect the needles to an electro-stimulator with intermittent pulsation for 10-20 minutes. Gradually increase the amount of stimulation. This method is applicable in the treatment of urinary retention.

3. Moxibustion

Points: Sanjiaoshu (U.B. 22), Shenshu (U.B. 23), Zhongji (Ren 3), Ciliao (U.B. 32)

Method: Use either moxibustion with moxa sticks or indirect moxibustion with ginger. Apply moxibustion with moxa sticks to each point for 3-5 minutes. Moxa cones on the ginger at each point should be 5-7 in number. Treat daily.

Remarks: Acupuncture is definitely effective in treating both retention of urine and incontinence of urine. It is important that the underlying causes should be determined and treated. If a full feeling is present in the urinary bladder, use caution to give shallow and slanted insertion, and not to puncture straightly and deeply.

REFERENCES:

1. Observed results of acupuncture in the treatment of the retention of urine after an obstetrical operation

Points: Taichong (Liv. 3), Sanyinjiao (Sp. 6), Yinlingquan (Sp. 9), and acupoints related to designated days and hours in terms of the Heavenly Stems and Earthly Branches; for a weak constitution, add Zusanli (St. 36).

Method: Insert the needles while twirling and rotating. After the needling sensation is obtained, retain the needles for 15 minutes with periodic manipulation, once every five minutes. Try to let the needling sensation extend upward to the thigh.

Results: The therapeutic result was obtained after 1-3 treatments.

(*Source:* Zhejiang Journal of Traditional Chinese Medicine, (10):17, 1964)

2. Observed results of acupuncture and cupping in the treatment of 43 cases of postpartum retention of urine

Points: Qugu (Ren 2), Zusanli (St. 36), Yinlingquan (Sp. 9), Sanyinjiao (Sp. 6)

Method: Puncture the points with even method. Retain the needles for 20 minutes. Then apply three cups on the transverse line close to Qihai (Ren 6) for 10 minutes.

Results: Generally speaking, after withdrawal of the needles, urination was possible within 20 minutes. Only a few cases needed another treatment.

(*Source:* Inner-Mongolia Traditional Chinese Medicine, 6(2):31, 1987)

3. Observed results of acupuncture in the treatment of 23 cases of retention of urine after hemorrhoid and anal fistula operation

Points: Zhibian (U.B. 54), Sanyinjiao (Sp. 6)

Method: When needling Zhibian (U.B. 54), insert the tip of the needle at an angle towards the medial, and let soreness, numbness and a distention sensation extend to the genitalia. The patient may then have a desire to pass urine. Puncture Sanyinjiao (Sp. 6), allowing the needling sensation to extend upward to the knee, medial aspect of the thigh or genitalia. Retain the needles for about 10 minutes with periodic manipulation, once every three minutes.

Results: One treatment was applied. Those cases which passed

192

urine in 30 minutes after the treatment numbered 18, and in 60 minutes, 4. No effect was produced in 1 case.

(*Source:* Shaanxi Journal of Traditional Chinese Medicine, 6(12):553, 1985)

4. Observed results of acupuncture in the treatment of 170 cases of retention of urine

Principal points: Qihai (Ren 6), Shenshu (U.B. 23)

Method: Subcutaneously insert Qihai (Ren 6) downward and join to Guanyuan (Ren 4), or subcutaneously insert Guanyuan (Ren 4) downward and join to Zhongji (Ren 3). Puncture with reducing method, retain the needle after the needling sensation is obtained. Needle Shenshu (U.B. 23) to a depth of 0.3-0.5 *cun* with reinforcing method.

Supplementary points: Shuidao (St. 28), Sanyinjiao (Sp. 6)

Method: Puncture bilateral Shuidao (St. 28) at an angle to the wall of urinary bladder, and puncture Sanyinjiao (Sp. 6) to a depth of 1.0-1.5 *cun*, or join horizontally to Taixi (K. 3) with moderate stimulation.

Results: Of 170 cases treated, an excellent effect (urination within half an hour) was produced in 86 cases, a better effect (urination from half an hour to two hours) in 75 cases, and no effect (no urination for more than two hours) in 9 cases.

(*Source:* Hebei Journal of Traditional Chinese Medicine, (1):45, 1986)

5. Clinical experience on indirect moxibustion with salt in treating 17 cases of postpartum urinary retention

Points and method: First, fill the umbilicus with cooked salt. Apply 0.3 cm thickness of Chinese onion paste on the salt. Then place a moxa cone on the paste. Renew another cone when the patient feels it scorching. Repeat the process until heat penetrates into the abdomen to cause urination. One day after, again apply 1-2 moxa cones for consolidation.

Results: Of 17 cases treated, 10 cases produced urine after 1 cone was applied, 6 cases after 2-4 cones, and 1 case after 7 cones in 2 days.

(*Source:* Journal of Integrated Traditional and Western Medicines, 5(11):692, 1985)

68. Urinary Infection

Principal points: Shenshu (U.B. 23), Pangguangshu (U.B. 28), Zhongji (Ren 3), Sanyinjiao (Sp. 6)

Method: Produce moderate or strong stimulation with filiform needles and use reducing method. To puncture Sanyinjiao (Sp. 6), the needling sensation must be strong and radiating up and down. Retain the needles for 20-30 minutes and manipulated intermittently. Treat once or twice daily.

Supplementary points:

Fever: Hegu (L.I. 4), Dazhui (Du 14)

Severe urodynia: Xingjian (Liv. 2), Zhongfeng (Liv. 4), Yinlingquan (Sp. 9)

Hematuria: Xuehai (Sp. 10), Taichong (Liv. 3), Ciliao (U.B. 32)

Chronic persistent recurrence: Guanyuan (Ren 4), Taixi (K. 3), with reinforcing method

All the other points are needled with even method.

Other therapies:

1. Ear acupuncture

Points: Urinary Bladder, Kidney, End of Inferior Helix Crus, Occiput, Lower Apex of Tragus

Method: Select 2-4 points each time. Bring about strong stimulation and retain the needles for 20-30 minutes. Treat daily.

2. Moxibustion

Points: Shenshu (U.B. 23), Pangguangshu (U.B. 28), Zhongji (Ren 3), Guanyuan (Ren 4), Ciliao (U.B. 32)

Method: Provide each point with mild moxibustion by means of moxa sticks for 3-5 minutes, or with indirect moxibustion by ginger for 5-7 cones. Apply moxibustion daily. This is beneficial to chronic pyelonephritis or chronic cystitis.

3. Wrist-and-ankle acupuncture

Points: Lower 1, bilateral

Method: Perform the routine operation of wrist-and-ankle acupuncture

Remarks: Acupuncture therapy has fair effect in treating urinary infection.

69. Urinary Stone

Principal points: Shenshu (U.B. 23), Pangguangshu (U.B. 28), Yinlingquan (Sp. 9), Sanyinjiao (Sp. 6), Weiyang (U.B. 39)

Method: During an attack of renal colic, puncture the points with strong stimulation and reducing method. Retain the needles with periodic manipulation, once every 5-10 minutes. Withdraw the needles until remission of pain. If there is no renal colic, apply moderate stimulation, reinforcing firstly and then reducing. Retain the needles for 20-30 minutes with periodic manipulation. Treat daily. Ten treatments constitute one course.

Supplementary points:

Stone in the upper urinary tract: Jingmen (G.B. 25), Tianshu (St. 25)

Stone in the lower urinary tract: Zhongji (Ren 3), Shuidao (St. 28)

Hemourine: Xuehai (Sp. 10)

Nausea and vomiting: Neiguan (P. 6), Zhongwan (Ren 12)

Constipation: Tianshu (St. 25), Zhigou (S.J. 6)

Deficient *yang* of the kidney: Guanyuan (Ren 4), Mingmen (Du 4), puncture with reinforcing method; also combined with moxibustion

Other therapies:

1. Electro-acupuncture

Points: Shenshu (U.B. 23), Sanyinjiao (Sp. 6)

Method: After insertion and the needling sensation is obtained, connect the needles to a high frequency pulse instrument with strong stimulation for 5-10 minutes. Treat daily. During an attack of renal colic, continue stimulation until remission of pain.

2. Ear acupuncture

Points: End of Inferior Helix Crus, Shenmen, Lower Apex of Tragus, Kidney, Ureter, Urinary Bladder

Method: Use filiform needles with strong stimulation. Retain the needles for 20-30 minutes. Treat daily, or use needle-embedding method.

3. Hydro-acupuncture

Points: Shenshu (U.B. 23), Guanyuan (Ren 4), Yinlingquan (Sp. 9), Zusanli (St. 36), Sanyinjiao (Sp. 6), Jiaoxin (K. 8), Fujie (Sp. 14), Qugu (Ren 2)

Method: Choose 2-4 points in each session. Inject 1-2 ml of 10% glucose solution into each point according to the routine procedure of hydro-acupuncture. Treat daily or once every other day.

Remarks: The above-mentioned therapies have certain lithagogue function and relieving pain function. The patient is encouraged to drink more water and do jumping exercises so as to help passing the stone.

REFERENCES:

1. Primary study on acupuncture in the treatment of 150 cases of urinary stone and renal colic

Principal points: Jingmen (G.B. 25), Shenshu (U.B. 23)

Supplementary points: Zusanli (St. 36), Sanyinjiao (Sp. 6), Ashi point

Method: The patient is in recumbent position with the knees flexed, and the affected leg is put above. Puncture Jingmen (G.B. 25) on the affected side. Join Shenshu (U.B. 23) to Jingmen (G.B. 25). Either Zusanli (St. 36) or Sanyinjiao (Sp. 6) can be chosen for treatment. After the needling sensation is obtained by moderate stimulation, retain the needles for 30 minutes with periodic manipulation, once every 3-5 minutes. Treat once or twice a day. Seven days' treatment is considered as one course. The interval between courses is 1-2 days.

Results:

Relieving pain: there were 108 cases in which colic pain was checked after needling for 5-20 minutes, 26 cases in which colic pain stopped after puncturing for 20-30 minutes and 16 cases in which colic pain was relieved after needling for 30-40 minutes. But, there were still 21 cases in which renal colic appeared again on that day, however, the colic pain was checked after repeated needling. So the effective rate in relieving pain reached 100 percent.

Lithagogue rate: There were 9 lithagogue cases after treatments for 3 days, 31 cases for 7 days, 37 cases for 8-14 days, and 11 cases for 21 days. The total lithagogue rate was 74 percent, with an average of 16.4 days.

(*Source:* Chinese Acupuncture & Moxibustion, (4):9, 1987)

2. Observed results of pressing ear points in the treatment of 41 cases of urinary stone

Points: Kidney, Urinary Bladder, Urethra, Ureter, Sanjiao, External Genitalia

Method: Apply vaccaria seeds on the points for pressure five times a day, 30 minutes in a session. Change the seeds after three days' application. Twenty minutes before the treatment, encourage the

196

patient to drink 250-500 ml of water and increase exercises so as to promote passing stones.

Results: There were 21 lithagogue cases. Among 41 cases, 11 cases were cured, marked effect was seen in 10 cases, improvement (the stone lowered 2-5 cm from the original place) in 8 cases, and no effect in 12 cases.

(*Source:* Journal of Traditional Chinese Medicine and Chinese Medica Materia of Jilin, (4):15, 1986)

70. Prostatitis

Principal points: a) Guanyuan (Ren 4), Sanyinjiao (Sp. 6); b) Qugu (Ren 2), Yinlingquan (Sp. 9)

Method: Use filiform needles with moderate stimulation and even movement method. Apply deep insertion on the abdomen to cause the needling sensation to extend slowly to the urethra. Retain the needles for 20-30 minutes with periodic manipulation, once every 10 minutes. Treat daily or once every other day. Ten treatments constitute one course. The above two groups can be used in rotation.

Supplementary points:

Fever: Dazhui (Du 14), Quchi (L.I. 11)

Urethral pain: Shuidao (St. 28)

Hemourine: Xuehai (Sp. 10), Yinbai (Sp. 1)

Bearing down sensation and distention pain in the lower abdomen or perineum: Dadun (Liv. 1), Ligou (Liv. 5)

Lower back pain: Zhishi (U.B. 52)

Seminal emission, impotence, or spermatorrhea: Guilai (St. 29). Puncture with reinforcing method, and combine moxibustion.

Difficult urination: Zhongji (Ren 3), Ciliao (U.B. 32)

Lassitude: Zusanli (St. 36), Gongsun (Sp. 4)

Deficient *yang* of the kidney: Mingmen (Du 4), Taixi (K. 3). Puncture with reinforcing method, and combine moxibustion.

Other therapies:

1. Ear acupuncture

Points: Prostate, Kidney, Intertragicus, Brain, End of Inferior Helix Crus

Method: Use filiform needles with moderate stimulation. Retain the needles for 20-30 minutes. Treat daily. Embedding needles can also

197

be used.

2. Laser acupuncture

Point: Huiyin (Ren 1)

Method: The patient is in supine position with the knees flexed. Expose Huiyin (Ren 1) on the perineum to the light given by the He-Ne laser machine. Treat daily for 5-10 minutes. Ten treatments constitute one course.

3. Cutaneous acupuncture

Points: Sanyinjiao (Sp. 6), Ququan (Liv. 8), Guanyuan (Ren 4), Qugu (Ren 2), Shuidao (St. 28), Jiaji points (Extra, from the 14th-21st vertebrae)

Method: Use cutaneous needles to tap the points gently until the local skin becomes congested. Treat once every other day. Ten treatments constitute one course. This method is applicable in the treatment of chronic prostatitis.

Remarks: Acupuncture and moxibustion therapies are quite effective in the treatment of prostatitis. With severe cases of acute prostatitis, other methods of treatment should be used.

REFERENCES:

1. Observed results of acupuncture in the treatment 80 cases of chronic prostatitis

Points: a) Guanyuan (Ren 4), Zhongji (Ren 3), Yinlingquan (Sp. 9), Sanyinjiao (Sp. 6); b) Huiyin (Ren 1), Shenshu (U.B. 23)

Method: Puncture 2 groups of points with reducing method. The needles are not retained. When needling Huiyin (Ren 1), insert a gauge No. 26 or No. 28 filiform needle, 3-4 *cun* in length, to a depth of 2-3 *cun*, until the patient feels soreness and a distention sensation around the perineum. Withdraw the needle after lifting and thrusting 3-5 times. Puncture Shenshu (U.B. 23) with a gauge No. 28 needle, 2 *cun* in length. Insert the tip of the needle towards the spine to a depth of 1 *cun*. Withdraw the needle until the local portion has soreness and a distention sensation. Treat daily or once every other day. Ten treatments constitute one course.

Results: Of 80 cases treated, 32 cases were cured, marked effect was evident in 17 cases, improvement in 15 cases, and no effect in 16 cases.

(*Source:* Chinese Acupuncture & Moxibustion, (2):19, 1987)

2. Observed results of needling the extra point in the treatment of

30 cases of chronic prostatitis

Point: Qianlixian (Extra, at the middle point between Huiyin, Ren 1, and the anus)

Method: Insert a gauge No. 28 needle to a depth of 1.5-2 *cun*. After the needling sensation is obtained, rotate the needle 2-3 times with small amplitude. Retain the needle for 20 minutes. Treat daily. Ten treatments constitute one course.

Results: Of 30 cases treated, 9 cases were cured, marked effect was evident in 15 cases, improvement in 3 cases, and no effect in 3 cases.

(*Source:* Zhejiang Journal of Traditional Chinese Medicine, 23(6):280, 1988)

71. Orchitis, Epididymitis

Principal points: Guanyuan (Ren 4), Sanyinjiao (Sp. 6), Guilai (St. 29)

Method: Empty the urinary bladder before puncturing the points on the abdomen with moderate stimulation. Retain the needles for 20-30 minutes. Treat daily. Ten treatments constitute one course.

Supplementary points:

Coldness and pain in the scrotum: Dadun (Liv. 1), Qugu (Ren 2), combined with moxibustion

Distention and pain in the swollen scrotum: Taichong (Liv. 3)

Chills and fever: Dazhui (Du 14), Quchi (L.I. 11)

Other therapies:

Ear acupuncture

Points: Liver, External Genitalia, Testis, Lower Apex of Tragus, Shenmen, Brain

Method: Choose 3-5 points in a session. Puncture with strong stimulation. Retain the needles for 20-30 minutes. Treat daily. Use ear points in rotation. Ten treatments constitute one course.

Remarks: Acupuncture and moxibustion are quite effective in the treatment of this illness. Proper rest should be ensured at its acute stage.

REFERENCES:

1. Observed results of applying a moxa cone at Yangchi (S.J. 4)

in the treatment of 204 cases of acute orchitis

Points and method: Place a moxa cone the size of a green bean at Yangchi (S.J. 4) for moxibustion. Use three cones in a session. Treat daily. Continue treatment for one week. There is no need to use other medication. If a high fever is present, fluids should be infused.

Results: All the cases were cured. The therapeutic result can be obtained from 10 hours to 7 days.

(*Source:* Journal of Traditional Chinese Medicine, 24(8):51, 1983)

2. Therapeutic result observation on suspended moxibustion in treating 84 cases of epididymitis

Principal points: Ashi point (on the swollen epididymis), Qihai (Ren 6), Xuehai (Sp. 10)

Supplementary points:

Qi stagnation with distention and pain: Shanzhong (Ren 17)

Blood stagnation with stabbing pain: Geshu (U.B. 17)

Deficient *qi* with bearing-down distention: Bilateral Zusanli (St. 36)

Yang deficiency with pain relieved by warmth: Guanyuan (Ren 4), Shenshu (U.B. 23)

Method: Treat once or twice a day. Ten treatments constitute one course. Three courses are needed.

Results: Of 84 cases treated, 46 cases were cured, 20 cases were nearly cured, marked effect was seen in 6 cases, improvement was seen in 5 cases, and no effect was evident in 7 cases. The total effective rate reached 91.7 percent.

(*Source:* Journal of Traditional Chinese Medicine, 26(12):39, 1985)

72. Nephritis

I. Acute nephritis

Principal points: Feishu (U.B. 13), Lieque (Lu. 7), Hegu (L.I. 4), Shuifen (Ren 9)

Method: Utilize filiform needles to produce moderate stimulation by means of reducing method and then retain the needles for 15-20 minutes. Treat daily and 10 times constitute one course.

Supplementary points:

Facial edema: Renzhong (Du 26)

Oliguria: Guanyuan (Ren 4), Qugu (Ren 2), Yinlingquan (Sp. 9), Sanyinjiao (Sp. 6)

Hematuria: Xuehai (Sp. 10)

Hypertension: Taichong (Liv. 3)

II. Chronic nephritis

Principal points: Pishu (U.B. 20), Shenshu (U.B. 23), Zusanli (St. 36), Shuifen (Ren 9)

Method: Utilize filiform needles to produce mild or moderate stimulation by means of reinforcing or even method, and then retained the needles for 20-30 minutes. Treat daily and 10 treatments constitute one course.

Supplementary points:

Edema with oliguria: Yinlingquan (Sp. 9), Sanyinjiao (Sp. 6)

Abdominal pain with loose stool: Tianshu (St. 25)

Hypertension: Hegu (L.I. 4), Taichong (Liv. 3)

Palpitation with insomnia: Shenmen (H. 7), Neiguan (P. 6)

Cough and asthma unable to lie horizontally: Chize (Lu. 5) with reducing method

Anuria: Qugu (Ren 2) with reducing method, and moxi Zhishi (U.B. 52)

Deficiency of both spleen and kidney: Qihai (Ren 6) with reinforcing method, the same as Pishu (U.B. 20), Shenshu (U.B. 23) and Zusanli (St. 36), with warm-needle moxibustion or suspending moxibustion by moxa sticks after the needling

Other therapies:

Ear acupuncture

Points: Kidney, Urinary Bladder, Lower Apex of Tragus, Intertragicus, Shenmen, Spleen

Method: Perform moderate stimulation with filiform needles which are retained for 20-30 minutes. Treat daily.

Remarks: Acupuncture therapy has certain effect in treating acute and chronic nephritises.

73. Impotence

Principal points: Shenshu (U.B. 23), Mingmen (Du 4), Qugu (Ren 2), Guanyuan (Ren 4), Sanyinjiao (Sp. 6), Yaoyangguan (Du 3)

Method: Puncture with moderate stimulation. Retain the needles for 15-20 minutes. Combine moxibustion after needling. Treat daily or once every other day.

Supplementary points:

Deficiency of the heart and spleen: Xinshu (U.B. 15), Shenmen (H. 7), moxi Baihui (Du 20) for 3-5 minutes

Flowing downward of damp-heat: Pangguangshu (U.B. 28), Ciliao (U.B. 32)

Other therapies:

1. Electro-acupuncture

Points: a) Baliao (U.B. 31-34), Rangu (K. 2); b) Guanyuan (Ren 4), Sanyinjiao (Sp. 6)

Method: Use the two groups of points in turn, and connect to the pulse current stimulator with low frequency for 3-5 minutes.

2. Hydro-acupuncture

Points: Guanyuan (Ren 4), Zhongji (Ren 3), Shenshu (U.B. 23)

Method: Inject 50 mg of Vitamin B_1 solution or 5 mg of testosterone propionate into the points. Treat once every 2-3 days. Four treatments constitute one course. Rotate solutions between treatments.

3. Ear acupuncture

Points: External Genitalia, Testis, Intertragicus, Brain, Shenmen

Method: Choose 2-3 points in a session. Puncture with moderate stimulation. Retain the needles for 5-15 minutes. Treat daily or once every other day. Ten treatments constitute one course.

Remarks: Acupuncture and moxibustion are of certain effect on the treatment of impotence. Sexual activity should not be advisable during treatments.

REFERENCE:

Observed results of using needle-embedding at Sanyinjiao (Sp. 6) in the treatment of 31 cases of impotence

Points: Bilateral Sanyinjiao (Sp. 6)

Method: While pressing Huiyin (Ren 1) with a finger of the left hand, insert the needle-embedding upward into Sanyinjiao (Sp. 6). After the needling sensation is obtained, fix the needle with adhesive tape for three days. Then instruct the patient to rest for three days after withdrawal of the needle.

Results: Of the 31 cases treated, 28 cases were cured, no effect in 3 cases.

(*Source:* Chinese Acupuncture & Moxibustion, (2):10, 1984)

202

74. Spermatorrhea

Principal points: Shenshu (U.B. 23), Guanyuan (Ren 4), Sanyinjiao (Sp. 6)

Method: Puncture with moderate stimulation. Treat daily or once every other day, or apply pulse current stimulator with low frequency to the above-mentioned points.

Supplementary points:

Accompanied by dreaming: Xinshu (U.B. 15), Shenmen (H. 7), Neiguan (P. 6)

Involuntary seminal emission: Zhishi (U.B. 52), Taixi (K. 3), Zusanli (St. 36), combined with moxibustion

Other therapies:

1. Cutaneous acupuncture

Points and method: Tap points along the Du and urinary bladder meridians on the lumbar sacral region, and points on the medial aspect of the lower limbs until the skin becomes reddish in color. Treat for 15 minutes, daily or once every other day.

2. Hydro-acupuncture

Points: Guanyuan (Ren 4), Zhongji (Ren 3)

Method: Insert the needle and let the needling sensation extend to the perineum (or penis), then inject 0.5-1.0 ml of Vitamin B_1 solution into each point. Treat once every other day. Ten treatments constitute one course.

3. Ear acupuncture

Points: Seminal Vesicle, Intertragicus, Liver, Kidney

Method: Choose 2-4 points in a session. Retain the needles for 10-30 minutes. Treat daily or once every other day, or embed the needles for 3-5 days.

4. Wrist-and-ankle acupuncture

Points: Lower 1, bilateral

Method: The routine procedure in wrist-and-ankle acupuncture.

REFERENCES:

1. Observed effectiveness of puncturing Huiyin (Ren 1) in the treatment of spermatorrhea and impotence

Point: Huiyin (Ren 1)

Method: Deeply puncture to a depth of 2 *cun* or more, and let the needling sensation of soreness and distention extend to the whole lower abdomen and further to the penis. This can obtain a very good therapeutic result. Retain the needle for half an hour.

Results: Of 9 cases treated, 8 cases were cured or showed marked effect. No effect (due to traumatic injury) was evident in 1 case.

(Source: Harbin Traditional Chinese Medicine, 7(4):27, 1964)

2. Observed results of acupuncture in the treatment of 212 cases of male sexual disfunction

Points: Qugu (Ren 2), Ciliao (U.B. 32), Yinlian (Liv. 11), moxi Dadun (Liv. 1), Shenque (Ren 8)

Supplementary points: Zusanli (St. 36), Neiguan (P. 6)

Method: Treat once every 2-3 days. Ten treatments constitute one course. Begin another course after 5-7 days' rest. To the patient whose response to the needling is dull, treat daily for the first three treatments. Sexual activity is not advisable in the first treating course.

Results: Of 212 cases treated, 161 cases were cured, marked effect was seen in 14 cases, improvement in 8 cases, and no effect in 29 cases. The total effective rate reached 86.3 percent.

(Source: Shanghai Journal of Acupuncture and Moxibustion, (3):4, 1985)

75. Male Infertility

Principal points: Guanyuan (Ren 4), Shenshu (U.B. 23), Mingmen (Du 4), Sanyinjiao (Sp. 6)

Method: Puncture with reinforcing method. Insert at Guanyuan (Ren 4) to a depth of 2 *cun*, and let the needling sensation extend to the penis or the perineum. Apply moderate stimulation to the points. Retain the needles for 20-30 minutes. Use moxibustion with moxa sticks after needling. Treat daily or once every other day. Ten treatments constitute one course.

Supplementary points: Zusanli (St. 36), Qihai (Ren 6), Zhishi (U.B. 52), Zhongji (Ren 3), Taixi (K. 3)

Other therapies:

1. Ear acupuncture

Points: External Genitalia, Testis, Brain, Intertragicus, Shenmen, Kidney

Method: Select 2-3 points in a session. Use filiform needles with moderate stimulation. Retain the needles for 20-30 minutes. Treat daily or once every other day. Ten treatments constitute one course.

2. Hydro-acupuncture

Points: Guanyuan (Ren 4), Shenshu (U.B. 23), Sanyinjiao (Sp. 6)

Method: According to the routine procedure, inject 0.5 ml of Vitamin B_1 solution into each point. Treat once every other day. Five treatments constitute one course.

Remarks: Male infertility is a stubborn disease. At present there is no effective therapy, but acupuncture and moxibustion are of certain effect to the treatment of the illness.

REFERENCES:

1. Observed results of indirect moxibustion with ginger in the treatment of 63 cases of azoospermia

Points: a) Dahe (K. 12), Qugu (Ren 2), Sanyinjiao (Sp. 6), Guanyuan (Ren 4), Zhongji (Ren 3), Shuidao (St. 28) or Guilai (St. 29); b) Baliao (U.B. 31, 32, 33, 34), Mingmen (Du 4), Shenshu (U.B. 23)

Method: Use the two groups of points in turn. Puncture gently with reinforcing method. Then apply indirect moxibustion with ginger or three moxa cones for the treatment.

Results: Among 63 cases, 52 cases were cured, improvement was evident in 9 cases, and no effect was seen in 2 cases.

(*Source:* Fujian Journal of Medicine and Medica Materia, 2(5):19, 1980)

2. Observed results of acupuncture and moxibustion in the treatment of 110 cases of absence of ejaculation

Principal points: Qugu (Ren 2), Yinlian (Liv. 11), Dadun (Liv. 1)

Supplementary points:

Weakness, poor appetite, irregular bowel movement: Zusanli (St. 36)

Insomnia: Baihui (Du 20), Neiguan (P. 6)

Impotence: Ciliao (U.B. 32), moxi Shenque (Ren 8)

Method: Treat once every 2-3 days. Ten treatments constitute one course. Puncture Qugu (Ren 2) and let the electro-stroke sensation extend to the urethra, apply strong stimulation to Yinlian (Liv. 11), and try to produce the sensation of distention and soreness. Apply moxibustion to Dadun (Liv. 1) for five minutes.

Results: Of 110 cases treated, normal ejaculation was obtained in 94 cases, 85.5 percent, with an average of 16 treatments. No effect was evident after 5 courses' treatment in 16 cases, 14.5 percent.

(*Source:* Journal of Traditional Chinese Medicine, 25(4):60, 1984)

76. Irregular Menstruation

Principal points: Guanyuan (Ren 4), Sanyinjiao (Sp. 6)

Method: Treat daily or once every other day, during the time when the woman is not menstruating. Manipulate the needles with moderate stimulation. Retain the needles for 20-30 minutes. If it is hypomenorrhea or menorrhagia, in the next treatment points can be needled during menstruation.

Supplementary points:

Qi stagnation and blood stasis: Taichong (Liv. 3), Ligou (Liv. 5), Shanzhong (Ren 17), Xuehai (Sp. 10), Hegu (L.I. 4)

Deficiency and cold in the lower *jiao*: Mingmen (Du 4), Shenshu (U.B. 23), Taixi (K. 3), combined with moxibustion

Deficient *qi* and blood: Zusanli (St. 36), Pishu (U.B. 20), Qihai (Ren 6), Ganshu (U.B. 18), Geshu (U.B. 17)

Heat in the blood: Taichong (Liv. 3), Xuehai (Sp. 10), Yinbai (Sp. 1)

Other therapies:

1. Ear acupuncture

Points: Uterus, Ovary, Intertragicus, Kidney, Liver

Method: Treat once every other day. Select 2-3 points for a treatment. Puncture with moderate stimulation. Retain the needles for 20-30 minutes, or simply embed.

2. Hydro-acupuncture

Points: Guanyuan (Ren 4), Pishu (U.B. 20), Shenshu (U.B. 23), Zusanli (St. 36), Sanyinjiao (Sp. 6), Tianshu (St. 25)

Method: Select 3-4 points for a treatment. Inject 0.5-1 ml of placenta liquid medicine into each point. Treat once every other day. Ten treatments constitute one course.

Remarks: Acupuncture therapy is quite effective in treating irregular menstruation. In general, 2-3 courses are needed for the treatment.

77. Dysmenorrhea

Principal points: Sanyinjiao (Sp. 6), Zhongji (Ren 3), Diji (Sp. 8), Taichong (Liv. 3)

Method: Start treatment 3-5 days prior to menstruation. Treat once every day. Retain the needles for 30-60 minutes with 2-3 periodic manipulations. If the pain is severe, puncture Sanyinjiao (Sp. 6) with strong stimulation for 20 minutes as well as periodic manipulations until the pain is lessened or alleviated.

Supplementary points:

Qi stagnation and blood stasis: Xuehai (Sp. 10), Qihai (Ren 6)

Stagnate coldness and dampness: Shenshu (U.B. 23), Ciliao (U.B. 32), Mingmen (Du 4). Warm needle or moxibustion can be used in combination.

Deficient *qi* and blood: Zusanli (St. 36), Geshu (U.B. 17), Pishu (U.B. 20), Qihai (Ren 6), Weishu (U.B. 21), combined with moxibustion

Other therapies:

1. Electro-acupuncture

Points: Guanyuan (Ren 4), Sanyinjiao (Sp. 6), Guilai (St. 29), Taichong (Liv. 3)

Method: Choose and connect two points, one on the body, the other on the lower limb. It is suitable to use a moderate frequency current with either dense or sparse-dense pulsation. When pain exists, apply 1-2 treatments daily with the current lasting 20-30 minutes.

2. Ear acupuncture

Points: Uterus, Intertragicus, End of Inferior Helix Crus, Kidney

Method: After routine sterilization, swiftly insert a filiform needle deeply and rotate for several minutes. Retain the needles for 20-30 minutes. Begin treatment three days prior to menstruation. Treat once every day until the flow has stopped. Or use needle-embedding or seed-embedding method. Ask the patient to press the embedded needles or seeds 2-3 times a day.

3. Moxibustion

Points: Guanyuan (Ren 4), Qugu (Ren 2), Sanyinjiao (Sp. 6), or Ashi points

Method: One or two days prior to menstruation, use a moxa stick to warm the points for 15-30 minutes until the patient is feeling comfortable. Treat 1-2 times a day.

4. Hydro-acupuncture.

Points and method: Inject 1 ml of 1% procaine solution subcutaneously at Shangliao (U.B. 31), and Ciliao (U.B. 32), following the routine procedure, once a day.

Remarks: The above-mentioned therapies are quite effective in alleviating pain. In cases of primary dysmenorrhea, manifestations in the majority patients will disappear after continuous treatments covering 2-4 menstruation circles. The patient should keep warm during the menstrual period and avoid eating raw or cold foods.

REFERENCES:

1. Observed results of ear acupuncture in the treatment of 30 cases of the primary dysmenorrhea

Points: Uterus, Intertragicus, Brain, End of Inferior Helix Crus

Method: Retain the needles for 15-30 minutes with 1-2 periodic manipulations, and 3-5 treatments constitute a course.

Results: Of 30 cases treated, marked effect was evident in 21 cases, and improvement was seen in 9 cases.

(*Source:* The Intermediate Medical Journal, (7):30, 1981)

2. Observed results of ear pressure in the treatment of 30 cases of dysmenorrhea

Principal points: Uterus, Liver, Gall Bladder, Kidney, Abdomen, Intertragicus, Lower Apex of Tragus, Lowering Blood Pressure Groove, Vagus Root

Supplementary points:

Vomiting: Stomach

Restlessness: Shenmen, Heart

Method: Secure vaccaria seeds at the above-mentioned points with adhesive tapes. Instruct the patient to press them more than 10 times each day.

Results: The pain disappeared in half a day in 18 cases. The pain stopped in a day in 7 cases. The pain was reduced in 4 cases, and no effect was evident in 1 case.

(*Source:* Hubei Journal of Traditional Chinese Medicine, (6):44, 1986)

3. Therapeutic result observation on acupuncture in the treatment of 49 cases of dysmenorrhea

1) Stagnated cold and blood stasis

Points: Qihai (Ren 6), Guilai (St. 29), Xuehai (Sp. 10), Ciliao

208

(U.B. 32), Sanyinjiao (Sp. 6), Shenshu (U.B. 23)

Method: Puncture with even movement method. Retain the needles for 30 minutes. Manipulate periodically once every five minutes. When the needles are withdrawn, add a moxa stick until the skin becomes reddish.

2) *Qi* stagnation in the liver

Points: Ciliao (U.B. 32), Tianshu (St. 25), Neiguan (P. 6), Diji (Sp. 8), Taichong (Liv. 3)

Method: Retain the needles for 30 minutes. Manipulate periodically once every 3-5 minutes.

3) Cold and deficient *qi* and blood

Points: Qihai (Ren 6), Guilai (St. 29), Shenshu (U.B. 23), Zhourong (Sp. 20), Xuehai (Sp. 10), Zusanli (St. 36), Sanyinjiao (Sp. 6)

Method: Use reinforcing method, while applying moxibustion to Qihai (Ren 6), Zusanli (St. 36), and Sanyinjiao (Sp. 6). Retain the needles for 20 minutes. Manipulate periodically once every five minutes. Generally speaking, begin treatment 7-10 days prior to menstruation, and treat once every other day until the flow has stopped.

Results: Of 49 cases treated, 42 were completely cured, remarkable effect was seen in 6 cases, and no effect in 1 case. The average number of treatments was 10.5.

(*Source:* Journal of Traditional Chinese Medicine, 24(8):8, 1983)

4. Observation of indirect moxibustion in the treatment of dysmenorrhea

Point: Zhongji (Ren 3)

Method: Place a moxa cone 1 cm in diameter on a slice of aconite at the point. After the cone was burned completely, renew cones until a 5-cm area of skin is redded. Apply a salve over the area. After a few hours blisters will appear. Let blisters be absorbed. This method is quite effective in treating deficient and cold type of dysmenorrhea.

(*Source:* Journal of Traditional Chinese Medicine, 6(12):36, 1985)

5. Observed results of plum-blossom needle in the treatment of 106 cases of dysmenorrhea

Points: Xingjian (Liv. 2), Yinbai (Sp. 1), Gongsun (Sp. 4), Taichong (Liv. 3), Sanyinjiao (Sp. 6), Guanyuan (Ren 4)

Method: Tap 70-90 times per minute. Treat once a day and 3 days prior to menstruation. During menstruation, ask the patient to avoid raw and cold foods.

Results: Full recovery was obtained in 30 cases, a remarkable effect was evident in 39 cases, improvement has seen in 25 cases and no effect was seen in 12 cases.

(*Source:* Journal of Traditional Chinese Medicine, (4):26, 1987)

6. Observed results of needling Sanyinjiao (Sp. 6) in the treatment of 50 cases of dysmenorrhea

Points: Sanyinjiao (Sp. 6), bilateral

Method: Insert the needles to a depth of 2-3 *cun*, with strong stimulation. Retain the needles for 20-30 minutes. Treat 2-5 days prior to menstruation and continue until the flow has stopped.

Results: Of 50 cases treated, during two menstruation periods manifestations disappeared in 38 cases.

(*Source:* Tianjin Medical Journal, 83(1), 1978)

78. Amenorrhea

Principal points: Sanyinjiao (Sp. 6), Guanyuan (Ren 4), Guilai (St. 29), Xuehai (Sp. 10)

Method: Apply moderate stimulation with filiform needles at the points. Retain the needles for 20-30 minutes with periodic manipulation. Treat daily or once every other day. Ten treatments constitute one course. Start another course after 3-5 days' rest.

Supplementary points:

1. Deficiency of *qi* and blood: Pishu (U.B. 20), Ganshu (U.B. 18), Zusanli (St. 36), Qihai (Ren 6)

2. *Qi* stagnation and blood stasis: Taichong (Liv. 3), Hegu (L.I. 4), Zhongji (Ren 3), Ciliao (U.B. 32), Dachangshu (U.B. 25)

3. Stagnated coldness and dampness: Mingmen (Du 4), Yaoyangguan (Du 3); combined with moxibustion

4. Palpitation: Neiguan (P. 6)

5. Fullness and distention in the chest and hypochondriac region, nipples, and lower abdomen: Qimen (Liv. 14), Zhigou (S.J. 6), Yanglingquan (G.B. 34)

Other therapies:

1. Cutaneous acupuncture

Points: Portions along the urinary bladder meridians and the Du meridian of the lumbar sacral region

Method: Apply moderate or gentle tapping with a plum-blossom needle at the area until the local skin exhibits redness. Treat once every other day.

2. Ear acupuncture

Points: Uterus, Intertragicus, Ovary, Shenmen, Brain, Liver, Spleen, Kidney

Method: Needle 3-4 points with moderate stimulation. Retain the needles for 30 minutes with periodic manipulation. Treat once every other day. Or use needle-embedding or seed-embedding method. Require the patient to press them three times a day.

3. Electro-acupuncture

Points: Tianshu (St. 25), Guilai (St. 29), Sanyinjiao (Sp. 6), Xuehai (Sp. 10)

Method: Select one point on the trunk and another on the lower limb and connect to an electro-stimulator. Use moderate frequency current with dense pulsation for 10-15 minutes. Treat once every other day.

Remarks: In general, acupuncture is quite effective in treating amenorrhea. However, with cases of secondary amenorrhea, the physician must be careful to determine the underlying cause and treat accordingly. Otherwise, poor therapeutic results can be expected.

79. Functional Uterine Bleeding

Principal points: Guanyuan (Ren 4), Sanyinjiao (Sp. 6), Yinbai (Sp. 1)

Method: Apply moderate stimulation with filiform needles at Guanyuan (Ren 4) and Sanyinjiao (Sp. 6). Retain the needles for 20-30 minutes with periodic manipulation. Moxi Yinbai (Sp. 1) with 5-7 moxa cones or use a moxa stick for 15-20 minutes. Treat once every day. Six treatments makes a course. With cases of excessive bleeding, moxi Yinbai (Sp. 1) with only one moxa stick during each treatment, but treat 3-4 times a day.

Supplementary points:

Heat in the blood: Dadun (Liv. 1) pricking blood out, Xuehai (Sp. 10), Quchi (L.I. 11)

Blood stasis: Taichong (Liv. 3), Diji (Sp. 8)

Qi stagnation: Taichong (Liv. 3), Zhigou (S.J. 6)

Yang and *qi* deficiency: Qihai (Ren 6), Zusanli (St. 36), Pishu (U.B. 20), Shenshu (U.B. 23), Mingmen (Du 4); combined with moxibustion

Other therapies:

1. Ear acupuncture

Points: Uterus, Intertragicus, Ovary, Liver, Kidney, Shenmen

Method: Select 3-4 points each session. Puncture with moderate stimulation. Retain the needles for 15-20 minutes. Start treatment three days prior to menstruation. Treat once every day. Points on opposite ear can be needled in turn. Or use needle-embedding or seed-embedding method. Ask the patient to press them 3-4 times a day.

2. Electro-acupuncture

Points: Guanyuan (Ren 4) in combination with Sanyinjiao (Sp. 6), Guilai (St. 29) in combination with Xuehai (Sp. 10)

Method: Select a pair of points and connect an electro-stimulator for a treatment. Use moderate or strong frequency current with dense pulsation for 20 minutes. Treat once or twice a day.

3. Head acupuncture

Points: Reproduction Area, bilateral

Method: Insert the needles 1.5 *cun* in length horizontally to the scalp. Rapidly twirl and rotate the needles on bilateral points continuously for 3-5 minutes. Retain the needles for 5 minutes, then twirl again for 3-5 minutes. Manipulate periodically 2-3 times. Or use electro-acupuncture with strong frequency current and dense pulsation for 20 minutes. Treat once every other day.

Remarks: Acupuncture therapy has an excellent effect in the treatment of this illness. If massive uterine bleeding in severe condition is present, other medication should be taken into consideration so as to avoid delaying effective treatment.

REFERENCE:

Observed results of a moxa stick applied to the treatment of functional uterine bleeding

Points : Yinbai (Sp. 1), Sanyinjiao (Sp. 6), Xuehai (Sp. 10), Guanyuan (Ren 4), Yamen (Du 15), Baihui (Du 20)

Method: Apply a moxa stick to each point for five minutes. Procedure starts from points on the lower part of the body progressing to points on the upper part of the body.

Results: The illness was completely cured after 1-4 treatments.

(*Source:* Guangxi Journal of Bare-footed Doctors, (3):32, 1976)

80. Leukorrhea

Principal points: Daimai (G.B. 26), Sanyinjiao (Sp. 6), Zhongji (Ren 3), Ciliao (U.B. 32)

Method: Use filiform needle with moderate stimulation. Retain the needles for 15-20 minutes. Moxibustion can be combined. Treat daily. Ten treatments constitute one course.

Supplementary points:

Dampness and deficiency of the spleen: Zusanli (St. 36), Pishu (U.B. 20); combined with moxibustion

Downward flowing of damp-heat: Yinlingquan (Sp. 9), Xingjian (Liv. 2)

Downward flowing of damp-cold: Yinbai (Sp. 1), Shenshu (U.B. 23), Guanyuan (Ren 4), Zusanli (St. 36); combined with moxibustion

Itching in the perineum: Ligou (Liv. 5), Taichong (Liv. 3)

Other therapies:

1. Ear acupuncture

Points: Uterus, Urinary Bladder, Intertragicus, Ovary, Liver, Spleen, Kidney

Method: Apply moderate stimulation at 3-4 points during each treatment. Retain the needles for 15-20 minutes. Treat daily or once every other day.

2. Electro-acupuncture

Points: Qihai (Ren 6) in combination with Sanyinjiao (Sp. 6)

Method: Connect electro-current for 5-10 minutes. Use moderate frequency. Treat daily.

Remarks: Acupuncture therapy is effective in treating this disease. If there is a red or yellow discharge, a thorough gynecological examination should be conducted promptly.

REFERENCES:

1. Observed results of acupuncture and moxibustion at Qugu (Ren 2) in the treatment of 30 cases of leukorrhea

Point: Qugu (Ren 2)

Method: Puncture the point 2.5-3 *cun* in depth with straight or slightly slanted insertion towards the perineum. It is better to let needle sensation radiate to the vagina. Retain the needle for an hour with periodic manipulation every 10 minutes. Treat once every three days. Two treatments constitute one course. If it is cold-damp leukorrhea, moxi the point in circle for half an hour with a moxa stick. If it is damp-heat leukorrhea, use acupuncture without moxibustion.

Results: Of 30 cases treated, full recovery was obtained in 27 cases and improved was seen in 3 cases.

(*Source:* Journal of Traditional Chinese Medicine, (5):17, 1987)

2. Observed results of needling and cupping in the treatment of 36 cases of leukorrhea.

Principal point: Ciliao (U.B. 32)

Supplementary points:

Itching in the perineum: Ligou (Liv. 5)

Cold-damp: moxi Mingmen (Du 4)

Damp-heat: Sanyinjiao (Sp. 6)

Method: Use a 2-2.5 *cun* filiform needle with the tip 45 degrees slanted downward to the lower limb. Quick insertion makes the needle sensation extend to the lower abdomen or the front perineum. Apply even movement method to cold-damp pattern. Retain the needles for 30 minutes. Periodically manipulate 2 times. For damp-heat pattern, use reducing method with lifting, thrusting, twirling and rotating. Apply cupping while the needles are in the points. Retain the needles for 15 minutes. Treat daily or once every other day. Seven treatments constitute one course. Begin another course after five days' rest.

Results: Of 36 cases treated, full recovery was obtained in 27 cases, and remarkable effect was evident in 9 cases.

(*Source:* Henan Traditional Chinese Medicine, (6):13, 1985)

81. Morning Sickness

Principal points: Neiguan (P. 6), Zusanli (St. 36), Gongsun (Sp. 4), Zhongwan (Ren 12)

Method: Use filiform needles with moderate stimulation. Retain the needles for 20-30 minutes with 2-3 periodic manipulations. Moxibustion can be also combined. In general, treat once every 1-2 days. With a severe case, it is possible to apply 2 treatments a day.

Supplementary points:

Disharmony between the liver and stomach, vomiting with bitter fluid: Taichong (Liv. 3), Yanglingquan (G.B. 34)

Phlegm and dampness in the middle *jiao*: Fenglong (St. 40), Yinlingquan (Sp. 9)

Fullness and stifling sensation in the chest and epigastric region: Shanzhong (Ren 17), horizontal insertion 0.5 *cun*, Jianli (Ren 11)

Other therapies:

Ear acupuncture

Points: Liver, Stomach, Shenmen, End of Inferior Helix Crus

Method: Use filiform needles with mild stimulation, and retain the needles for 10-25 minutes. Treat once every day. Ten treatments constitute one course. The needle-embedding or seed-embedding method can be used instead. Ask the patient to press them 3-4 times a day.

Remarks: Acupuncture therapy with no side-affect is very effective in the treatment of this disease. It is not advisable to needle many points in a single treatment and manipulation should be mild. In case of severe vomiting with dehydration, other medication should be taken into consideration.

REFERENCE:

Observed results of Vitamin B_1 point injection in the treatment of 124 cases of morning sickness

Points: Bilateral Shenmen of ear point

Method: Inject 0.1 ml of Vitamin B_1 solution into Shenmen by using a gauge No. 4.5 hypodermic needle. In general, one injection is enough, however, if symptom occurs, inject again.

Results: Of 124 cases treated, full recovery was obtained in 119 cases, and improved was evident in 5 cases.

(*Source:* Journal of Traditional Chinese Medicine, (5):53, 1987)

82. Malposition of Fetus

Point: Zhiyin (U.B. 67)

Method: During treatment, ask the patient to loosen her belt and clothes at the waist, and position the patient either sitting on the chair or laying on the bed. Hold a moxa stick about 3 cm above the surface of the point. The thermal stimulation lasts 15-20 minutes each time. Treat once or twice a day. Four treatments constitute one course. It is possible to apply moxa sticks at Zhiyin (U.B. 67) bilaterally, separately or simultaneously.

Remarks: Moxibustion is quite effective in correcting malposition of fetus, especially for second or subsequent pregnancies. Malposition of fetus induced by some organic deformity cannot be treated by this method and it is not advisable to adopt this method to the treatment of habitual abortion or toxemia of pregnancy.

REFERENCES:

1. Observed results of acupuncture and moxibustion applied to Zhiyin (U.B. 67) in treating 246 cases of malposition of fetus

Point: Zhiyin (U.B. 67)

Method: Use a 0.5 *cun* filiform needle to puncture the point to a depth of 0.1-0.2 *cun* with upward slanted insertion. Apply even movement method. The patient will experience a sensation of soreness, numbness, and distention or pain around the point. Retain the needle for 15 minutes. Before treatment, ask the patient to empty her bladder and loose clothing at the waist. After treatment, require her to moxi herself at Zhiyin (U.B. 67) for 10-15 minutes, then go to sleep. Treat once every day. Seven treatments constitute one course.

Results: Of 246 cases treated, full recovery with normal delivery was obtained in 211 cases and no effect was evident in 35 cases.

(*Source:* Henan Traditional Chinese Medicine, (6):12, 1985)

2. Study on direct moxibustion applied to Zhiyin (U.B. 67) in correcting 402 cases of malposition of fetus

Point: Zhiyin (U.B. 67)

Method: The patient is in laying position with knees flexed. Place and burn two cones about 0.04 gram each at Zhiyin (U.B. 67), bilaterally. When they are completely burned, remove ashes and renew cones until small blisters are formed. Then apply salves over the areas to prevent an infection. For pregnancies of less than 35 weeks, treat once a week. Use 5-7 cones in a session. Four treatments constitute one course. For pregnancies of more than 36 weeks, treat twice a week. Nine cones are required for the treatment. Four treatments constitute one course.

Results: Of 402 cases treated, 341 cases were corrected (among them, corrected by moxibustion once: 227 cases; twice: 83 cases; three times: 23 cases; four times: 8 cases). No effect was evident in 61 cases.

(*Source:* Chinese Acupuncture & Moxibustion, (3):17, 1981)

3. Therapeutic result observation on vaccaria seeds on the ear in correcting 169 cases of malposition of fetus

Points: Uterus, End of Inferior Helix Crus, Brain, Liver, Spleen, Abdomen

Method: Apply vaccaria seeds on ears in rotation for 3-4 days. Instruct the patient to press the seeds for about 15 minutes after meals, and press once in half supine position before sleep.

Results: Of 169 cases treated, those which were successful after 1-3 treatments were 138 cases, of which 111 cases received only one treatment. The total success rate was 81.7 percent.

(*Source:* Zhejiang Journal of Traditional Chinese Medicine, 23(2):83, 1988)

83. Inertia of Uterus (Prolonged Labor)

Principal points: Sanyinjiao (Sp. 6), Zhiyin (U.B. 67), Hegu (L.I. 4)

Method: Puncture Sanyinjiao (Sp. 6) and Hegu (L.I. 4) with moderate stimulation. Apply moxibustion at Zhiyin (U.B. 67). Retain the needles for 30-60 minutes with periodic manipulation.

Supplementary points:

Palpitation and shortness of breath: Neiguan (P. 6), Zusanli (St. 36)

Severe abdominal pain: Taichong (Liv. 3)

Other therapies:

1. Ear acupuncture

Points: Uterus, Brain, Intertragicus, Kidney, Urinary Bladder

Method: Use filiform needles with moderate stimulation. Manipulate periodically once every 3-5 minutes until the baby is delivered.

2. Electro-acupuncture

Points: Zusanli (St. 36), Sanyinjiao (Sp. 6), Taixi (K. 3), Taichong (Liv. 3)

Method: Select two points. After you have punctured them and a needling sensation is obtained, connect with the electro-stimulator. Choose either the sparse-dense or the intermittent pulsation. The current duration depends on symptoms.

Remarks:

Acupuncture therapy is quite effective in the treatment of inertia of uterus. It can strengthen the uterus in contraction and promote the normal delivery. But it is not advisable for prolonged labor due to deformity of uterus and contracted pelvis.

As to retention of placenta after childbirth, or subinvolution of uterus with uterine bleeding or lower abdominal dull pain, Zusanli (St. 36), Sanyinjiao (Sp. 6), and Qihai (Ren 6) can be moxied with moxa sticks. The therapeutic result is excellent.

REFERENCES:

1. Observation on acupuncture in the treatment of 30 cases of prolonged labor

Points: Hegu (L.I. 4), Sanyinjiao (Sp. 6)

Method: Apply the combined manipulation of lifting, thrusting twirling and rotating, after insertion and the needling sensation is obtained. Try to let the needling sensation go upward. Then connect with an electro-stimulator. The frequency used depends on the patient's tolerance. Treat twice a day. Retain the needles for two hours. During the first treatment, needles can be withdrawn after the uterus contraction becomes normal.

Results: Normal delivery with normal postpartum uterus contraction right after needling occurred in 2 cases. Normal delivery within 10 minutes occurred in 13 cases, within 11-30 minutes in 11 cases, within 31-60 minutes in 3 cases and within 2 hours in 1 case.

The duration between puncturing and delivery, 2 hours and 55 minutes in 1 case, 5 hours in 1 case, 5-10 hours in 22 cases and 10-15 hours in 6 cases. The amount of vaginal bleeding reached 30-350 ml. Placentas were all delivered within 35 minutes.

(*Source:* Henan Traditional Chinese Medicine, 7(2):22, 1987)

2. Observed results of ear acupuncture in the treatment of 7 cases of prolonged labor

Points: Uterus, Abdomen, Lumbosacral Vertebrae, Brain, End of Inferior Helix Crus

Method: Needle one ear with periodic manipulation once every three minutes until the baby is delivered.

Results: The babies were all delivered within 10-45 minutes.

(*Source:* Journal of Traditional Chinese Medicine, (4):27, 1984)

3. Observed results of acupuncture in the treatment of 2 cases of postpartum placenta retention with massive bleeding

Points: Hegu (L.I. 4), Sanyinjiao (Sp. 6), Dazhong (K. 4)

Method: For case 1, Hegu (L.I. 4), Sanyinjiao (Sp. 6), and Dazhong (K. 4) were punctured bilaterally with strong stimulation. Needles were retained for half an hour with periodic manipulation once every five minutes until the bleeding was checked and placenta deliv-

218

ered. For case 2, the same method was used. The bleeding was reduced but not checked. Then direct moxibustion, about ten moxa cones used, was applied at Dadun (Liv. 1). The bleeding was completely stopped and the placenta was delivered after one hour.

(*Source:* Zhejiang Journal of Traditional Chinese Medicine, 7(10):4, 1964)

84. Insufficient Lactation

Principal points: Shanzhong (Ren 17), Rugen (St. 18), Shaoze (S.I. 1)

Method: Puncture Rugen (St. 18) to a depth of 1 *cun* with its tip upward transverse insertion, and needle Shanzhong (Ren 17) with 0.5-1 *cun* transverse insertion until needling sensation extends to each breast. Apply mild or moderate stimulation to the points. Retain the needles for 30 minutes. Treat daily. Four treatments constitute one course. Mild moxibustion with moxa sticks can be combined.

Supplementary points:

Deficient *qi* and blood: Pishu (U.B. 20), Ganshu (U.B. 18), Zusanli (St. 36); combined with moxibustion

Qi stagnation in the liver: Taichong (Liv. 3), Neiguan (P. 6), Qimen (Liv. 14)

Other therapies:

1. Ear acupuncture

Points: Chest, Intertragicus, End of Inferior Helix Crus, Spleen, Stomach

Method: Use filiform needles with moderate stimulation. Retain the needles for 20 minutes. Treat once every day, or two ears are needled in turn, treating twice a day.

2. Cutaneous acupuncture

Points: From the places 2 *cun* lateral to the third thoracic vertebrae to the places 2 *cun* lateral to the fifth thoracic vertebrae, area around the breasts and intercostal regions

Method: Tap vertically along the two lines lateral to the thoracic vertebrae from the upper part to the lower part. Tap 4-5 times for each line. Then tap 5-7 times along the left and right intercostal spaces. On the breasts, tap from the areola mammae, radiating to the bottom; but apply circular tapping to the areola mammae. Mild stimulation is advisable. Avoid strong stimulation so as not to injure the skin. Treat daily.

3. Hydro-acupuncture

Points: Shanzhong (Ren 17), Rugen (St. 18), Ganshu (U.B. 18), Pishu (U.B. 20), Zusanli (St. 36)

Method: Mix 100 mg of Vitamin B$_1$ into 2 ml of 0.5% procaine. Then inject 0.3-0.5 ml of mixed solution into each point. Inject daily.

Remarks: Acupuncture is relatively effective in the treatment of insufficient lactation at the early stage.

REFERENCES:

1. Observed results of acupuncture in treating 94 cases of insufficient lactation

Points: Ashi points, Shanzhong (Ren 17), Neiguan (P. 6)

Method: Ashi points are mostly located on 3 *cun* superior, or inferior, or lateral to the nipple. In the treatment, slantly insert the tip of the needle 0.5-0.7 *cun* towards the nipple. Do not retain the needles. In a case with deficiency, apply reinforcing method to Shanzhong (Ren 17) and Neiguan (P. 6). In a case with excess syndrome, apply reducing method to Shanzhong (Ren 17) and Neiguan (P. 6). Treat daily.

Results: Of 94 cases treated, 70 cases were completely cured, 17 cases were evidently effective, and 7 cases showed no effect.

(*Source:* Jilin Traditional Chinese Medicine, (6):21, 1985)

2. Observed results of face acupuncture in treating 100 cases of insufficient lactation

Point: Yingruxue (located at the meeting place between 1.1 cm lateral superior to the inner canthus and 1.3 cm inferior to Zanzhu, U.B. 2)

Method: Apply a 15-degree slanted insertion to reach the periosteum. Point the tip of needle to the opposite shoulder.

Results: Of 100 cases treated, some effect was evident in 89 cases, and no effect was evident in 11 cases.

(*Source:* Henan Traditional Chinese Medicine, (3):36, 1981)

3. Observed results of acupuncture in promoting lactation

Point: Lieque (Lu. 7)

Method: Insert horizontally to a depth of 0.3 *cun*. Keep on twirling until the patient experiences the needling sensation.

Results: Generally speaking, lactation could be promoted by one treatment, and the accompanied symptom of distention and pain in the breast should disappear.

(*Source:* Nursing Journal, (3):115, 1978)

85. Delactation

Principal points: Foot-Linqi (G.B. 41), Guangming (G.B. 37)

Method: Use a filiform needle with mild or moderate stimulation. Retain the needles for 15-20 minutes. Apply a moxa stick after needling. Duration of moxibustion to each point is 10 minutes. Treat daily, and 3-5 continuous treatments are needed.

Other therapies:

Cutaneous acupuncture.

Points: Xinshu (U.B. 15), Ganshu (U.B. 18), Shanzhong (Ren 17), Rugen (St. 18)

Method: Apply a plum-blossom needle to tap with moderate stimulation until local mild congestion is formed. Treat daily.

Remarks: Acupuncture is quite effective in the treatment of delactation.

REFERENCE:

Observed results of acupuncture in the treatment of 26 cases of delactation

Points: Zusanli (St. 36), Neiguan (P. 6)

Method: Puncture Zusanli (St. 36), and Neiguan (P. 6) straightly.

Results: In 21 cases, lactation was checked 2-3 days after treatment, and distention and pain in the breast also disappeared. In 3 cases, combined with other medication, a complete cure was obtained. After one needling treatment, 2 cases did not continue further treatment.

(*Source:* Shaanxi Journal of Traditional Chinese Medicine, 2(4):21, 1981)

86. Chronic Pelvic Inflammation

Principal points: Guanyuan (Ren 4), Sanyinjiao (Sp. 6), Shuidao (St. 28)

Method: Ask the patient to empty her bladder before acupuncture treatment. Puncture Guanyuan (Ren 4) and Shuidao (St. 28) to get the needling sensation extending to the perineum. Retain the needles for 30 minutes with 2-3 periodic manipulations. Treat daily or once every other day. Fifteen treatments constitute one course. Begin the next course after rest for 3-5 days.

Supplementary points:

Accumulation of damp-heat: Ciliao (U.B. 32), Yinlingquan (Sp. 9)

Stagnated cold-damp: Guanyuan (Ren 4), Shuidao (St. 28); combined with moxibustion

Stagnated blood: Diji (Sp. 8), Fushe (Sp. 13), Qichong (St. 30). Moxibustion is added to the points on the lower abdomen.

Soreness, heavy sensation and pain in the lumbar region: Shenshu (U.B. 23), Ciliao (U.B. 32), Weizhong (U.B. 40)

Other therapies:

1. Cutaneous acupuncture

Points: Jiaji points (Extra, from L3 to S3), portion on the lower abdomen traveled by meridians of the Ren, kidney, stomach and spleen

Method: Take Jiaji points (Extra, L3-S3) along the lumbo-sacral regions as the main points, and tap with a plum-blossom needle. Choose points on the lower abdomen traveled by the above-mentioned meridians as the supplementary points. Tap with moderate stimulation until the local skin turns red in color. Treat once every other day.

2. Ear acupuncture

Points: Pelvic, Uterus, Lower Apex of Tragus, Ovary, Intertragicus, Liver, Spleen, Kidney

Method: Choose 2-4 points in a session. Use filiform needles with moderate stimulation. Retain the needles for 20-30 minutes and with periodic manipulation. Treat daily or once every other day. The method of needle-embedding and seed-embedding can also be used.

3. Hydro-acupuncture

Points: Weibao (Extra), Guanyuan (Ren 4), Qihai (Ren 6), Pishu (U.B. 20), Shangliao (U.B. 31), Shenshu (U.B. 23), Sanyinjiao (Sp. 6), Zusanli (St. 36)

Method: Select 2-4 points in a treatment. Use 25 mg of Vitamin B$_1$ mixed with normal saline into a 5-ml solution. A 0.5-ml injection is needed for each point. Treat daily.

4. Electro-acupuncture

Points: Weibao (Extra), Guilai (St. 29), Sanyinjiao (Sp. 6), Yinlingquan (Sp. 9)

Method: Pair points on the abdomen with points on the lower limbs, and then connect with the electro-stimulator after the needling sensation is obtained. Use sparse-dense pulsation with a frequency which the patient can tolerate. The current operates for 20-30 minutes in a session. Treat once every other day.

Remarks: Acupuncture has certain effectiveness in the treatment of this illness. Most cases are hard to be cured rapidly. It is better to combine other medication to enhance the therapeutic result.

REFERENCES:

1. Observation on He-Ne laser at acupoints in treating 60 cases of chronic pelvic inflammation

Points:

For deficient *yang* in the spleen and kidney: Zigong (Extra), Xuehai (Sp. 10), Zusanli (St. 36), Sanyinjiao (Sp. 6), all bilateral, Zhongji (Ren 3)

For *qi* stagnation in the liver: Zigong (Extra), Ganshu (U.B. 18), both bilateral, Qihai (Ren 6)

For mass in the abdomen: Zigong (Extra), Shenshu (U.B. 23), Xuehai (Sp. 10), all bilateral, Qihai (Ren 6)

Method: A Model CE-2 He-Ne laser is used with wavelength 6328 Å, output power 3-5 mw, laser diameter 1.5-2 mm, and laser distance 2-5 cm. Irradiate each point for five minutes. Irradiation in a treatment should be less than 20 minutes. Treat daily or once every other day, and 10-15 treatments constitute one course. Begin another course after 7-10 days' rest.

Results: Of 60 cases treated, 21 cases were wholly recovered, marked effect was evident in 20 cases, improvement in 15 cases, and no effect in 4 cases.

(*Source:* Chinese Acupuncture & Moxibustion, 3(1):40, 1983)

2. Observed results of indirect moxibustion with ginger in treating 71 cases of chronic pelvic inflammation

Principal points: Qihai (Ren 6), Zhongji (Ren 3), Guilai (St. 29)

Supplementary points: Dachangshu (U.B. 25), Ciliao (U.B. 32)

Method: Use three moxa cones for the indirect moxibustion with ginger.

Results: Of 71 cases treated, full recovery was obtained in 35 cases, marked effect was evident in 19 cases, improvement was seen in 16 cases and 1 case exhibited no effect.

(*Source:* Journal of Traditional Chinese Medicine, (6):36, 1986)

3. Study on acupuncture in treating 108 cases of chronic cervicitis
Point: Lower 1
Method: Insert to a depth of 1-1.5 *cun*. Retain the needle for half an hour. Treat daily. Ten treatments constitute one course.
Results: Of 108 cases treated, 56 cases (51.9 percent) were completely cured. Positive effect was evident in 32 cases (29.6 percent), and no effect was obtained in 20 cases (18.5 percent). The total effective rate was 81.5 percent.
(*Source:* Journal of Integrated Traditional and Western Medicines, 7(12):753, 1987)

87. Pruritus of Vulva

Principal points: Zhongji (Ren 3), Sanyinjiao (Sp. 6), Xialiao (U.B. 34)
Method: Use filiform needles with moderate stimulation. Retain the needles for 20-30 minutes with periodic manipulation. Treat daily. Ten treatments constitute one course.
Supplementary points:
Severe itching: Qugu (Ren 2), Ququan (Liv. 8)
Trichomonal vaginitis: Ligou (Liv. 5)
Other therapies:
1. Ear acupuncture
Points: Shenmen, Brain, End of Inferior Helix Crus, Intertragicus, External Genitalia, Liver, Spleen, Kidney
Method: Select 2-3 points in a session. Use filiform needles with strong stimulation. Retain the needles for 20-30 minutes. Treat daily. Needle-embedding or seed-embedding method can also be used. Ask the patient to press them 3-4 times a day.
2. Hydro-acupuncture
Points: Qugu (Ren 2), Sanyinjiao (Sp. 6), Yinlian (Liv. 11), Yinjiao (Ren 7), Ciliao (U.B. 32), Xialiao (U.B. 34)
Method: Select one point on the abdomen and one point on the back together with Sanyinjiao (Sp. 6) in a session. Inject 0.2-0.3 ml of 100 μg/ml Vitamin B_{12} solution into each point. Treat once every other day. Ten treatments constitute one course.
Remarks: Acupuncture is quite effective in treating this disease. But the patient is required to keep the local area clean.

REFERENCE:

Observation on acupuncture in treating 56 cases of chronic pruritus of vulva

Points: Qichong (St. 30), Zhongji (Ren 3), Huiyin (Ren 1), Yinlingquan (Sp. 9), Sanyinjiao (Sp. 6), Zhaohai (K. 6), Taichong (Liv. 3)

Method: Use a combination of lifting, thrusting, twirling and rotating with small amplitude, but rapid insertion. No lifting and thrusting at Huiyin (Ren 1). Retain the needles for 30 minutes after the needling sensation is obtained. Treat twice a week. Ten treatments constitute one course.

Results: The number of courses ranged from 1 to 7, but the average was 2 courses. Of 56 cases treated, 29 cases were basically cured, marked effect was evident in 10 cases, improvement in 15 cases and no effect in 2 cases. The total effective rate reached 96.4 percent.

The total number of cases with skin lesions was 39. Among 39 cases, 6 cases fully recovered, marked effect was evident in 6 cases, improvement in 11 cases and no effective in 16 cases. The total effective rate reached 59 percent.

(Source: Chinese Acupuncture & Moxibustion, (3):7, 1985)

88. Prolapsed Uterus

Principal points: Baihui (Du 20), Weibao (Extra), Zigong (Extra), Sanyinjiao (Sp. 6), Qugu (Ren 2)

Method: Needle Baihui (Du 20) in combination with moxibustion, and puncture Weibao (Extra) to a depth of 2 cun in a slanted insertion along the inguinal groove. Let the needle sensation extend to the perineum so the uterus may have a contracting feeling. When needling Zigong (Extra) and Qugu (Ren 2), point tips of needles to the symphysis pubis, and let the needling sensation radiate to the perineum. Retain the needles for 30 minutes with periodic, moderate or strong manipulation. Treat daily or once every other day. Ten treatments constitute one course. Begin another course after 5-7 days' rest.

Supplementary points:

Qi deficiency: Zusanli (St. 36), Qihai (Ren 6), Taixi (K. 3); combined with moxibustion

Damp-heat: Yinlingquan (Sp. 9), Taichong (Liv. 3)

Other therapies:
1. Electro-acupuncture

Points: Weibao (Extra), Zigong (Extra), Guanyuan (Ren 4), Zhongji (Ren 3), Sanyinjiao (Sp. 6), Zusanli (St. 36)

Method: Puncture Weibao (Extra), Zigong (Extra), Guanyuan (Ren 4) and Zhongji (Ren 3), and point the tips of needles to the symphysis pubis, letting the needling sensation extend to the perineum. Use the electro-stimulator for 15-30 minutes with the frequency at 20-30 times per minute and intermittent or sparse-dense pulsation. Treat once every other day. Ten treatments constitute one course. Begin another course after seven days' rest.

2. Ear acupuncture

Points: Uterus, Kidney, Brain, External Genitalia, End of Inferior Helix Crus

Method: Use filiform needles with moderate stimulation. Retain the needles for 20 minutes and apply periodic manipulation. Use current for 15 minutes after connecting the needles with the electro-stimulator. Treat once every other day. Needle-embedding or seed-embedding method can also be used. Ask the patient to press them 3-4 times a day.

3. Head acupuncture

Points: Bilateral Leg Motor and Sensory Area, Reproduction Area

Method: Insert a filiform needle 1.5 *cun* in length horizontally to the scalp. Retain the needles for 20 minutes with twice periodic swift twirling and rotating. Each periodic manipulation lasts 2-3 minutes or connect the needles with the electro-stimulater for 20 minutes. Treat daily or once every other day. Ten treatments constitute one course. Begin another course after rest for 3-5 days.

4. Hydro-acupuncture

Points: Weidao (Extra), Zigong (Extra), Guanyuan (Ren 4), Zusanli (St. 36), Sanyinjiao (Sp. 6), Baliao (U.B. 31-34)

Method: Select 3-4 points for a session. Give a 2 ml of 10% glucose injection at each point. Treat once every other day. Ten treatments constitute one course.

Remarks: Acupuncture therapy is effective in the treatment of mild cases of prolapsed uterus. Before puncturing points on the abdomen, the patient's urinary bladder should be emptied, and the prolapsed uterus must be pushed back into the vagina. After the needles are withdrawn, ask the patient to take a half-hour rest on the bed to enhance the therapeutic result. It is important the patient should have proper rest and avoid heavy work during treatments.

89. Hysteromyoma

Principal points: Zhongji (Ren 3), Guilai (St. 29), Sanyinjiao (Sp. 6), Taichong (Liv. 3), Fenglong (St. 40)

Method: Use filiform needles with moderate stimulation and even movement method. Insert at Zhongji (Ren 3) and Guilai (St. 29) to a depth of 3-4 *cun*. Let the needling sensation extend to the perineum. Treat once every other day. Ten treatments constitute one course.

Supplementary points:

Excessive menses in amount and deep red in color: Xuehai (Sp. 10), Xingjian (Liv. 2)

Excessive menses in amount and light red in color: Qihai (Ren 6), Zusanli (St. 36); combined with moxibustion

Deficiency of the liver and kidney: Ganshu (U.B. 18), Shenshu (U.B. 23), Guanyuan (Ren 4); combined with moxibustion

Other therapies:

Ear acupuncture

Points: Uterus, Ovary, Intertragicus, Kidney

Method: Use filiform needles with moderate stimulation. Retain the needles for 20-30 minutes. Treat daily or once every other day, and 5-10 treatments constitute one course.

Remarks: Acupuncture is certainly effective in the treatment of hysteromyoma.

REFERENCES:

1. Observation on acupuncture in treating 346 cases of hysteromyoma

Points: Zigong (Extra), bilateral, Qugu (Ren 2), Henggu (K. 11)

Method: Puncture Zigong (Extra) to a depth of 0.8-1.0 *cun* with slanted insertion. Puncture Qugu (Ren 2) and Henggu (K. 11) to a depth of 0.6-0.8 *cun* with straight insertion. The above-mentioned points can be used in turn and in combination with points of the back and lower limbs. Urine should be emptied before needling Qugu (Ren 2) and Henggu (K. 11). Pt. Brain can be taken as the supplementary ear point. Generally speaking, use even movement method. Retain the needles for 15-20 minutes after the needling sensation is obtained. Treat once every other day. Ten treatments constitute one course.

Results: The least number of treatments needed was 10, while the most treatments needed was over 40.

The rate of complete cure was 83.2 percent. Those nearly cured accounted for 11.3 percent. The 2/3 belittled rate was 5 percent. The total effective rate reached 100 percent. The following table indicates the curable results:

Size of myoma	Cases	Treatments	Results				
			Cured	Nearly cured	2/3 belittled	No effect	Effective rate (%)
Hen egg size	12	10−11	11	1			100
Duck egg size	85	10−25	82	3			100
Goose egg size	102	10−30	93	6	3		100
Fist size	115	20−40	94	15	6		100
Child's head size	32	20−40	8	14	10		100
Total	346		288	39	19		100

(Source: Acupuncture and Moxibustion of China (1):27, 1986)

2. Observed results of acupuncture in treating 20 cases of hysteromyoma

Main points: Neiguan (P. 6), Zhaohai (K. 6), 3-4 local points around myoma

Secondary points:

Poor constitution: Zusanli (St. 36), Sanyinjiao (Sp. 6)

Soreness in the lumbar region and bearing-down sensation in the lower abdomen: Guanyuan (Ren 4)

Indigestion: Zhongwan (Ren 12), Hegu (L.I. 4), Gongsun (Sp. 4)

Method: Puncture straightly to a depth of 0.6-0.8 *cun* with even method. Retain the needles for 15-30 minutes. Treat once every two days. Seven treatments constitute one course.

Results: A cure (the myoma disappeared, the size of uterus became normal) was obtained in 15 cases, marked effect (the myoma reduced, the size of uterus became normal) was evident in 3 cases and improvement (the myoma reduced to 2/3, the size of uterus was close to the normal) was seen in 2 cases. The treatments ranged from 7 to 40 in number.

228

(*Source:* Shanxi Traditional Chinese Medicine, 4(2):47, 1988)

90. Female Sterility

Principal points: Guanyuan (Ren 4), Sanyinjiao (Sp. 6), Zusanli (St. 36), Zigong (Extra)

Method: Use filiform needles with moderate stimulation, and even method. Retain the needles for 20-30 minutes. Combine moxibustion with moxa sticks. Treat once every other day. Ten treatments constitute one course. Begin another course after seven days' rest.

Supplementary points:

Deficiency and cold in the lower *jiao*: Shenshu (U.B. 23), Zhongji (Ren 3); combined with moxibustion

Deficiency of the liver and kidney: Zhaohai (K. 6), Xuehai (Sp. 10), Ganshu (U.B. 18)

Phlegm-dampness obstructed in the uterus: Yinlingquan (Sp. 9), Fenglong (St. 40), Zhongliao (U.B. 33)

Other therapies:

Ear acupuncture

Points: Uterus, Ovary, Intertragicus, Brain, Kidney

Method: Select 2-3 points in a session. Use filiform needles with moderate stimulation. Retain the needles for 15-30 minutes. Treat daily. Ten treatments constitute a course. Needle-embedding or seed-embedding method can also be used.

Remarks: Acupuncture therapy has certain effectiveness in the treatment of functional sterility.

REFERENCES:

1. Observed results of acupuncture in treating primary sterility

Points: Zhongji (Ren 3), Sanyinjiao (Sp. 6), Dahe (K. 12)

Method: Begin acupuncture 12 days prior to menstruation. Treat once every day with even method. Continue treatments for three days. Retain the needles for 15 minutes.

Results: The total number of cases was 15. All women, whose ages ranged from 24 to 29, were without pregnancies after being married for 2-5 years. After acupuncture treatment over 2-3 menstrual cycles, all had become pregnant.

(*Source:* Jiangxi Journal of Traditional Chinese Medicine, (5):40,

1986)

2. The summary of acupuncture combined with Chinese herbal medicine in treating 50 cases of non-ovulation

Points: Zhongji (Ren 3), Dahe (K. 12), Xuehai (Sp. 10), Sanyinjiao (Sp. 6), Diji (Sp. 8)

Method: Choose 3-4 points in a session. Puncture those points for three continuous days between two menstrual periods. Retain the needles for 20-30 minutes. If irregular menstruation is also a symptom, Chinese herbal medicine can be taken as supplementary medication.

Results: Through the treatment over 1-7 menstrual cycles, pregnancy occurred in 28 cases, ovulation in 17 cases and no effect was evident in 5 cases.

(*Source:* Jiangxi Journal of Traditional Chinese Medicine, (4):33, 1981)

91. Hyperplasia of Mammary Gland

Principal points: Jianjing (G.B. 21), Shanzhong (Ren 17), Zulinqi (G.B. 41), Rugen (St. 18), Wuyi (St. 15)

Method: Produce moderate or strong stimulation with filiform needles and apply the even method. Thrust at Rugen (St. 18) and Wuyi (St. 15) 1-2 *cun* horizontally towards the center of the breast. Retain the needles for 20-30 minutes and manipulate every 10 minutes. Treat daily or once every other day. Ten times constitute one course.

Supplementary points:

Distending pain of the breast: Taichong (Liv. 3)

Irregular menstruation: Sanyinjiao (Sp. 6)

Stuffiness in the chest and irritability: Neiguan (P. 6)

Deficiency of *qi* and blood: Zusanli (St. 36) and Qihai (Ren 6), with reinforced needling and combined with moxibustion

Yin deficiency of liver and kidney: Ganshu (U.B. 18) and Shenshu (U.B. 23), with reinforced needling

Other therapies:

Ear acupuncture

Points: Chest, Intertragicus, Liver, Ovary

Method: Apply moderate stimulation with filiform needles. Retain the needles for 30 minutes. Treat daily. Needle-embedding method can be used.

230

Remarks: There has been no satisfactory method discovered so far to treat the hyperplasia of mammary gland. Acupuncture has certain effect in treating this disease but other therapies should be combined in the treatment.

REFERENCES:

1. Observation on the short-term therapeutic effect and inquiry on the mechanism of acupuncture in treating hyperplasia of mammary gland

Principal points: a) Wuyi (St. 15), Shanzhong (Ren 17), Hegu (L.I. 4); b) Tianzong (S.I. 11), Jianjing (G.B. 21), Ganshu (U.B. 18)

Supplementary points:

Flaring of liver fire: Hegu (L.I. 4) is replaced by Taichong (Liv. 3) and Xiaxi (G.B. 43)

Yin deficiency of liver and kidney: Ganshu (U.B. 18) is replaced by Taixi (K. 3)

Deficiency of *qi* and blood: Ganshu (U.B. 18) and Hegu (L.I. 4) are replaced by Pishu (U.B. 20) and Zusanli (St. 36)

Irregular menstruation: Sanyinjiao (Sp. 6)

Stuffiness in the chest: Waiguan (S.J. 5)

Method: Puncture Wuyi (St. 15) obliquely at an angle of 25 degrees towards the lateral side. Needle Shanzhong (Ren 17) horizontally downward; thrust Jianjing (G.B. 21) horizontally forward; and insert Tianzong (S.I. 11) obliquely downward to the lateral side. The depth of needling in these three points is always 1.5 *cun*. After the arrival of *qi*, retain the needles for 30 minutes during which 2-3 other points can be punctured. Points of the two groups can be alternated. Treat daily and 30 treatments constitute one course. There is a 3-4 days' interval between every two courses and usually 3-4 courses are needed.

Results: There were 500 patients treated. The total effective rate was 94.6 percent.

(*Source:* Journal of Traditional Chinese Medicine, 28(1):47, 1987)

2. Observed results of 32 cases of hyperplasia of the mammary gland treated with microwave acupuncture

Principal points: a) Rugen (St. 18), Yanglingquan (G.B. 34); b) Yingchuang (St. 16), Shanzhong (Ren 17). The two groups can be alternated.

Supplementary points:

Syndrome of stagnation of *qi* and accumulation of phlegm:

Fenglong (St. 40), or Zusanli (St. 36)

Syndrome of stagnation of *qi* and blood: Xuehai (Sp. 10), or Geshu (U.B. 17)

Method: Employ a Model DBJ-1 microwave acupuncture apparatus. At the beginning treat for 20 minutes at each point, and decrease to 15 minutes each when the symptoms were relieved. Treat daily or once every other day. Ten treatments constituted one course, and a 5-7 days' break is necessary after two consecutive courses. Suspend treatment during menstruation.

Results: After 2-5 courses, 10 cases were cured, the lumps and pain all disappeared. Marked effect was evident in 11 cases, the lumps lessened more than half in size and the pain disappeared, or the lumps were resolved and the pain remained, but was alleviated. Some effect was seen in 8 cases, the lumps lessened less than half in size and the pain was alleviated or disappeared, and 3 failed, both the lumps and pain were not distinctly improved.

(*Source:* Shanghai Journal of Acupuncture and Moxibustion, (2):7, 1987)

3. Observed results of 25 cases of masculine hyperplasia of mammary gland treated with moxibustion

Principal points: Ruzhong (St. 17) on the affected side, Zusanli (St. 36) bilateral

Supplementary points:

Syndrome of liver fire: Zusanli (St. 36) is replaced by Taichong (Liv. 3)

Syndrome of *qi* and blood deficiency: Qihai (Ren 6)

Syndrome of *yin* deficiency in liver and kidney: Zusanli (St. 36) is replaced by Taixi (K. 3)

Method: Perform moxibustion with moxa sticks once daily. Ten treatments constitute one course and there is a 3-day interval between 2 courses. During each treatment, syndromes of liver *qi* stagnation and liver-fire flaring are reduced for 20 minutes and syndromes of *qi* and blood deficiency and *yin* deficiency in liver and kidney are reinforced for 40 minutes.

Results: Of 25 cases treated, 13 cases were cured, 6 showed marked effect, 4 were improved and 2 failed.

(*Source:* Shanghai Journal of Acupuncture and Moxibustion, 6(3):30, 1987)

232

92. Acute Mastitis

Principal points: Jianjing (G.B. 21), Rugen (St. 18), Zusanli (St. 36), Shaoze (S.I. 1)

Method: To puncture the points, insert a needle 2 *cun* in length at Jianjing (G.B. 21) subcutaneously towards the acromion to bring on strong sensation. Never thrust Rugen (St. 18) too deep, but 0.5 *cun* transversely upward along the surface of the breast. Provide moderate or strong stimulation at all points, and retain the needles for 30 minutes, manipulating every 5-10 minutes. Treat daily, but 2-3 times a day for severe cases. Moxibustion is applicable on all the points.

Supplementary points:

Fever: Quchi (L.I. 11), Hegu (L.I. 4)

Liver *qi* stagnation: Qimen (Liv. 14), Taichong (Liv. 3), Shanzhong (Ren 17)

Other therapies:

Ear acupuncture

Points: Chest, Intertragicus, Lower Apex of Tragus

Method: Use filiform needles to thrust the points and produce strong stimulation, and then retain the needles for 20-30 minutes. Treat daily.

Remarks: Acupuncture therapy has fair effect in treating acute mastitis which has not become suppurative. The effect will be more satisfactory if medication is incorporated.

REFERENCES:

1. Observed results of 53 cases of acute mastitis treated with acupuncture

Points: Taichong (Liv. 3), Liangqiu (St. 34)

Method: Retain the needles for 25-30 minutes and manipulate 2-4 times. Treat daily.

Results: Of the 53 cases treated, 38 cases were cured with 1 treatment, 13 were cured with 2 treatments and 2 were cured with 3 treatments.

(*Source:* Journal of Traditional Chinese Medicine and Chinese Medica Materia of Jilin, (2):32, 1988)

2. Clinical summary on 1,000 cases of acute mastitis treated with bleeding at acupoints

Points: Mid-mammary type: Gaohuangshu (U.B. 43), Pohu

(U.B. 42), Shentang (U.B. 44)

Supramammary type: Gaohuangshu (U.B. 43), Pohu (U.B. 42), Fufen (U.B. 41)

Submammary type: Gaohuangshu (U.B. 43), Shentang (U.B. 44), Yixi (U.B. 45)

Method: Select the points from the affected side, and bleed with a three-edged needle. Let out three drops of blood from each point, and treat daily. For those with chills and fever, supplement Dazhui (Du 14) and Taodao (Du 13) with the bleeding method.

Results: Of 1,000 cases treated, 970 cases were cured, making up 97 percent; 18 cases (1.8 percent) showed some effectiveness but with the residual of hard lump, and 12 cases (1.2 percent) failed with suppuration.

(*Source:* Chinese Acupuncture & Moxibustion, (3):5, 1981)

3. Observed results of 70 cases of acute mastitis treated with acupuncture at Neiguan (P. 6)

Point: Neiguan (P. 6)

Method: After the arrival of *qi*, manipulate the needle continuously and require the patient to gently press the lump. When the pain is alleviated, retain the needle for 10-15 minutes and manipulate a few times.

Results: Of 70 cases treated, 61 cases were cured with 1 treatment, and 9 were cured with 2 treatments.

(*Source:* Chinese Acupuncture & Moxibustion, (3):8, 1986)

4. Observed results of 79 cases of mastitis treated with acupuncture and massage at Quchi (L.I. 11)

Point: Quchi (L.I. 11)

Method: Insert to a depth of 1.5-2 *cun* at Quchi (L.I. 11), and produce strong stimulation for one minute by rapidly lifting, thrusting and rotating the needle. The most satisfactory results will be gained, if the needling sensation can be propagated up to the shoulder. After removing the needle, hold up the elbow joint of the affected side with your left hand and massage at the point with the thumb of your right hand to heighten the therapeutic effect.

Results: All the cases were cured with 1-3 treatments.

(*Source:* Chinese Acupuncture & Moxibustion, (6):55, 1987)

5. Observed results of 124 cases of acute mastitis treated with acupuncture

Points: Jianjing (G.B. 21) on the affected side, or bilateral in severe cases

Method: Thrust the point perpendicularly to a depth of 0.5-1 *cun* and retain the needle for 20 minutes. In addition, divide the distance from Daling (P. 7) to Quze (P. 3) on the course of pericardium meridian into 7 equal parts, and bleed, with a three-edged needle, 1-3 drops of blood from each.

Results: Among 86 cases of unilateral mastitis, 41 were cured (body temperature became normal and, the local mass was resolved all in one day), 37 showed marked effect (symptoms were notably improved, the local mass was resolved by more than half and the cure was obtained in 2-3 days), 7 showed some effect (symptoms improved, the mass was resolved by less than half, and the cure was obtained in 4-5 days), and 1 failed (no cure was obtained after 5 treatments). Among the 38 cases of bilateral mastitis, 20 were cured, 12 showed marked effect, and 6 showed some effect. The total effective rate was 99.2 percent.

(*Source:* Shanghai Journal of Acupuncture and Moxibustion, (1):16, 1986)

6. Observed results of 47 cases of acute mastitis treated with moxibustion on Shanzhong (Ren 17) and poking method at Tianzong (S.I. 11)

Points and method: Provide indirect moxibustion with garlic at Shanzhong (Ren 17) with 5-7 cones to make the skin flush in the local region. Then, use the tip of the right thumb to press and poke Tianzong (S.I. 11) on the affected side with fairly strong stimulation. Repeat the poking a number of times. Treat twice daily.

Results: Of 47 cases treated, 43 cases were cured, 3 showed marked effect and 1 showed improvement.

(*Source:* Journal of Traditional Chinese Medicine, 22(8):11, 1981)

93. Infantile Convulsion

I. Acute convulsion

Principal points: Zhongchong (P. 9), Renzhong (Du 26), Hegu (L.I. 4), Taichong (Liv. 3).

Method: During the attack of the convulsion, first thrust Renzhong (Du 26) and bleed Zhongchong (P. 9) with a thick filiform needle or a three-edged needle. Then puncture Hegu (L.I. 4) and

Taichong (Liv. 3) with filiform needles and stimulate for a short while by lifting, thrusting and rotating. The needles are not retained, but after the needles are removed, a small amount of blood should be squeezed out from the needle holes.

Supplementary points:

High fever: Dazhui (Du 14), Quchi (L.I. 11), or Quze (P. 3), Weizhong (U.B. 40), with bleeding method

Lockjaw: Jiache (St. 6)

Convulsion of limbs: Houxi (S.I. 3), Neiguan (P. 6), Shenmai (U.B. 62), Yanglingquan (G.B. 34)

Opisthotonos: Shenzhu (Du 12), Fengchi (G.B. 20)

Unconsciousness: Yongquan (K. 1)

Whooping sound in the throat: Fenglong (St. 40), Lieque (Lu. 7)

Convulsion caused by sudden fright: Shenmen (H. 7)

II. Chronic convulsion

Principal points: Baihui (Du 20), Hegu (L.I. 4), Taichong (Liv. 3), Guanyuan (Ren 4), Zusanli (St. 36)

Method: Produce moderate or mild stimulation with filiform needles. Do not retain the needles or retain the needles for only 20 minutes. Treat daily.

Supplementary points:

Yang deficiency in spleen and kidney: Pishu (U.B. 20), Shenshu (U.B. 23) with mild moxibustion by means of moxa sticks after the needling; or indirect moxibustion with ginger at Qihai (Ren 6) for 10 cones

Yin deficiency in liver and kidney: Taixi (K. 3), Ququan (Liv. 8)

Other therapies:

Ear acupuncture

Points: Shenmen, End of Inferior Helix Crus, Brain, Occiput, Heart, Liver

Method: Produce strong stimulation with filiform needles. Retain the needles for 60 minutes, manipulating every 10 minutes. Bleeding Ear Apex can be done to those with persistent hyperpyrexia. This therapy is appropriate to the acute convulsion.

Remarks: Acupuncture therapy has good effect in alleviating infantile convulsions, however, other therapeutic measures must be combined when treating severe cases.

REFERENCES:

Clinical summary of 100 cases of infantile hyperpyrexia treated with acupuncture and bleeding method

Principal points: First Fengchi (G.B. 20) and Dazhui (Du 14), then Quchi (L.I. 11) and Hegu (L.I. 4)

Supplementary points:

High fever: Shixuan (Extra), and Ear Apex, both are bled with a three-edged needle to produce five drops of blood

Convulsion: Baihui (Du 20), Yintang (Extra)

Vomiting: Zhongwan (Ren 12), Tianshu (St. 25), Qihai (Ren 6), Shangjuxu (St. 37)

Sore throat: Shaoshang (Lu. 11), Yamen (Du 15)

Cough, asthma with excessive sputum: Feishu (U.B. 13), Tiantu (Ren 22), Chize (Lu. 5), Fenglong (St. 40)

Whooping cough: Feishu (U.B. 13), Sifeng (Extra)

Parotitis: Jiaosun (S.J. 20), Ashi points

Lassitude and constitutional weakness: Guanyuan (Ren 4), Zusanli (St. 36)

Method: Needle twice daily.

Results: All the cases showed an abatement of fever. The average number of treatments was 2.32.

(*Source:* New Journal of Traditional Chinese Medicine, (10):32, 1986)

94. Infantile Malnutrition

Principal points: Sifeng (Extra), Zhongwan (Ren 12), Zusanli (St. 36), Pishu (U.B. 20), Weishu (U.B. 21)

Method: After strict sterilization, prick Sifeng (Extra) with a thick filiform needle or a three-edged needle. Swiftly insert the needle to a depth of 2-3 mm according to the build of the child, and after the withdrawal of the needle, squeeze a small amount of liquid out of the needle hole. Treat once every other day and five treatments constitute one course. Puncture the other points superficially with filiform needles and gentle stimulation. The needles are not retained. Mild moxibustion with a moxa stick can be offered after the needling. Treat daily.

Supplementary points:

Vomiting: Neiguan (P. 6)

Tidal fever: Dazhui (Du 14)

Abdominal distention with loose stool: Tianshu (St. 25), Qihai (Ren 6)

Cold limbs: Qihai (Ren 6)

Sleeplessness: Jianshi (P. 5)

Parasites: Baichongwo (Extra)

Other therapies:

1. Cutaneous acupuncture

Points: Pishu (U.B. 20), Weishu (U.B. 21), Sanjiaoshu (U.B. 22), Jiaji points (Extra) from seventh thoracic vertebrae to fifth lumbar vertebrae, Zusanli (St. 36), Sifeng (Extra)

Method: Use skin needles to produce mild stimulation until the skin is flushed in the local region. Treat daily.

2. Moxibustion

Points: Pishu (U.B. 20), Zusanli (St. 36), Zhongwan (Ren 12), Tianshu (St. 25), Sifeng (Extra)

Method: Provide 3-5 moxa cones at each point, twice daily.

Remarks: Puncturing Sifeng (Extra) has fairly good effect in treating infantile malnutrition, so attention should be paid to it. The method of finger-pressure and kneading paraspinal muscles also has good effect in the treatment of this disease, thus can be combined in the clinic.

REFERENCES:

1. Treatment of simple infantile indigestion with acupuncture

Principal points: Zusanli (St. 36), Hegu (L.I. 4), Tianshu (St. 25), Guanyuan (Ren 4)

Supplementary Points: Pishu (U.B. 20), Sanyinjiao (Sp. 6)

Method: Shallowly needle to a depth of 0.1-0.2 *cun* in children under three years. Rotate the handle of the needle repeatedly 30 times and then remove the needle.

Results: The cure rate reached 93.3 percent and average number of treatments was 2.08.

(*Source:* Journal of Anhui College of Traditional Chinese Medicine, (2):140, 1959)

2. Observed results of 21 cases of infantile malnutrition treated with acupuncture

Points and method: Use a three-edged needle to prick the palmar aspect of the first interphalangeal joint of the middle finger. Squeeze out a small amount of blood or yellow liquid. Treat once every four days and five treatments constitute one course.

Results: Of 21 cases treated, 15 were cured with a 2-month period of treatment and 6 were cured with a 6-month period of treatment.

(*Source:* Journal of Traditional Chinese Medicine, 21(8):52, 1980)

95. Infantile Diarrhea

Principal points: Sifeng (Extra), Tianshu (St. 25), Zhongwan (Ren 12), Zusanli (St. 36)

Method: Prick Sifeng (Extra) with a filiform needle and squeeze out a slight amount of yellow transparent liquid from the point. Puncture the other points with the needles twisted in, and after the arrival of *qi* further rotate the needles for 10-20 seconds then withdraw, or retain the needles in Tianshu (St. 25), Zhongwan (Ren 12) and Zusanli (St. 36) for 5-10 minutes. Treat once or twice daily.

Supplementary points:

Syndrome of damp-heat: Quchi (L.I. 11), Neiting (St. 44), Yinlingquan (Sp. 9)

Syndrome of food retention: Jianli (Ren 11), Lineiting (Extra)

Invasion of exogenous wind-cold: Hegu (L.I. 4), Waiguan (S.J. 5)

Persistent diarrhea due to spleen *yang* deficiency: Pishu (U.B. 20), Shenshu (U.B. 23), Mingmen (Du 4), applying mild moxibustion with a moxa stick for 5-10 minutes after the needling

Severe fever: Dazhui (Du 14), Hegu (L.I. 4)

Vomiting: Neiguan (P. 6), Shangwan (Ren 13)

Abdominal distending pain: Xiawan (Ren 10), Hegu (L.I. 4)

Cold limbs: Guanyuan (Ren 4), applying mild moxibustion with a moxa stick for 5-10 minutes or indirect moxibustion with ginger for 3-5 cones

Other therapies:

1. Moxibustion

Points: Guanyuan (Ren 4), Shenque (Ren 8), Zhongwan (Ren 12)

Method: When the child is sleeping soundly, perform mild moxibustion with a moxa stick. To start with, set the fire 5 cm away from the skin, and after 3-5 minutes, move the fire closer to the point but not less than the distance of 3 cm. Perform moxibustion first at Zhongwan (Ren 12) then moved down to Shenque (Ren 8) and

Guanyuan (Ren 4).Twenty minutes of treatment is necessary at Zhongwan (Ren 12) and Shenque (Ren 8), and 30-50 minutes at Guanyuan (Ren 4).

2. Ear acupuncture

Points: Stomach, Spleen, Large Intestine, Small Intestine, Pancreas, Gall Bladder, End of Inferior Helix Crus, Shenmen

Method: Select 2-3 points for each treatment. Twist filiform needles in for about one minute, then withdraw, or retain the needles for 30-60 minutes. Treat daily.

3. Hydro-acupuncture

Points: Zusanli (St. 36), Dachangshu (U.B. 25), and moxi Shenque (Ren 8)

Method: Use 1 ml of Vitaminum B₁ complex plus an equal quantity of injection water. Inject 1 ml of the solution into Zusanli (St. 36) and Dachangshu (U.B. 25) contralaterally with the routine operating method of hydro-acupuncture. Treat daily and alternate the points of the two sides. Simultaneously combine mild moxibustion with a moxa stick at Shenque (Ren 8) for about five minutes. The disease can be cured with 1-2 treatments.

4. Laser irradiation at acupoints

Point: Shenque (Ren 8)

Method: Employ a He-Ne laser with a wavelength of 6328Å, power at 3 mw, and the diameter of the light spot at about 2 mm. Treat daily, 10-15 minutes each time and three times constitute one course.

Remarks: The above methods are simple but have quick effect in treating infantile diarrhea. Medication should be incorporated promptly to those with dehydration so as to avoid aggravating the disease.

REFERENCES:

1. Summary of the treatment of 700 cases of infantile diarrhea with acupuncture

Points and method: Treat bilateral Tianshu (St. 25) with reinforcing method and Changqiang (Du 1) with sparrow-pricking reducing method. Do not retain the needles. Treat daily.

Results: Of 700 cases treated, 612 cases (87.4 percent) were cured with 1-2 treatments, 52 cases (7.4 percent) basically recovered after 3 treatments, and 36 cases (5.1 percent) were unchanged after 3 attempts.

(*Source:* The Intermediate Medical Journal, (2):52, 1987)

2. Observed results of 14 cases of infantile diarrhea treated with

needling at Changqiang (Du 1)

Point: Changqiang (Du 1)

Method: Insert the needle to a depth of 0.5-0.8 *cun* and withdraw after stimulating by quickly rotating in small amplitude for two minutes. Treat daily.

Results: Of 14 cases treated, 9 cases had no more diarrhea after only 1 treatment, 4 cases had no diarrhea after 2-3 treatments, and 1 case was unchanged.

(*Source:* Shanghai Journal of Acupuncture and Moxibustion, 6(1):14, 1987)

3. Observed results of 560 cases of infantile diarrhea treated with moxibustion at the 12th thoracic vertebrae

Point: Middle point of the 12th thoracic vertebrae

Method: Apply moxibustion at the middle point of the 12th thoracic vertebrae until the skin is flushed.

Results: Of 560 cases treated, 498 cases (88.9 percent) were cured; 54 (9.6 percent) were improved; and 8 (1.4 percent) were unchanged. The total effective rate was 98.6 percent.

(*Source:* Chinese Acupuncture & Moxibustion, (3):22, 1987)

4. Clinical observation on the treatment of 100 cases of infantile diarrhea with acupuncture

Points: Sifeng (Extra), Zhongwan (Ren 12), Tianshu (St. 25), Qihai (Ren 6), or Zusanli (St. 36), Sanyinjiao (Sp. 6)

Method: Combine acupuncture with moxibustion, do not retain the needles, and treat daily.

Results: Of 100 cases treated, 95 cases were cured with only 1 treatment and the total effective rate was 99 percent.

(*Source:* Chinese Acupuncture & Moxibustion, (5):14, 1984)

5. Treatment of chronic infantile diarrhea with rush-pith moxibustion

Points and method: Soak the rush pith with vegetable oil at one end, then ignite and moxi at Changqiang (Du 1). Usually after one treatment, there will be no more diarrhea. If the diarrhea relieved, offer one more treatment 3-5 days later.

(*Source:* Zhejiang Journal of Traditional Chinese Medicine, 15(8):258, 1980)

96. Infantile Enuresis

Principal points: Guanyuan (Ren 4), Zhongji (Ren 3), Sanyinjiao (Sp. 6), Yiniaodian (Extra, 1 *cun* below Xiajuxu, St. 39)

Method: Needle the points on the abdomen obliquely downward to conduct the needling sensation down to the genital region. Apply mild or moderate stimulation and retain the needles for 10-20 minutes. Treat daily or once every other day, and 10 treatments constitute one course. Mild moxibustion with a moxa stick can be offered after the needling or moxibustion can be used alone.

Supplementary points:

Deficiency of *qi*: Zusanli (St. 36), Qihai (Ren 6)

Dream-disturbed sleep: Shenmen (H. 7)

Difficulty of waking up from the sleep: Baihui (Du 20), Shenmen (H. 7)

Frequent micturition: Baihui (Du 20), Ciliao (U.B. 32)

Other therapies:

1. Ear acupuncture

Points: Kidney, Urinary Bladder, Central Rim, Brain, Intertragicus, Urethra, Occiput

Method: Select 3-4 points for each treatment and perform strong stimulation with filiform needles. Retain the needles for 30-60 minutes. Treat daily and five treatments constitute one course. There is a one-week interval between two courses. To treat severe cases, the needle-embedding method can be employed and the needles are retained for 3-5 days. Or the seed-embedding method can be also used, which can be changed in 5-7 days.

2. Cutaneous acupuncture

Points: Guanyuan (Ren 4), Qihai (Ren 6), Qugu (Ren 2), Shenshu (U.B. 23), Sanyinjiao (Sp. 6), and Jiaji points (Extra) from the 11th thoracic vertebrae to the sacral vertebrae

Method: Tap repeatedly with a cutaneous needle until the skin is flushed. Treat daily.

3. Wrist-and-ankle acupuncture

Points: Lower 1, bilateral

Method: Apply the routine method of wrist-and-ankle needling.

4. Head acupuncture

Points: Leg Motor and Sensory Area, Reproduction Area

Method: Apply the routine operation of head acupuncture. Repeatedly manipulate the needles for 10-15 minutes.

5. Laser irradiation on acupoints

Points: Qugu (Ren 2), Zhongji (Ren 3), Guanyuan (Ren 4), Henggu (K. 11), Guilai (St. 29), Sanyinjiao (Sp. 6)

Method: Select 2-4 points for each treatment and radiate each point for 5-10 minutes. Treat once every other day, and 5-10 treatments constitute one course.

Remarks: Acupuncture has fair effect in the treatment of infantile enuresis. This disease is liable to recur, so 3-5 more treatments should be offered even it is cured so as to consolidate the effectiveness.

Require the patient to empty the bladder before needling at Guanyuan (Ren 4), Zhongji (Ren 3), etc., which are located in the lower abdomen.

REFERENCES:

1. Observed results of 14 cases of infantile enuresis treated by needling Baihui (Du 20) and Sishencong (Extra)

Points and method: Needle Baihui (Du 20) and Sishencong (Extra) obliquely with the tip of the needle reaching the periosteum to obtain the sensation of distention and heaviness.

Results: Of 14 cases treated, 10 were cured, and 4 improved. The effectiveness was acquired after 2-3 treatments.

(*Source:* Shaanxi Journal of Traditional Chinese Medicine, 4(6):14, 1983)

2. Observed results of treating enuresis by needling the little toe

Points: The mid-point of the first transverse crease under the little toe (bilateral)

Method: When the tip of the needle reaches the bone, twist the needle in an oblique angle until the patient feels localized sharp pain and a hot distending sensation in the lower abdomen. Retain the needles for 30 minutes and manipulate every 10 minutes or connect with an electro-apparatus. Treat daily or once every other day, and 10 treatments constitute one course.

Results: Of 5 cases treated, all were cured.

(*Source:* Jiangxi Journal of Traditional Chinese Medicine, (1):45, 1983)

3. Report on 230 cases of enuresis treated with acupuncture at Guanyuan (Ren 4) and Sanyinjiao (Sp. 6)

Points: Guanyuan (Ren 4), Sanyinjiao (Sp. 6)

Method: Swiftly insert filiform needles to produce moderate stimulation, and retain the needles for 20-30 minutes after the arrival of *qi*. Treat twice weekly and 10 treatments constitute one course.

Results: Of 230 cases treated, 92 cases were cured, 29 showed marked effect, 78 were improved, and 31 were unchanged. The total effective rate was 86.5 percent.

(*Source:* Jiangxi Journal of Traditional Chinese Medicine, (6):35, 1983)

4. Observed results of 131 cases of enuresis treated with needle-embedding method

Points: Lieque (Lu. 7), Sanyinjiao (Sp. 6), both bilateral

Method: After sterilizing the skin, obliquely insert an intradermal needle into the point and fix with adhesive plaster after the arrival of soreness, distention and a numb sensation. Retain the needles for 4 days in summer but 7-10 days in winter and spring.

Results: Among 131 cases, 105 cases had no enuresis or only occasionally after treating for one month.

(*Source:* Zhejiang Journal of Traditional Chinese Medicine, 15(8):365, 1980)

97. Infantile Polysialia

Principal points: Jiache (St. 6), Dicang (St. 4), Chengjiang (Ren 24), Hegu (L.I. 4)

Method: Swiftly insert a gauge 30 filiform needle (0.32 mm in diameter) 1 *cun* in length into the point. Ensure the insertion is superficial. Then apply the vibrating method by lifting and thrusting the needle for one minute and remove the needle after that. Treat daily and six treatments constitute one course. Retain the needles for 10-20 minutes if the child is willing to accept it.

Supplementary points:

Indigestion: Zusanli (St. 36), Zhongwan (Ren 12)

Stomatitis: Quchi (L.I. 11), Zusanli (St. 36)

Other therapies:

1. Ear acupuncture

Points: Mouth, Tongue, Spleen, Lower Apex of Tragus

Method: Select two points on one ear only, and thrust with filiform needles. Then rotate for about one minute. Do not retain the needles. Treat daily on alternate ears. Five treatments constitute one course, with a 5-day interval if a second course is needed. If the child is afraid of the needling, ear acupressure is also applicable with seeds, which should be changed every 3-5 days.

2. Hydro-acupuncture

Points: Jiache (St. 6), Dicang (St. 4), Chengjiang (Ren 24), Hegu (L.I. 4)

Method: Select 2-3 points for each treatment. Inject 0.2-0.3 ml of Vitamin B$_1$ (10 mg/ml) into each point, once every other day. Ten treatments constitute one course.

Remarks: The above methods have fair effect in treating infantile polysialia, but the effectiveness is unsatisfactory for polysialia due to cerebral dysgenesis. If there is a definite primary disease, the active measures should be taken simultaneously.

REFERENCE:

Effectiveness of infantile polysialia treated with acupuncture

Points: Jiache (St. 6), Dicang (St. 4), Hegu (L.I. 4), Tianzhu (U.B. 10), Lianquan (Ren 23), Quchi (L.I. 11)

Method: Apply swift insertion and moderate vibration of lifting and thrusting the needle.

Results: After 2-4 treatments, the symptoms disappeared, and after 10 treatments, 5 cases were cured, 3 showed marked effect, 1 was slightly improved and 1 was unchanged.

(*Source:* Journal of Traditional Chinese Medicine, (4):27, 1961)

98. Infantile Hernia

Principal points: Dadun (Liv. 1), Guilai (St. 29), Guanyuan (Ren 4), Tituo (Extra), Baihui (Du 20)

Method: Provide moderate stimulation by filiform needles with even method. It is not necessary to retain the needles. If the child is not cooperative, but withdraw after a couple of minutes manipulation. Those who are cooperative can have 30-minute retention. Moxibustion can be done at Baihui (Du 20) with a moxa stick for 5-10 minutes during the retention or after the withdrawal. Treat daily or once every other day and 10 treatments constitute one course.

Supplementary points:

Deficiency of *qi*: Zusanli (St. 36), Qihai (Ren 6), reinforced with needling and moxibustion

Deficient cold: Mingmen (Du 4), reinforced with needling and moxibustion

Excruciating lower abdominal pain: Taichong (Liv. 3), Ququan (Liv. 8)

Other therapy:

Moxibustion

Points: a) Sanyinjiao (Sp. 6) of the healthy side, Guilai (St. 29) of the affected side; b) Sanjiaojiuxue (Extra)

Method: Select either of the two groups. When the first group is used, provide moxibustion at one point in each treatment and alternate two points. Perform the moxibustion with 5-7 wheat-sized moxa cones directly on the point, and three days later, repeat the same procedure on the other point. Two treatments constitute one course, with a two-week interval between courses. To employ the second group, perform suspending moxibustion with a moxa stick over the point for 10 minutes, once or twice daily.

Remarks: Acupuncture in combination with moxibustion, or sole moxibustion therapy, has fairly good effect in treating infantile hernia. Surgical operation should be recommended for the severe cases.

REFERENCES:

1. The cure of seven cases of infantile incarcerated hernia by acupuncture

Points: Zusanli (St. 36), Sanyinjiao (Sp. 6)

Method: Stimulate by lifting, thrusting and rotating the needles after the arrival of *qi* and do not retain the needles.

Results: The time of the retraction of hernia content was 5 minutes for 1 case, 10 minutes for 1 case, 20 minutes for 1 case, 30 minutes for 1 case, and 50-60 minutes for 3 cases. Among them, a hot compress was combined for 3 cases.

(*Source:* Journal of Traditional Chinese Medicine, (8):5, 1964)

2. Observed results of the treatment of 43 cases of inguinal hernia and incarcerated hernia with acupuncture

Principal points: Dadun (Liv. 1), bilateral

Supplementary points: Guanyuan (Ren 4), Shenque (Ren 8), Xuehai (Sp. 10)

Method: Needling Dadun (Liv. 1) is sufficient for those with mild symptoms but moxibustion should be incorporated at Guanyuan (Ren 4) and Shenque (Ren 8) for 10-15 minutes for severe cases. Needle supplementary point Xuehai (Sp. 10) for those with distinct symptoms of blood stagnation. Needles are not retained in children.

Results: Of 43 cases treated, 38 were cured, 4 were improved and 1 remained unchanged.

(*Source:* Chinese Acupuncture & Moxibustion, (2):2, 1986)

99. Sequela of Poliomyelitis

Principal points: Ganshu (U.B. 18), Shenshu (U.B. 23), Yaoyangguan (Du 3), Yanglingquan (G.B. 34), Xuanzhong (G.B. 39), Taixi (K. 3), Quchi (L.I. 11), Zusanli (St. 36)

Method: Select 3-4 points for each treatment and employ the reinforcing technique with filiform needles. Superficial needling and mild stimulation are appropriate for those with good needling sensation, while for those with a dull sensation or even difficultly obtaining the arrival of *qi*, strong stimulation is essential, with repeated manipulation of needles so as to strengthen the needling sensation. To treat the dislocation of joints, provide mild moxibustion with a moxa stick over every point after the needling, and combine cupping at the place of the dislocated joint. Warm-needle moxibustion is applicable to muscular atrophy. For those with cold limbs and purplish skin, moxibustion should be used.

Supplementary points:

a) Paralysis of the upper limb

Difficulty raising the shoulder: Jianjing (G.B. 21), Jianyu (L.I. 15), Binao (L.I. 14)

Dislocation of the shoulder joint: Jianyu (L.I. 15), Jianliao (S.J. 14), Jugu (L.I. 16)

Motoring impairment of the elbow: Chize (Lu. 5), Quze (P. 3), Shousanli (L.I. 10)

Difficulty intorting and extorting the hand: Shousanli (L.I. 10), Yangchi (S.J. 4), Yangxi (L.I. 5), Houxi (S.I. 3), Sidu (S.J. 9), Shaohai (H. 3)

Wrist drop: Waiguan (S.J. 5), Yanggu (S.I. 5)

Difficulty flexing the fingers: Jianshi (P. 5), Neiguan (P. 6), Lingdao (H. 4)

247

Difficulty extending the fingers: Hegu (L.I. 4), Waiguan (S.J. 5), Zhigou (S.J. 6).

b) Paralysis of the lower limb

Difficulty raising the leg: Biguan (St. 31), Huantiao (G.B. 30), Futu (St. 32), Jiaji points (Extra) from L1 to L5; Fengshi (G.B. 31), Yinshi (St. 33)

Dislocation of the hip joint: Huantiao (G.B. 30), Juliao (G.B. 29), Biguan (St. 31)

Motoring impairment of the knee: Yinshi (St. 33), Liangqiu (St. 34), Shangjuxu (St. 37), Dubi (St. 35)

Back of knee: Chengfu (U.B. 36), Weizhong (U.B. 40), Chengshan (U.B. 57)

Foot drop: Xiajuxu (St. 39), Jiexi (St. 41)

Strephenopodia: Kunlun (U.B. 60), Qiuxu (G.B. 40), Fuyang (U.B. 59)

Strephexopodia: Shangqiu (Sp. 5), Taixi (K. 3), Sanyinjiao (Sp. 6)

Paralysis of the abdominal muscles: Liangmen (St. 21), Tianshu (St. 25), Daimai (G.B. 26)

Other therapies:

1. Ear acupuncture

Points: Shenmen, Brain, Cervical Vertebrae, Thoracic Vertebrae, Lumbosacral Vertebrae

Method: Use 3-4 points for each treatment, perform moderate stimulation, and retain the needles for 30 minutes. Treat daily.

2. Cutaneous acupuncture

Points: Paralysis of the upper limb: Du meridian (from the nape down to fourth thoracic vertebrae), Hand-Yangming and Hand-Taiyang meridians of the affected arm, Quchi (L.I. 11), Waiguan (S.J. 5)

Paralysis of the lower limb: Du meridian (lumbosacral region), urinary bladder meridian (lumbosacral region), and Foot-Yangming and Foot-Jueyin meridians of the affected leg

Paralysis of the abdominal muscles, Foot-Yangming, Foot-Taiyin and Foot-Shaoyang meridians

Method: Tap with the cutaneous needle along the above-mentioned meridians until the local region is flushed. Treat daily.

3. Electro-acupuncture

Points: Consulting the points for body acupuncture in terms of the location of the paralysis.

Method: Select 3-4 points for each treatment. After the arrival of *qi*, connect the apparatus with the needles to give the highest stimulation the patient can tolerate. Treat daily or once every other day, 5-15 minutes each time.

Remarks: Sequela of poliomyelitis can be treated with acupuncture. The effectiveness is fair for a fresh case but unsatisfactory for a chronic case. When the motoring function has recovered to a certain degree, functional training should be appropriately strengthened and require the patient to pay attention to his posture so as to prevent the deformity of joints caused by overexertion and improper postures.

100. Pertussis

1. Initial cough

Principal points: Fengmen (U.B. 12), Lieque (Lu. 7), Hegu (L.I. 4), Fenglong (St. 40)

Method: Provide moderate stimulation with filiform needles, and treat daily.

Supplementary points:

Chills and fever but no sweating: Dazhu (U.B. 11), Dazhui (Du 14), Waiguan (S.J. 5), and moxi Fengmen (U.B. 12)

Severe cough: Tiantu (Ren 22)

Itching and red throat: Shaoshang (Lu. 11) with bleeding method

2. Spasmodic cough

Principal points: Dazhui (Du 14), Kongzui (Lu. 6), Chize (Lu. 5), Fenglong (St. 40), Sifeng (Extra)

Method: Prick Sifeng (Extra) with a thick filiform needle and squeeze a little yellow or white mucus out. Bleed Dazhui (Du 14) and combine cupping. Puncture the other points to a shallow depth, but do not retain the needles. With those children who are cooperative, retain the needles for 10-20 minutes. Treat once or twice daily.

Supplementary points:

Long-lasting cough with the pain in the chest and costal region: Qimen (Liv. 14) with superficial or oblique insertion but no retention of the needle, Zhigou (S.J. 6), Yanglingquan (G.B. 34)

Cough with vomiting: Neiguan (P. 6) with superficial needling but swift withdrawal of the needle

Nasal bleeding: Yingxiang (L.I. 20) with the needle going

obliquely towards the ala nasa, and Shangxing (Du 23) with needle thrusting subcutaneously downward

3. Convalescence

Principal points: Feishu (U.B. 13), Pishu (U.B. 20), Taiyuan (Lu. 9), Zusanli (St. 36)

Method: Perform reinforcing method with filiform needles and shallow insertion. Do not retain the needles. With those who are cooperative retain the needles for 10-20 minutes. Treat daily or once every other day.

Supplementary points:

Qi deficiency in lung and spleen with forceless cough: Qihai (Ren 6), Guanyuan (Ren 4), with mild moxibustion by means of a moxa stick

Anorexia with loose stool: Zhongwan (Ren 12), Tianshu (St. 25)

Cold limbs: Guanyuan (Ren 4), with mild moxibustion by means of a moxa stick or moxa cones

Other therapies:

1. Ear acupuncture

Points: Lung, Trachea, Shenmen, End of Inferior Helix Crus, Ear-asthma

Method: Produce moderate stimulation with filiform needles which however are not retained. Needle 2-3 points each time and alternate ears. Treat daily.

2. Cutaneous acupuncture

Points: Du meridian (nape and back regions), Dazhui (Du 14), Zhongwan (Ren 12), Neiguan (P. 6), Taiyuan (Lu. 9), Fenglong (St. 40)

Method: Tap the nape and back regions of the Du meridian and the other points with a cutaneous needle several times in repetition to cause the skin to become flushed in the local areas. Treat daily.

3. Cupping

Points: Fengmen (U.B. 12), Feishu (U.B. 13), Pishu (U.B. 20), Zhongfu (Lu. 1), Shanzhong (Ren 17)

Method: Use cups in small diameter for on-and-off cupping alternating between back and chest. Treat daily, 5-10 minutes each time.

4. Pricking method

Point: Shenzhu (Du 12)

Method: After sterilizing the local region, prick the point with a three-edged needle until causing bleeding, and then suck with a small diame-

250

ter cup for 5-10 minutes. Treat once every other day.

Remarks: Acupuncture therapy has fair effect in the treatment of this disease. Pricking Sifeng (Extra) can prevent the worsening of symptoms in the short term.

REFERENCE:

Report on 240 cases of pertussis treated with acupuncture

Principal points: Fengmen (U.B. 12), Feishu (U.B. 13), Dingchuan (Extra), Tiantu (Ren 22)

Supplementary points: Yuji (Lu. 10), Shaoshang (Lu. 11), Fenglong (St. 40), Quchi (L.I. 11)

Method: Treat daily or once every other day. Four treatments constitute one course with 2-5 days' break between courses.

Results: Of the 240 cases treated with acupuncture alone, 194 were cured, 21 showed marked effect, 19 improved, and 6 remained unchanged. The total effective rate was 97.5 percent.

101. Parotitis

Principal points: Yifeng (S.J. 17), Jiache (St. 6), Hegu (L.I. 4)

Method: Provide the former two points with moderate stimulation while intensely stimulating the distant points to conduct the needling sensation up and down. Retain the needles for 20-30 minutes, and treat daily.

Supplementary points:

Fever: Dazhui (Du 14), Quchi (L.I. 11)

Sore and swelling of the throat: Shaoshang (Lu. 11), Shangyang (L.I. 1) bled with a three-edged needle

Headache: Fengchi (G.B. 20), Taiyang (Extra), Touwei (St. 8)

Complication of orchitis: Xuehai (Sp. 10), Ququan (Liv. 8), Xingjian (Liv. 2), Sanyinjiao (Sp. 6), Qugu (Ren 2), Wuli (Liv. 10)

Other therapies:

1. Rush pith moxibustion

Point: Jiaosun (S.J. 20)

Method: Cut the hair short at the location of Jiaosun (S.J. 20) on the affected side. After sterilizing the skin, ignite a rush pith soaked with vegetable oil and swiftly place on the point. Immediately lift after a crack is heard when the fire touches the skin. Usually the swelling can be resolved with only one moxibustion treatment. However, this can be repeated the next day in case the swelling is not fully resolved. There will be a millet-like wound due to the fire at the locus of the moxibustion. The wound should be kept clean to prevent infection. Usually it will automatically heal in a couple of days without any special treatment.

2. Cutaneous acupuncture

Points: Jiache (St. 6), Yifeng (S.J. 17), Hegu (L.I. 4), Waiguan (S.J. 5), Lieque (Lu. 7), Jiaji points (Extra) from first to fourth thoracic vertebrae, Erjian (L.I. 2)

Method: Tap mildly and moderately with a cutaneous needle until the skin becomes flushed in the local area. Treat daily or once every other day.

3. Ear acupuncture

Points: Parotid Gland, Cheek, Brain, Ashi point

Method: Apply strong stimulation with filiform needles. Retain the needles for 20 minutes with manipulation during retention. Treat daily.

Remarks: Acupuncture has fair effect in treating this disease. To use rush pith moxibustion, the point should be located accurately, the soaking of oil should be appropriate and the operation should be skilled, otherwise the effect will be unsatisfactory and the patient will be tortured. During the epidemic of this disease, needling Hegu (L.I. 4) in healthy children can play a role in prevention.

REFERENCES:

1. Observed results of the treatment of parotitis with moxibustion at Pt. Ear Apex

Point: Ear Apex on the affected side

Method: Utilize a rush pith and one end is soaked with vegetable oil (the soaking is up to 0.5 *cm* of the pith). After the ignition, swiftly put the rush pith on the point and apply mild pressure. Then immediately lift the pith and the fire should have died out, but a clear crack can burst as a sign of successful operation. Treat daily.

Results: Of 78 cases treated, 19 cases had the symptoms such as the swelling of the parotid gland resolved in 2 days, 21 cases had the resolution in 3 days, 32 cases in 4 days, and 6 cases in 5 days.

(*Source:* Chinese Acupuncture & Moxibustion, (3):56, 1987)

2. Observation on the therapeutic effect of 329 cases of epidemic parotitis treated with transient cauterization at Jiaosun (S.J. 20)

252

Point: Jiaosun (S.J. 20)

Method: Soak a match stick wrapped with a little absorbent cotton with vegetable oil, and after igniting, transiently cauterize at Jiaosun (S.J. 20) on the affected side. Lift out immediately. No more repetition is made. If the focus is bilateral, Jiaosun (S.J. 20) on both sides should be cauterized. Treat daily.

Results: All the cases were cured, and the duration of treatment ranged from 1 to 4 days, 3 days in average.

(*Source:* Journal of Anhui College of Traditional Chinese Medicine, 4(4):42, 1985)

3. Clinical observation on 1,080 cases of epidemic parotitis treated with acupuncture

Points: Hegu (L.I. 4), Yifeng (S.J. 17), Lieque (Lu. 7)

Method: Use reducing technique and retain the needles for 20 minutes.

Results: Of 1,080 cases treated, 310 cases were cured with only one treatment, 538 cases with two treatments and 232 with three treatments.

(*Source:* The Intermediate Medical Journal, 23(2):52, 1988)

4. Treatment of 350 cases of epidemic parotitis with bleeding therapy

Principal point: Shaoshang (Lu. 11)

Supplementary point: Hegu (L.I. 4)

Method: Bleed Shaoshang (Lu. 11) with a three-edged needle and squeeze 3-6 drops of blood out. Then needle Hegu (L.I. 4) with even technique but do not retain the needles. Treat daily.

Results: Resolution of all the symptoms, such as painful swelling of the parotid gland, is considered as a cure. Of 350 cases treated, 165 cases were cured with only one treatment, 142 were cured with two treatments and 43 with three treatments.

(*Source:* Chinese Acupuncture & Moxibustion, (2):14, 1987)

5. Observed results of the treatment of epidemic parotitis by needling Shousanli (L.I. 10)

Points: Shousanli (L.I. 10), bilateral

Method: Apply perpendicular needling to a depth of 1-1.5 *cun* with moderate stimulation.

Results: Usually the cure can be obtained with only one treatment, and two dosages of universal relief decoction for disinfection can be combined in severe cases.

(*Source:* Hunan Journal of Medicine and Medica Materia, (2):19, 1981)

6. Observation on the therapeutic effect of epidemic parotitis treated with bleeding method at ear point

Point: Ear Apex on the affected side

Method: Apply bleeding method once daily.

Results: Of 30 cases treated, 22 cases were cured within 3 days, 6 cases within 3-6 days, and 2 cases only after 6 days, which were regarded as failures.

(*Source:* Tianjin Journal of Traditional Chinese Medicine, (6):20, 1987)

102. Conjunctivitis

Principal points: Jingming (U.B. 1), Taiyang (Extra), Hegu (L.I. 4), Fengchi (G.B. 20)

Method: In puncturing Jingming (U.B. 1), ask the patient to close his eyes. Then gently push the eyeball laterally and fix with one finger. Slowly insert the needle to a depth of 1 *cun* between the orbit and the nose. No twirling, rotating, lifting or thrusting is advisable, do not retain the needle. Prick Taiyang (Extra) to produce a few drops of blood. Needle Hegu (L.I. 4) and Fengchi (G.B. 20) with moderate stimulation. Retain the needles for 15-20 minutes. Generally speaking, select Jingming (U.B. 1) and Taiyang (Extra) on the affected side as well as bilateral Hegu (L.I. 4) and Fengchi (G.B. 20) for the treatment. Treat daily. Five treatments constitute one course.

Supplementary points:

Invasion of exogenous wind-heat: Shaoshang (Lu. 11), pricking a few drops of blood out

Excessive fire in the liver and gall bladder: Xingjian (Liv. 2), Taichong (Liv. 3), puncturing with reducing method

Headache: Shangxing (Du 23), Yintang (Extra)

Fever: Quchi (L.I. 11), causing blood out with a thick filiform needle or a three-edged needle

Prolonged redness of eye: Geshu (U.B. 17), Neiguan (P. 6)

Other therapies:

1. Ear acupuncture

Points: Eye, Liver, Ear Apex, Eye 1, Eye 2

Method: Apply moderate stimulation with filiform needles. Retain the needles for 30 minutes with periodic manipulation. Prick some blood out at Ear Apex. Treat daily.

2. Moxibustion

Point: Opposite Ear Apex in relation to the affected eye

Method: Apply a moxa stick at the point until a mild hot sensation is felt, and 10-15 minutes are needed for a treatment. Treat daily.

3. Cutaneous acupuncture

Points: Portion around orbital ridge, lateral temporal region, Fengchi (G.B. 20).

Method: Use a plum-blossom needle to tap rather strongly and quickly (four times/second) until the local area becomes reddish in color. Treat daily.

4. Pricking and cupping

Points: Taiyang (Extra), Yuyao (Extra), vein at back of the ear

Method: Use a filiform needle or three-edged needle to prick blood out at Taiyang (Extra). Then apply a small cup on the point for 1-3 minutes. Squeeze out a few drops of blood after pricking Yuyao (Extra). Apply massage to the ear first so as to cause slight venous pooling. This makes the veins easier to see. Then use a three-edged needle to prick the vein to allow a few drops of blood to escape. This bloodletting method can be used alone, or in combination. Treat daily, and 1-3 treatments are needed. This method is suitable to the treatment of acute conjunctivitis.

Remarks: Acupuncture therapy is quite effective in the treatment of this illness.

REFERENCES:

1. Observed results of acupuncture in treating seven cases of acute conjunctivitis

Points: Jingming (U.B. 1), Tongziliao (G.B. 1), Hegu (L.I. 4), Ear Apex

Method: Puncture with strong stimulation. Retain the needles for 20 minutes. Cause bleeding at bilateral Ear Apex. Treat daily. Continue for three treatments.

Results: The cured rate was 100 percent.

(*Source:* Chinese Acupuncture & Moxibustion, (3):42, 1982)

2. Observed results of ear acupuncture as the main method in treating 64 cases of hemorrhagic conjunctivitis

Points: Jingming (U.B. 1), Ear Apex, Eye

Method: Puncture Jingming (U.B. 1) to a depth of 0.4-0.6 *cun*. Retain the needle for 15 minutes. Use Pt. Ear Apex for blood-letting and Pt. Eye for seed-embedding.

Results: Of 64 cases treated, 44 were cured by one treatment. The total effective rate reached 100 percent.

(*Source:* Shanghai Journal of Acupuncture and Moxibustion, (3):26, 1987)

3. Observed results of puncturing Taiyang (Extra) in combination with cupping in treating 27 cases of overflowed lacrimation

Point: Taiyang (Extra)

Method: Insert straightly to a depth of 1 *cun*. Retain the needle for 20-30 minutes after the needling sensation is obtained. Apply cupping at Taiyang (Extra) for 15-20 minutes right after withdrawal of the needle. After cupping, apply an adhesive plaster which functions in relieving pain affected by invasion of dampness.

Results: Of 27 cases treated, 21 were cured by 1 treatment, 1 was cured by 2 treatments, 3 showed some improvement and 2 showed no effect.

(*Source:* Journal of Traditional Chinese Medicine, 25(3):60, 1984)

4. Observed results of acupuncture in treating 52 cases of electric ophthalmitis

Points: Taiyang (Extra), Zanzhu (U.B. 2), Inner-Yingxiang (Extra)

Method: Prick Inner-Yingxiang (Extra) with a three-edged needle to let a few drops of blood out. Treat daily.

Results: Of 52 cases treated, 49 cases were cured, and 3 cases showed improvement.

(*Source:* Chinese Acupuncture & Moxibustion, (3):27, 1986)

103. Hordeolum (Stye)

Principal points: Taiyang (Extra), Hegu (L.I. 4), Quchi (L.I. 11)

Method: With either a thick filiform needle or a three-edged needle, bleed Taiyang (Extra) to produce 2-3 drops of blood. Apply reducing method at Hegu (L.I. 4) and Quchi (L.I. 11) with moderate stimulation. Retain the needles for 20-30 minutes. Treat daily.

Supplementary points:

Swelling on the inner canthus at the board of upper eyelid: Zanzhu (U.B. 2), Jingming (U.B. 1)

Swelling on the outer canthus at the board of upper eyelid: Sizhukong (S.J. 23), Tongziliao (G.B. 1)

Swelling at the middle way of upper eyelid: Yangbai (G.B. 14), Yuyao (Extra)

Swelling at the board of lower eyelid: Chengqi (St. 1), Sibai (St. 2)

Invasion by exogenous wind-heat: Shaoze (S.I. 1), pricking to produce a few drops of blood

Excessive heat in the spleen and stomach: Neiting (St. 44)

Chronic stye: Zusanli (St. 36), Pishu (U.B. 20), combining with moxibustion

Other therapies:

1. Cupping

Point: Dazhui (Du 14)

Method: After local sterilization, prick Dazhui (Du 14) to cause a few drops of blood, then apply a cup for 5-10 minutes. Treat daily.

2. Ear acupuncture

Points: Eye, Liver, Spleen, Ear Apex

Method: Use filiform needles with moderate stimulation. Retain the needles for 15-20 minutes. Treat daily. Apply blood-letting at Ear Apex. For a chronic case, embed vaccaria seeds with adhesive tape at the ear points.

3. Pricking

Points: On scapular areas

Method: Small papules, reddish in color, may be found at two scapular areas. After routine sterilization, prick these reddish papules and cut the subcutaneous tissue fiber. Choose papules on the right scapular area for a stye on the left eye, and papules on the left scapular area for a stye on the right eye.

Remarks: Acupuncture therapy is very effective in the treatment of hordeolum. However, squeezing the stye too early may cause infection.

REFERENCES:

1. Observed results of embedding intradermal needles on the ear points in treating 47 cases of hordeolum

Principal point: Eye

Supplementary points: Liver, Shenmen, Brain

Method: Apply embedding with intradermal needles.

Results: Of 47 cases treated, 35 were cured. The total effective rate was 97.5 percent.

(*Source:* Chinese Acupuncture & Moxibustion, (2):8, 1986)

2. Observed results of blood-letting at Ganshu (U.B. 18) in treating 12 cases of relapsed hordeolum

Point: Ganshu (U.B. 18) on the affected side

Method: Puncture with slanted downward insertion a gauge 26 or 28 needle to a depth of 0.4-0.6 *cun*. Apply reducing method with strong stimulation. After withdrawing the needle, squeeze out a drop of blood.

Results: Treat once a week, with all 12 cases cured in 3 treatments. The effective rate reached 100 percent.

(*Source:* Chinese Acupuncture & Moxibustion, (3):27, 1985)

3. Observed results of pricking the third toe, bilaterally, in treating 10 cases of stye

Points: Tip of the third toe, bilaterally

Method: Prick with a three-edged needle to produce 3-5 drops of blood.

Results: Of 10 cases treated, 9 cases were cured by one treatment. Only 1 case was cured after subsequent treatments.

(*Source:* New Journal of Traditional Chinese Medicine, (2):40, 1984)

104. Ptosis of Upper Eyelid (Blepharoptosis)

Principal points: Zanzhu (U.B. 2), Sizhukong (S.J. 23), Yangbai (G.B. 14), Kunlun (U.B. 60)

Method: Insert horizontally from Zanzhu (U.B. 2) and Sizhukong (S.J. 23) to Yuyao (Extra). Horizontally puncture downward at Yangbai (G.B. 14) to a depth of 1 *cun*. Retain the needles for 20-30 minutes with periodic manipulation. Apply moxibustion with a moxa stick at the local region after withdrawing the needles. Treat daily.

Supplementary points:

Deficient *qi* in the spleen: Zusanli (St. 36), Qihai (Ren 6), Pishu (U.B. 20), combining with moxibustion

Deficient *yang* in the spleen and kidney: Pishu (U.B. 20), Shenshu (U.B. 23), Zusanli (St. 36), combining with moxibustion

Traumatic injury: Geshu (U.B. 17), Fengchi (G.B. 20)

Headache: Shangxing (Du 23), Taiyang (Extra)
Other therapies:
1. Cutaneous acupuncture
Points: The pathways of the urinary bladder and kidney meridians on the affected side of the head, orbital muscle
Method: Use a plum-blossom needle to tap from the upper part to the lower part, and from the medial to the lateral. Apply mild stimulation to the eye region, but moderate stimulation to the head region until the skin becomes reddish in color. Treat once every other day.
2. Moxibustion
Point: Dabao (Sp. 21)
Method: Apply non-scar moxibustion with 5-7 cones in a session. Instruct the patient to massage the upper part of the eyebrow and push it upward for 10 minutes, twice a day. After such massage, the patient should apply a hot compress with a towel for 3-5 minutes. Treat once every other day. Acupuncture can be combined.
Remarks: Acupuncture and moxibustion are quite effective in the treatment of blepharoptosis due to oculomotor paralysis, myasthenia gravis, traumatic injury, trachoma, etc. However, in cases of congenital blepharoptosis, an operation is needed.

REFERENCES:
1. Clinical observation on electro-acupuncture in treating 17 cases of ptosis of upper eyelid
Principal points: Yangbai (G.B. 14), superior orbital nerve
Supplementary points:
Musculus rectus medialis paralysis: Jingming (U.B. 1)
Musculus rectus lateralis paralysis: Tongziliao (G.B. 1)
Inferior oblique muscle paralysis: Qiuhou (Extra), Zanzhu (U.B. 2), Chengqi (St. 1), Ganshu (U.B. 18), Pishu (U.B. 20), Shenshu (U.B. 23)
Method: Retain the needles for 20 minutes. Set the frequency and stimulation to the tolerance of the patient but causing maximum contraction of the eyelid. Then reduce the frequency and stimulation gradually. Treat daily. Ten treatments constitute one course, and 1-14 courses are needed for treatment.
Results: Of 17 cases treated, 12 were cured, 1 case was nearly cured, 2 cases showed marked effect, 1 case showed some improvement

and no effect was evident in 1 case.

(*Source:* Liaoning Journal of Traditional Chinese Medicine, (12):29, 1983)

2. Observed results of acupuncture in treating 24 cases of myasthenia gravis of musculi oculi

Principal points: Zanzhu (U.B. 2), Yangbai (G.B. 14), Yuyao (Extra)

Supplementary points: Zusanli (St. 36), Sanyinjiao (Sp. 6), Taiyang (Extra), Sibai (St. 2). For double vision, add Jingming (U.B. 1) and Fengchi (G.B. 20)

Method: Apply shallow insertion for mild stimulation, selecting 4-5 points each time, and alternating the points. Provide Zusanli (St. 36) and Sanyinjiao (Sp. 6) with moxibustion after needling. Treat daily.

Results: All the cases were cured. Usually, 10-30 treatments were needed.

(*Source:* Shandong Journal of Traditional Chinese Medicine, (2), 1984)

105. Night Blindness

Principal points: Jingming (U.B. 1), Zanzhu (U.B. 2), Fengchi (G.B. 20), Chengqi (St. 1), Guangming (G.B. 37), Hegu (L.I. 4), Qiuhou (Extra)

Method: Slowly and gently twirl and insert at points around eyes, after insertion, no lifting, thrusting, twirling or rotating should be used at points of Jingming (U.B. 1), and Qiuhou (Extra). Do not retain the needles. Use a cotton ball to press for one minute as soon as the needle is withdrawn, so as to avoid a subcutaneous hemorrhage. Moderate stimulation can be used for the other points. Retain the needles for 20-30 minutes. Treat daily or once every other day. Ten treatments constitute one course.

Supplementary points:

Yin deficiency of the liver and kidney: Ganshu (U.B. 18), Shenshu (U.B. 23), Taixi (K. 3)

Yang deficiency of the spleen and kidney: Pishu (U.B. 20), Shenshu (U.B. 23), Mingmen (Du 4), combining with warm-needle or moxibustion

Deficient *qi* and blood: Zusanli (St. 36), Sanyinjiao (Sp. 6), adding moxibustion after needling

Headache and dizziness: Shangxing (Du 23), Taiyang (Extra), Baihui (Du 20)

Palpitation and insomnia: Shenmen (H. 7), Neiguan (P. 6)

Other therapies:

1. Ear acupuncture

Points: Eye, Liver, Kidney, Heart, Spleen

Method: Select 2-3 points in a session. Use the above-mentioned points in turn with moderate stimulation. Retain the needles for 30 minutes with periodic manipulation. Treat once every other day. Ten treatments constitute one course.

2. Hydro-acupuncture

Points: Ganshu (U.B. 18), Shenshu (U.B. 23), Pishu (U.B. 20), Danshu (U.B. 19), Zusanli (St. 36), Zhaohai (K. 6)

Method: Choose 2-3 points in a session. Inject 0.5 ml of 100 mg/ml Vitamin B_1 solution into each point. Treat once every other day. Fifteen treatments constitute one course.

Remarks: Acupuncture is quite effective in the treatment of this illness. In combination with conventional or herbal medicine it can shorten the length of recovery and enhance the therapeutic result.

REFERENCE:

Observed results of acupuncture in treating night blindness

Points: Zanzhu (U.B. 2), Sizhukong (S.J. 23), Hegu (L.I. 4), Sibai (St. 2), Yuyao (Extra), Quchi (L.I. 11)

Method: Treat daily.

Results: Of 4 cases treated, recovery was completely achieved after 3-4 treatments.

(*Source:* Jiangxi Journal of Traditional Chinese Medicine, (2):32, 1960)

106. Color Blindness

Principal points: Jingming (U.B. 1), Qiuhou (Extra), Zanzhu (U.B. 2), Guangming (G.B. 37), Fengchi (G.B. 20)

Method: Apply slowly rotated insertion at the points around the eye. Withdraw the needle to the subcutaneous region, and then pull it out rapidly. Press with a cotton ball for one minute to avoid bleeding.

No twirling, rotating, lifting or thrusting should be applied at Jingming (U.B. 1). Do not retain the needle. When Qiuhou (Extra) is punctured, gently push the eyeball upward, and slowly puncture the point straightly along the orbital ridge to a depth of 0.5-1.5 *cun*. Do not lift, thrust or retain the needle. Moderate stimulation can be applied to the other points. Retain the needles for 20-30 minutes. Treat daily or once every other day. Ten treatments constitute one course.

Supplementary points:

Deficiency of the liver and kidney: Ganshu (U.B. 18), Shenshu (U.B. 23)

Deficient *qi* and blood: Pishu (U.B. 20), Zusanli (St. 36), adding moxibustion after needling

Dizziness and tinnitus: Taixi (K. 3), Sanyinjiao (Sp. 6)

Dryness of eyes: Yingu (K. 10), Ququan (Liv. 8)

Distention of eyes: Geshu (U.B. 17), Neiguan (P. 6), Taiyang (Extra)

Other therapies:

1. Ear acupuncture

Points: Eye, Liver, Kidney

Method: Use filiform needles with mild stimulation. Retain the needles for 20 minutes. Treat daily or once every other day. Ten treatments constitute one course. Or use needle-embedding or seed-embedding method.

2. Cutaneous acupuncture

Points: Zanzhu (U.B. 2), Sibai (St. 2), Sizhukong (S.J. 23), Yangbai (G.B. 14), Fengchi (G.B. 20), Ganshu (U.B. 18), Shenshu (U.B. 23), Dazhui (Du 14)

Method: Apply mild stimulation to the points around the eye, but moderate stimulation for the other points. Treat daily. Ten treatments constitute one course.

3. Electro-acupuncture

Points: Tongziliao (G.B. 1), Sizhukong (S.J. 23), Zanzhu (U.B. 2), Yangbai (G.B. 14), Fengchi (G.B. 20), Guangming (G.B. 37), Hegu (L.I. 4), Zusanli (St. 36)

Method: Connect one point around the eye pairing with one point of the limb with the electro-stimulator. Use sparse-dense or intermittent pulsation with moderate stimulation to the tolerance of the patient for 10-20 minutes in a session. Treat daily. Ten treatments constitute one course. Begin another course after five days' rest.

4. Hydro-acupuncture

Points: Yifeng (S.J. 17), Taiyang (Extra), Fengchi (G.B. 20), Ganshu (U.B. 18), Zusanli (St. 36)

Method: Choose 2-3 points for each session. The above-mentioned points can be used in turn. Inject 0.5 ml of 100 mg/ml Vitamin B_1 solution into each point. Treat once every other day. Ten treatments constitute one course.

Remarks: Acupuncture has certain effect to the treatment of color blindness. Usually, 3-5 courses are needed for treatment. In addition to local points around the eye, selecting the points based on differentiation of syndromes is most important in treating the root cause.

REFERENCE:

Clinical observation on electro-acupuncture in treating 200 cases of color blindness

Points: a) Jingming (U.B. 1), Sizhukong (S.J. 23), Tongziliao (G.B. 1), Shangguan (G.B. 3), Zusanli (St. 36); b) Qiuhou (Extra), Zanzhu (U.B. 2), Yiming (Extra), Hegu (L.I. 4); c) Yangbai (G.B. 14), Yuyao (Extra), Taiyang (Extra), Fengchi (G.B. 20), Taichong (Liv. 3) or Foot-Linqi (G.B. 41)

Method: Puncture bilaterally. Every day select one group of points for a session. Use the three groups in turn. For the purpose of reinforcing or reducing, needle most of points with twirling and rotating only. Apply reinforcing method to points on the limbs, and even method to points around or near the eye. A Model G-6805 electro-stimulator, made in Shanghai, is often adopted with intermittent pulsation for 15-20 minutes. Set the frequency to the tolerance of the patient. Treat daily. Ten treatments constitute one course. Begin another course after 3-6 days' rest.

Results: The total effective rate for short-term therapeutic result reached 94 percent, with 47 percent cured, 28 percent showing marked effect and 19 percent improving.

(*Source:* New Journal of Traditional Chinese Medicine, (7):40, 1983)

107. Myopia (Near sightedness)

Points: Jingming (U.B. 1), Zanzhu (U.B. 2), Chengqi (St. 1),

Fengchi (G.B. 20), Hegu (L.I. 4), Guangming (G.B. 37)

Method: After instructing the patient to close his eyes, gently push the eyeball laterally and away from Jingming (U.B. 1), and fix it with your finger. Then slowly insert the needle between the orbit and the nose to a depth of 0.5-1 *cun*. While the needle is inserted, no lifting, thrusting, twirling or rotating should be applied. Do not retain the needle. Puncture Chengqi (St. 1) with slanted insertion towards the inner canthus. Needle Fengchi (G.B. 20) to a 1-1.5 *cun* depth towards the opposite eyeball and let the needling sensation extend to the temple and eye. Retain the needles for 15-30 minutes. Treat daily or once every other day. Ten treatments constitute one course.

Supplementary points:

Deficiency of the liver and kidney: Ganshu (U.B. 18), Shenshu (U.B. 23), Taixi (K. 3), combining with moxibustion

Deficient *qi* and blood: Zusanli (St. 36), Sanyinjiao (Sp. 6), combining with moxibustion

Dizziness, blurred vision: Baihui (Du 20), Taiyang (Extra)

Other therapies:

1. Ear acupuncture

Points: Eye, Liver, Kidney

Method: Use filiform needles with moderate stimulation. Retain the needles for 20-30 minutes. Treat once every other day. Ten treatments constitute one course. Or, apply vaccaria seeds with a piece of adhesive tape to the ear point. Instruct the patient to press them once in the morning and once in the evening. Three minutes of pressure is needed for each point. The adhesive tape and seeds should be changed once a week.

2. Cutaneous acupuncture

Points: Zanzhu (U.B. 2), Sizhukong (S.J. 23), Sibai (St. 2), Yangbai (G.B. 14), Taiyang (Extra), Fengchi (G.B. 20)

Method: Tap points around the eye gently with a plum-blossom needle. Apply moderate stimulation to Fengchi (G.B. 20) until local reddish color appears in the skin. Treat daily. Ten treatments constitute one course. Or use an electric plum-blossom needle. Point prescription is the same.

Remarks: Acupuncture therapy is quite effective in the treatment of myopia, especially pseudomyopia in children and adolescents. In order to consolidate the therapeutic result, eye-massage care can be used in combination. Instruct the patient to massage Fengchi (G.B.

20), Taiyang (Extra), Yangbai (G.B. 14), Chengqi (St. 1), Zanzhu (U.B. 2), 2-3 points each time and each point for 3-5 minutes. Treat once or twice a day.

REFERENCES:

1. Observed results of puncturing Qiuhou (Extra) in treating 210 cases of myopia

Point: Qiuhou (Extra)

Method: If the case involves myopia in one eye, puncture Qiuhou (Extra) on the healthy side. With myopia in both eyes, puncture Qiuhou (Extra) first on the side where the symptoms are mild, then on the severe side. Do not retain the needle with a patient who is sensitive or fainting, but apply twirling and rotating gently to a severe case. Retain the needles for 30 minutes. For those who exhibit a dull response and poor vision, apply strong stimulation. Treat daily. Twelve treatments constitute one course. Begin another course after three days' rest.

Results: In general, a positive effect can be obtained after 1-2 courses.

(*Source:* Guangxi Journal of Traditional Chinese Medicine, (3):46, 1981)

2. Observation of the long-term therapeutic result of low voltage electro-acupuncture in treating 100 cases of myopia

Points: Chengqi (St. 1), lower Jingming (U.B. 1), Yanglao (S.I. 6), Hegu (L.I. 4)

Method: After insertion and the needling sensation obtained, connect the needles with a Model EDE-1 electro-stimulator. For the treatment of myopia, use low voltage and retain the needles for 15 minutes. Treat daily. Ten treatments constitute one course.

Results: In cases the treatment was ceased for one year after over 10 treatments, marked effect (vision test showed 5 lines more than that before treatment) was seen in 42 eyes. Improvement (vision test showed 2 lines more than that before treatment) was evident in 97 eyes. No effect was seen in 61 eyes. The total effective rate was 69.5 percent. When the treatment was ceased for 3 years, marked effect was seen in 12 eyes. Improvement was evident in 37 eyes and no effect was seen in 151 eyes. The total effective rate was 24.5 percent.

(*Source:* Shanghai Journal of Acupuncture and Moxibustion, (2):25, 1987)

3. Observed results of wrist-and-ankle acupuncture in treating 151

cases of myopia

Point: Upper 1

Method: Choose the bilateral points for myopia in both eyes, but one point on the affected side for myopia in one eye. The needle insertion should not cause pain. If there is pain due to the insertion, withdraw the needle to the continuous region and then reinsert. Retain the needle for an hour. Instruct the patient to look at a place faraway while the needle is in the point. Treat daily. Ten treatments constitute one course. Begin another course after rest for five days. Usually 2-3 courses are needed for treatment.

Results: The therapeutic standard: cured is when vision through treatment reaches 1.0 degree or more; marked effect is when vision increases 3 lines more but below 1.0 degree; improvement is when vision increases 1-2 lines; no effect is when vision remains unchanged.

Of 151 cases (299 eyes) treated, 17 eyes (5.7 percent) were cured, marked effect was evident in 97 eyes (32.4 percent), improvement was seen in 139 eyes (46.5 percent), and no effect was seen in 46 eyes (15.4 percent). The total effective rate was 84.6 percent.

(*Source:* Shanghai Journal of Acupuncture and Moxibustion, (4):11, 1987)

4. Observed results of pressing ear points in treating 99 cases of myopia

Points: Heart, Liver, Eye, Eye 1, Eye 2

Method: Apply vaccaria seeds with adhesive tapes at the points. Instruct the patient to press them several times in the morning, at noon, and in the evening. Vaccaria seeds and adhesive tapes should be changed once every two days. Both ears can be applied in turn. Eight treatments constitute one course.

Results: After 1-2 courses of treatment, cases with vision that reached more than 1.0 degree occupied 18.8 percent; cases with vision that increased 3 lines but lower than 1.0 degree occupied 25.4 percent; and cases with vision that increased 2 lines occupied 35.4 percent. The total effective rate was 79.6 percent.

(*Source:* Jiangsu Chinese Medical Journal, 7(12):21, 1986)

108. Strabismus

Principal points:

Esotropia (musculus rectus lateralis paralysis): Qiuhou (Extra), Taiyang (Extra), Sizhukong (S.J. 23), Hegu (L.I. 4)

Exotropia (musculus rectus medialis paralysis): Jingming (U.B. 1), Sibai (St. 2), Zanzhu (U.B. 2), Fengchi (G.B. 20)

Method: In puncturing Qiuhou (Extra), push the eyeball gently upward and slowly insert the needle along the infraorbital ridge to a depth of 0.5-1 *cun*. Withdraw the needle after the needling sensation of distention and soreness is obtained. Do not retain the needle. Straightly insert at Taiyang (Extra) to a depth of 0.5-1 *cun*. Puncture Sizhukong (S.J. 23) joining Yuyao (Extra) with 0.5-1 *cun* insertion. Apply straight insertion to a depth of 0.5-1 *cun* at Hegu (L.I. 4). In needling Jingming (U.B. 1) gently push the eyeball laterally and away from the point. Straightly insert the needle along the orbital ridge to a depth of 0.5-1 *cun*. No twirling, rotating, lifting or thrusting is allowed. Withdraw the needle after the sensation of distention and soreness is obtained. Do not retain the needle. Apply straight insertion to a depth of 0.3 *cun* at Sibai (St. 2). Insert slanted downward to a depth of 0.3-0.5 *cun* at Zanzhu (U.B. 2) in the direction of Jingming (U.B. 1). Gently press the point for several minutes after withdrawing the needle. In general, retain the needles for 10-15 minutes. Treat daily. Ten treatments constitute one course.

Supplementary points:
Esotropia: Tongziliao (G.B. 1)
Exotropia: Yintang (Extra)
Other therapies:
Electro-acupuncture
Points:
Exotropia: Jingming (U.B. 1), Hegu (L.I. 4)
Esotropia: Tongziliao (G.B. 1), Hegu (L.I. 4)
Method: Use sparse-dense, or intermittent electric pulsation with moderate stimulation for 10-15 minutes. Treat daily or once every other day. Ten treatments constitute one course. Begin another course after 3-5 days' rest.

Remarks: Acupuncture and electro-acupuncture have certain effect in the treatment of strabismus, especially short-term strabismus duration.

REFERENCES:

1. Based on differentiation of syndromes, using plum-blossom needle in treating 103 cases of common strabismus

Principal points: Zhengguang (Extra, at the middle point between Zanzhu, U.B. 2, and Yuyao, Extra, inferior to the superior orbital ridge), Zhengguang 2 (Extra, at the middle point between Sizhukong, S.J. 23, and Yuyao, Extra, inferior to the superior orbital ridge)

Supplementary points:

Deficient blood in the liver: Fengchi (G.B. 20), Ganshu (U.B. 18), Danshu (U.B. 19), Neiguan (P. 6), Baihui (Du 20)

Deficient *qi* in the spleen: Pishu (U.B. 20), Weishu (U.B. 21), Zhongwan (Ren 12), Baihui (Du 20), Fengchi (G.B. 20), Neiguan (P. 6), Zusanli (St. 36)

Deficiency of the kidney: Shenshu (U.B. 23), Fengchi (G.B. 20), Ganshu (U.B. 18), Danshu (U.B. 19), Dazhui (Du 14), and two sides along the lumbar vertebrae

Eye's position nearly restored: Zhengguang (Extra), Zhengguang 2 (Extra), Fengchi (G.B. 20), two sides along T8-T12 and lumbar vertebrae, Baihui (Du 20), Ganshu (U.B. 18), Danshu (U.B. 19), Pishu (U.B. 20), Shenshu (U.B. 23), Zhongwan (Ren 12) or Dazhui (Du 14)

Method: Connect a plum-blossom needle to an electro-stimulator with the highest frequency which the patient can tolerate. Tap evenly at the area 0.5-1.5 *cun* around each point 20-50 times. Treat once every other day. Fifteen treatments in a month constitute one course. Begin another course after 15 days' rest.

Results: Among 182 eyes in 103 cases, 57 eyes recovered, 101 eyes showed marked effect, 21 eyes were improvement and 3 eyes displayed no effect. The total effective rate was 98.3 percent.

(*Source:* Chinese Acupuncture & Moxibustion, 4(2):11, 1984)

2. Therapeutic result observation on acupuncture in treating 10 cases of strabismus

Points:

Exotropia: Zanzhu (U.B. 2), Yuyao (Extra), or middle point of eyebrow

Esotropia: Tongziliao (G.B. 1), the end of eyebrow, Sizhukong (S.J. 23)

Method: 10-15 treatments constitute one course.

Results: Among 3 mild cases, all were cured. Among 3 medium cases, 1 was cured, 1 was improved, and 1 showed no effect. Among 4 severe cases, 1 was cured, 1 showed marked effect, 1 was improved, and 1 showed no effect.

(*Source:* Fujian Journal of Traditional Chinese Medicine, 1(1):32, 1981)

3. Clinical observation on acupuncture in treating 18 cases of double vision (diplopia) due to ophthalmo-paralysis

Points:

Musculus rectus medialis paralysis: Jingming (U.B. 1) with reinforcing method, Zanzhu (U.B. 2) joining Yuyao (Extra), Yintang (Extra) with reducing method

Musculus rectus lateralis paralysis: Taiyang (Extra) with reinforcing method, Tongziliao (G.B. 1) joining Yuyao (Extra), Anmian (Extra) with reducing method

Musculus rectus inferior paralysis: Chengqi (St. 1) with reinforcing method, Sibai (St. 2), Taiyang (Extra) with reducing method

Musculus rectus superior paralysis: Shangming (Extra, also named Shangchengqi), Yangbai (G.B. 14), Yintang (Extra), Yuyao (Extra)

Method: Retain the needles for 45 minutes after the needling sensation is obtained. Treat daily or once every other day. Fifteen treatments constitute one course.

Results: Of 18 cases treated, 16 were cured and the remaining 2 showed improvement.

(*Source:* Yunnan Journal of Traditional Chinese Medicine, 2(4):32, 1981)

109. Optic Atrophy

Principal points: Jingming (U.B. 1), Qiuhou (Extra), Fengchi (G.B. 20), Hegu (L.I. 4)

Method: Puncture Fengchi (G.B. 20) to a depth of 1-1.5 *cun*, applying slanted insertion. The tip of the needle should be pointed to the direction of the opposite eyeball. Try to let the needling sensation extend to the eye's region. Puncture Qiuhou (Extra) with straight insertion. Before the treatment, instruct the patient to look upward. Then secure the eyeball from below with a finger, and slowly insert the needle along the orbital ridge to a depth of 1-1.5 *cun*. Let the needling sensation extend throughout the eye. Do not lift, thrust, twirl or rotate the needle. No retaining is allowed. When puncturing Jingming (U.B. 1), first instruct the patient to close his eyes, and gently push the eyeball laterally and away from the point, holding it with one finger. Then slowly insert the needle between the orbit and the nose bone to a depth of 1-1.5 *cun*. Do not lift, thrust, twirl or rotate the needle. Retaining the needle is not advisable. Puncture Fengchi (G.B. 20) and Hegu (L.I. 4), and retain the needles for 20-30 minutes. Treat once every other day. Ten treatments constitute one course.

Supplementary points:

Yin deficiency in the liver and kidney: Ganshu (U.B. 18), Shenshu (U.B. 23), combining with moxibustion

Yang deficiency of the spleen and kidney: Pishu (U.B. 20), Shenshu (U.B. 23), Zusanli (St. 36), with reinforcing method, and combining with moxibustion

Qi stagnation in the liver: Shanzhong (Ren 17), Taichong (Liv. 3), Guangming (G.B. 37)

Qi stagnation and blood stasis: Geshu (U.B. 17), Neiguan (P. 6)

Deficient blood in the heart: Shenmen (H. 7), Geshu (U.B. 17), Xinshu (U.B. 15)

Distention of eyes: Guanchong (S.J. 1), pricking to cause bleeding

Insomnia or dreamful sleep: Shenmen (H. 7)

Other therapies:

1. Cutaneous acupuncture

Points: Eye area, Jiaji points (Extra) from T5-T12, Ganshu (U.B. 18), Shenshu (U.B. 23), Fengchi (G.B. 20)

Method: Tap gently around the eye area, and the other points with moderate stimulation. Treat once every other day.

2. Hydro-acupuncture

Points: Zusanli (St. 36), Sanyinjiao (Sp. 6), Guangming (G.B. 37), Ganshu (U.B. 18)

Method: Inject 0.5 ml of 0.015 mg/ml Vitamin B_{12} solution into each point. Treat once every other day. Ten treatments constitute one course.

3. Ear acupuncture

Points: Eye, Liver, Brain

Method: Use filiform needles, with moderate stimulation. Retain the needles for 10-15 minutes. Treat daily or once every other day. Ten treatments constitute one course. Needle-embedding can also be used.

Remarks: Acupuncture has certain effect on the treatment of optic atrophy. Generally speaking, continuous treatments are needed for 3-6 months.

270

The blood vessels around the eyes are abundant, and the tissues are very loose. Puncturing Jingming (U.B. 1), Qiuhou (Extra) or the other points around eyes may cause internal bleeding or a black eye, but will not affect the vision. After 1-3 weeks, it will vanish. To avoid bleeding, the needle should be inserted slowly with no lifting or thrusting. Bleeding can be stopped by applying pressure at the point for 1-2 minutes after the needle is withdrawn.

REFERENCES:

1. Observed results of needling Qiuhou (Extra) in treating 38 cases of optic atrophy

Points: Qiuhou (Extra), combined with Yiming (Extra)

Method: Insert at Qiuhou (Extra) to a depth of 1.5-2 *cun*, and at Yiming (Extra) to a depth of 1 *cun*. Retain the needles for five minutes. Treat daily. Ten treatments constitute one course. Begin another course after five days' rest.

Results: More than 1.0-degree vision increase was seen in 9 eyes. Marked effect was evident in 11 eyes, improvement in 25 eyes, and no effect in 20 eyes.

(*Source:* Journal of Traditional Chinese Medicine, 29(5):48, 1988)

2. Therapeutic result analysis on electro-acupuncture applied at Xingming (Extra) in treating 150 cases of eye disorders

Points: Xingming 1 (Extra, middle way between the posterior inferior part of the auricle and the skin crease behind the earlobe or 0.5 *cun* anterior and superior to the depression between the mastoid of temporal bone and the posterior border of mandibular branch), Xingming 2 (Extra, on the forehead, 0.5 *cun* lateral to the place which is 1 *cun* directly above the lateral end of eyebrow)

Method: Insert at a 45-degree angle to a depth of 1-1.5 *cun* at Xingming 1 (Extra). Insert horizontally towards the forehead to a depth of 0.5-0.8 *cun* at Xingming 2 (Extra).

Results: Among 150 cases with 14 kinds of eye disorders, a cure was obtained in 71 eyes, marked effect in 73 eyes, improvement in 80 eyes and no effect in 9 eyes. The total effective rate reached 96.13 percent.

Remarks: This method is not only effective in treating frequently encountered eye disorders, but also stubborn eye disorders, such as: optic atrophy, optical fundus disorders, vitreous opacity, strabismus, amblyopia and ametropia.

(*Source:* Shanxi Traditional Chinese Medicine, "Additional Publication of Acupuncture and Moxibustion," (7), 1981)

3. Therapeutic result analysis on acupuncture in treating 74 cases of central serious retinopathy

Points: Yifeng (S.J. 17) joining Qubin (G.B. 7), Sizhukong (S.J. 23)

Method: Puncture with even method and let the needling sensation extend to the eye region. Then connect the needles with the electro-stimulator for 20-30 minutes. Choose two points on the affected side, or bilateral sides if both eyes are affected. Use two points in turn. Treat three times a week. Ten treatments constitute one course. The interval between two courses is three days.

Results: Among 90 eyes, 42 eyes were cured, marked effect was seen in 16 eyes, improvement in 24 eyes, and no effect in 8 eyes.

(*Source:* Chinese Acupuncture & Moxibustion, 4(1):8, 1984)

4. Observed results of using a plum-blossom needle in treating three cases of sudden blindness

Principal points: Jingming (U.B. 1), Zanzhu (U.B. 2), Yuyao (Extra), Sizhukong (S.J. 23), Tongziliao (G.B. 1), Taiyang (Extra), Chengqi (St. 1)

Supplementary points: Ear Pts. Liver, Kidney, Eye; Yiming (Extra), Hegu (L.I. 4), massaging on Binao (L.I. 14)

Method: Tap with the plum-blossom needle.

Results: All three cases were cured by one treatment.

(*Source:* New Journal of Traditional Chinese Medicine, (4):35, 1984)

5. Clinical observation on acupuncture in treating 20 cases of cortical psychic blindness

Points: a) Jingming (U.B. 1), Sibai (St. 2), Taichong (Liv. 3); b) Zanzhu (U.B. 2), Fengchi (G.B. 20), Guangming (G.B. 37), Hegu (L.I. 4)

Method: Use the two groups in turn. Treat daily. Apply reinforcing method at Jingming (U.B. 1), Sibai (St. 2) and Zanzhu (U.B. 2), and puncture the other points with the even method.

Results: All were cured by 6-17 treatments.

(*Source:* Chinese Acupuncture & Moxibustion, 4(3):13, 1984)

110. Tympanitis

Principal points: Tinggong (S.I. 19), Yifeng (S.J. 17), Qiuxu (G.B. 40), Hegu (L.I. 4)

Method: Select points around the ear on the affected side, and bilateral points on the limbs for the treatment. Use filiform needles with strong stimulation and reducing method. Retain the needles for 20-30 minutes. For acute tympanitis, treat daily. For chronic tympanitis, treat daily or once every other day.

Supplementary points:

Excessive heat: Dazhui (Du 14), Quchi (L.I. 11)

Headache: Taiyang (Extra), Shangxing (Du 23)

Flaring-up of fire of the gall bladder: Fengchi (G.B. 20), Foot-Linqi (G.B. 41), Waiguan (S.J. 5)

Excessive dampness and deficiency of the spleen: Zusanli (St. 36), Yinlingquan (Sp. 9), with reinforcing method, and combining with moxibustion

Other therapies:

1. Ear acupuncture

Points: Kidney, Internal Ear, External Ear, Intertragicus, Occiput

Method: Puncture with moderate stimulation. Retain the needles for 20-30 minutes. Treat daily. If there is fever present, cause bleeding at the small veins behind the ear.

2. Moxibustion

Point: Yifeng (S.J. 17)

Method: Light the moxa stick at one end and hold about 1 *cun* from the surface of the skin. Burn the moxa stick until the skin becomes warm and reddish in color. Before the treatment, use sterilized cotton balls to clean pus and fluid in external auditory canal, wash with instillation of hydrogen peroxide solution, and clean again with sterilized cotton ball. Then apply moxibustion with the moxa stick. After moxibustion, place a piece of drainage tissue in the ear for evacuation of pus. Duration of moxibustion is about one minute in a session. Treat daily.

3. Hydro-acupuncture

Points: Yifeng (S.J. 17), Ermen (S.J. 21), Tinggong (S.I. 19), Fengchi (G.B. 20), Waiguan (S.J. 5), Taiyang (Extra)

Method: Select 1-2 points around the ear in a session, combined with the point on the upper limb. Inject 1 ml of 0.5% procaine hydrochloride solution into each point. Treat once or twice a day.

Remarks: Acupuncture and moxibustion are quite effective in the treatment of tympanitis.

REFERENCES:

1. Clinical therapeutic result observation on He-Ne laser light on acupoints in treating 70 cases of acute tympanitis

Principal points: Tinghui (G.B. 2), Yifeng (S.J. 17), Zusanli (St. 36), Qiuxu (G.B. 40)

Supplementary points: Ermen (S.J. 21), Quchi (L.I. 11), Taixi (K. 3), Ashi point on the ear cochlea

Method: Choose 2-4 points unilaterally or bilaterally in a session. Before treating, clean pus and fluid in external auditory canal by instilling 2% hydrogen peroxide solution. Use the Model 795-B He-Ne laser stimulator with two tubes, wavelength 6328Å, laser power output 10 mw, light diameter 1.5 mm, and at a distance of 20 cm from acupoints. Radiate each point for five minutes. Ten treatments constitute one course. Two consolidation treatments are needed after recovery from chronic tympanitis in the acute stage.

Results: Among 70 cases with 100 ears affected by tympanitis, 75 ears were cured, improvement was evident in 20 ears and no effect was seen in 5 ears. The effective rate was 95 percent, the cure rate reached 75 percent.

(*Source:* Chinese Acupuncture & Moxibustion, (5):9, 1987)

2. Therapeutic observation on ear acupuncture in treating 34 cases of chronic tympanitis with pus

Points: Mouth, Tragic Apex, Middle Conchae, Internal Ear

Method: Insert cutaneous needles to a depth of 3-5 mm, then fix them with adhesive tape. Instruct the patient to press Pt. Mouth 3-5 times a day. Generally speaking, pus and fluid in the ear disappear after 2-7 treatments. Then apply another three treatments for consolidation.

Results: Of 51 ears treated, 44 ears were cured, improvement was evident in 4 ears and no effect was seen in 3 ears.

(*Source:* Chinese Acupuncture & Moxibustion, 5(5):15, 1985)

111. Tinnitus, Deafness

Principal points: Yifeng (S.J. 17), Tinghui (G.B. 2), Xiaxi (G.B.

43), Hand-Zhongzhu (S.J. 3)

Method: Puncture Tinghui (G.B. 2) first. Ask the patient to open his mouth, and then insert the needle straight into a depth of 1 *cun*. Withdraw the needle after the needling sensation is obtained. Puncture Yifeng (S.J. 17) with straight insertion to a depth of about 1 *cun*. Try to get the sensation of soreness and numbness in the ear while needling. Puncture Xiaxi (G.B. 43) and Hand-Zhongzhu (S.J. 3) with moderate stimulation. Retain the needles for 30 minutes with periodic manipulation. Treat daily or once every other day.

Supplementary points:

Invasion by exogenous wind: Waiguan (S.J. 5), Hegu (L.I. 4)

Excessive fire in the liver and gall bladder: Xingjian (Liv. 2), Foot-Linqi (G.B. 41)

Deficient essence in the kidney: Shenshu (U.B. 23), Taixi (K. 3)

Deficient *qi* in the middle *jiao*: Pishu (U.B. 20), Zusanli (St. 36), combining with moxibustion

Dizziness and vertigo: Baihui (Du 20), Fengchi (G.B. 20)

Spermatorrhea and impotence: Zhishi (U.B. 52), Qugu (Ren 2)

Other therapies:

1. Ear acupuncture

Points: Brain, Intertragicus, Liver, Kidney

Method: Select points on the affected side or bilateral points. Use filiform needles with strong stimulation, or connect with an electro-stimulator. Retain the needles for 30-60 minutes. Treat daily or once every other day. Approximately 15-20 treatments constitute one course. Needle-embedding can also be used.

2. Hydro-acupuncture

Points: Fengchi (G.B. 20), Yifeng (S.J. 17), Ermen (S.J. 21), Tinggong (S.I. 19), Waiguan (S.J. 5), Sanyinjiao (Sp. 6)

Method: Choose 1-2 points on the head and one point on the limb in a session. The above-mentioned points can be selected in turn for the treatment. Inject 0.5-1.5 ml of 0.1-0.25% procaine hydrochloride solution into each point. Treat daily. Ten treatments make one course. Begin another course after a week's rest.

3. Head acupuncture

Points: Vertigo and Hearing Area, bilateral

Method: Puncture horizontally to the scalp with rapidly insertion. Twirling may be continued for 5-10 minutes. Then retain the needles for 30 minutes. Treat once every 2-3 days.

Remarks: Acupuncture has certain effect to the treatment of this illness, the shorter the duration of the illness, the better result. As to tinnitus deafness resulted from some underlying cause with general manifestations, the primary cause must be carefully determined and treated accordingly.

Acupuncture therapy is also effective in the treatment of deaf-mutism. It may enable some patients to restore their hearing and speaking abilities. The treating principle is to treat deafness before mutism. After hearing ability has been restored in a certain degree, further speech training should follow.

For the treatment of mutism, select Lianquan (Ren 23), Neck-Futu (L.I. 18), Tongli (H. 5), Hegu (L.I. 4), and needle with strong stimulation. Retain the needles for 30 minutes. Treat once every other day. Continue treatments for 1-3 months. Besides ear acupuncture, electro-acupuncture, hydro-acupuncture or moxibustion can be taken into consideration to enhance the therapeutic result. In general, after treatments, the patient with a slight hearing ability can obtain a better result.

REFERENCE:

Therapeutic result observation on acupuncture in treating 37 cases of sudden deafness

Points: Shenshu (U.B. 23), Yifeng (S.J. 17), Waiguan (S.J. 5), Tinghui (G.B. 2)

Method: Apply even method. After the needling sensation is obtained, connect the needles to the electro-stimulator for 20-40 minutes. Select four points on the affected side for a problem in one ear, and choose any bilateral two points out of the four points in turn for disorders effecting both ears. Treat six times a week. Twelve treatments constitute one course. Begin another course after rest for two days.

Results: Of 37 cases with 45 ears treated, 26 ears were cured, marked effect was seen in 8 ears, improvement was evident in 8 ears and no effect was seen in 3 ears.

(*Source:* Chinese Acupuncture & Moxibustion, 6(1):28, 1986)

112. Deaf Mutism

Principal points:

For deafness: Tinggong (S.I. 19), Tinghui (G.B. 2), Ermen (S.J.

276

21), Yifeng (S.J. 17)

For mutism: Yamen (Du 15), Lianquan (Ren 23), Tongli (H. 5)

Supplementary points: Hand-Zhongzhu (S.J. 3), Waiguan (S.J. 5), Hegu (L.I. 4).

Method: Treat deafness before mutism. As hearing ability is improved, combine speech training. Select points around the ear as the main points. Select 1-2 points in a session. The above-mentioned points can be used in turn. Insert the needle to a depth of 1.5-2 *cun* after instructing the patient to open his mouth. For children, carefully apply proper insertion to a depth of 1-1.5 *cun* with moderate stimulation. Either do not retain the needles, or retain the needles for 15-20 minutes. Select one supplementary point with moderate stimulation for the treatment. Treat daily, and 10-15 treatments constitute one course. Continue another treatment after 3-7 days' rest.

Other therapies:

1. Electro-acupuncture

Points: Same as above

Method: Use an electro-stimulator with low frequency and moderate stimulation after the needling sensation has been obtained. Treat daily. Each session lasts 10-15 minutes.

2. Head acupuncture

Points: Vertigo and Hearing Area, Speech Area

Method: Follow the routine procedure of head acupuncture.

3. Hydro-acupuncture

Points: Tinggong (S.I. 19), Head-Wangu (G.B. 12), Fengchi (G.B. 20), Yifeng (S.J. 17), Xinshu (U.B. 15), Ganshu (U.B. 18), Shenshu (U.B. 23)

Method: Choose 3-4 points in a session. Inject 0.3-0.5 ml of 10 mg/ml Vitamin B_1 or 15 μg/ml Vitamin B_{12} into each point. Treat once every other day. Ten treatments constitute one course.

Remarks: Acupuncture therapy is effective in the treatment of deaf-mutism, a minority of patients may achieve even better results. Patients with slight hearing ability can be cured by acupuncture treatment. Besides acupuncture, speech training is also a very important measure for the treatment. When Yamen (Du 15) is punctured, accurate location, correct angle, proper depth of insertion and careful manipulation are advisable.

REFERENCE:
Observed results of electro-acupuncture in treating 115 cases of deaf-mutism
Points: Ermen (S.J. 21), Tinggong (S.I. 19), Tinghui (G.B. 2), Tingling (Extra), Tingming (Extra), Yifeng (S.J. 17), Waiguan (S.J. 5), Hegu (L.I. 4), Hand-Zhongzhu (S.J. 3)
Method: The above nine points are divided into three groups. Choose one group of points and connect to an electro-stimulator with three sockets for 30 minutes. Rapidly puncture 1-2 points among Yamen (Du 15), Shanglianquan (Extra), Lianquan (Ren 23), Fengchi (G.B. 20) and Zengyin (Extra). Do not retain the needles. Treat daily. Ten treatments constitute one course. Begin speech training when the patient can hear a loud voice. At the same time continue treatment for consolidation.
Results: Among 99 patients whose age ranged from 2.5 to 20 years old after received two courses' treatments, improvement was seen in 72 cases, the effective rate reaching 72.7 percent. Among 11 patients whose age ranged from 21 to 30 years old, improvement was seen in 7 cases, the effective rate reaching 63.67 percent. Among 5 patients whose age ranged from 31 to 33 years old, improvement was seen in 3 cases, the effective rate reached 60 percent.
(*Source:* Chinese Acupuncture & Moxibustion, (6):46, 1986)

113. Acute Tonsillitis

Principal points: Shaoshang (Lu. 11), Hegu (L.I. 4), Biantaoti (Extra)
Method: Prick Shaoshang (Lu. 11) with a thick filiform needle and cause slight bleeding. Puncture Hegu (L.I. 4) with periodic manipulation, so as to strengthen the needling sensation. Retain the needles for 30 minutes. Treat daily.
Supplementary points:
Fever: Dazhui (Du 14), Quchi (L.I. 11)
Severe sore throat: Yuji (Lu. 10), Shaoze (S.I. 1)
Other therapies:
1. Moxibustion
Point: Jiaosun (S.J. 20)
Method: Apply moxibustion with a burning oiled rush directly

278

over the point. Hair around the point should be parted and the acupoint should be completely exposed. Generally speaking, a cure can be obtained in one treatment.

2. Ear acupuncture

Points: Pharynx and Larynx, Helix 4, Helix 6, Ear Apex, veins on the back of ear

Method: When needling veins on the back of ear, massage the auricle so as to cause slight venous pooling. Use a thick filiform needle to prick once or twice on the vein to let 2-3 drops of blood out. Also prick Ear Apex to cause 2-3 drops of blood. Treat daily. Or select Pharynx and Larynx, Helix 4, and Helix 6, using filiform needles with strong stimulation. Retain the needles for 30-60 minutes. Treat once or twice a day.

3. Blood-letting therapy

Points: Shaoshang (Lu. 11), Shangyang (L.I. 1)

Method: Use a three-edged needle or a thick filiform needle to prick and let a few drops of blood out. Treat daily, and 2-3 treatments constitute one course.

Remarks: Acupuncture and moxibustion therapies can obtain relatively good results in the treatment of acute tonsillitis. The blood-letting therapy can get especially quick results in the treatment. As to chronic tonsillitis in acute attack, acupuncture and moxibustion therapies are also quite effective in improving the symptoms, but the complete recovery requires prolonged treatments.

REFERENCES:

1. Observed results of puncturing Xishang (Extra) in treating 168 cases of acute tonsillitis

Point: Xishang (Extra, 3 *cun* above Ximen, P. 4)

Method: Rapidly insert the needle to a depth of 1-1.5 *cun*, applying a strong reducing method, and rotate with large amplitude. Let the needling sensation of numbness, soreness and distention extend to the shoulder and neck regions. Slowly withdraw the needle after two minutes. Treat once every eight hours in the first day. Then once daily. Hegu (L.I. 4) and Quchi (L.I. 11) may be used as the secondary points.

Results: The cure rate reached 91.65 percent.

(*Source:* Tianjin Medical Journal, (12):608, 1975)

2. Observed results of acupuncture in treating 50 cases of acute

tonsillitis

Point: Shousanli (L.I. 10)

Method: Choose Shousanli (L.I. 10) on the affected side for the treatment. It is better to let the needling sensation extend to the isthmus of fauces.

Results: Of 50 cases treated, 23 were cured by 1 treatment, 14 by 2, 10 by 3 and no effect was seen in 3 cases. Generally speaking, pain was immediately checked after the needle insertion and rotation.

(*Source:* Chinese Acupuncture & Moxibustion, (3):6, 1987)

3. Therapeutic result observation on acupuncture in treating 200 cases of acute tonsillitis

Points: Local area (on the affect side)

Method: Prick the tonsil in 2-4 spots with a three-edged needle to let a few drops of blood out.

Results: Fever was reduced by 1 treatment in 124 cases, and fever was reduced after 2 treatments in 76 cases.

(*Source:* Hebei Journal of Traditional Chinese Medicine, (2):16, 1988)

4. Observed results of bleed-letting by a three-edged needle in treating 28 cases of tonsillitis

Points: Shangyang (L.I. 1), Shaoshang (Lu. 11), Hegu (L.I. 4)

For high fever: add Yongquan (K. 1)

Method: Prick to allow a few drops of blood out at bilateral Shangyang (L.I. 1) and Shaoshang (Lu. 11).

Results: The cure standard includes: pain was checked in 6-15 minutes, normal temperature restored in 6-8 hours, pus absorbed or disappeared in 24-48 hours, and leukocyte reduced from 16,400 to 6,200. The cured rate by 1 treatment was 100 percent.

(*Source:* Chinese Acupuncture & Moxibustion, (5):20, 1984)

114. Laryngopharyngitis

Principal points: Lianquan (Ren 23), Tiantu (Ren 22), Hegu (L.I. 4)

Method: When needling Lianquan (Ren 23), insert the needle towards the root of the tongue to a depth of 0.5-0.8 *cun*. First, insert perpendicularly to a depth of 0.2 *cun* at Tiantu (Ren 22). Then point the needle downward along the posterior side of the manubrium sterni to a depth of 1-1.5 *cun*. Do not puncture too deeply, or do not puncture slantly to the left or the right. No retaining is allowed. Puncture Hegu (L.I. 4) with strong stimulation. Retain the needles at Hegu (L.I. 4) for 30-60 minutes. Treat daily. In cases of acute laryngopharyngitis, treat twice daily.

Supplementary points:

Invasion by exogenous wind and heat: Shaoshang (Lu. 11), Shangyang (L.I. 1), bleeding with a three-edged needle or thick filiform needle

Excessive heat in the lung and stomach: Neiting (St. 44), Yuji (Lu. 10), Xuanji (Ren 21)

Chronic laryngopharyngitis due to *yin* deficiency in the lung and kidney: Taixi (K. 3), Zhaohai (K. 6), Feishu (U.B. 13)

Qi stagnation and blood stasis: Jianshi (P. 5), Sanjian (L.I. 3)

Sudden hoarseness, itching and slight pain in the throat, running nose: Lieque (Lu. 7), Tongli (H. 5)

Headache: Shangxing (Du 23), Taiyang (Extra)

Cough: Chize (Lu. 5), Lieque (Lu. 7)

Nasal obstruction, running nose: Yingxiang (L.I. 20), Nose-Heliao (L.I. 19)

Other therapies:

1. Ear acupuncture

Points: Pharynx and Larynx, Lung, Trachea, Neck

Method: For an acute case, puncture with moderate stimulation and rotate for 2-3 minutes. Retain the needles for an hour. Treat daily. For chronic cases, puncture with mild stimulation. Retain the needles for 30-60 minutes. Treat daily. Ten treatments constitute one course.

2. Laser acupuncture

Point: Zengyin (Extra, the depression lateral to the thyroid cartilage)

Method: Select bilateral Zengyin (Extra) and connect with the He-Ne laser machine in erect position. Set laser power output at 1.5 mw, red light diameter at 0.5 cm and power supply at 0-10 mA. The patient should be in recumbent position. The distance between the light source and the acupuncture point is about 20 cm. Radiate each point for one minute. Treat daily. Ten treatments constitute one course. The interval between courses is 3-5 days. This is applicable to a patient with chronic laryngopharyngitis.

Remarks: Acupuncture is quite effective in the treatment of acute laryngopharyngitis. As to chronic laryngopharyngitis, it has certain effect. Laser acupuncture can do much better, but the courses needed will be rather long.

115. Hoarseness

Principal points: Lianquan (Ren 23), Tianding (L.I. 17), Daying (St. 5), Neck-Futu (L.I. 18), Yuji (Lu. 10)

Method: Puncture with moderate stimulation, applying reducing or even method. Retain the needles for 20-30 minutes. Treat daily or once every other day. Ten treatments constitute one course.

Supplementary points:

Sore throat: Erjian (L.I. 2)

Fever: Hegu (L.I. 4), Quchi (L.I. 11)

Fever due to *yin* deficiency: Taixi (K. 3), Zhaohai (K. 6)

Invasion by exogenous wind: Fengchi (G.B. 20), Waiguan (S.J. 5)

Fire transformed from *qi* stagnation: Taichong (Liv. 3)

Sudden loss of voice: Tongli (H. 5)

Other therapies:

1. Ear acupuncture

Points: Lung, Pharynx and Larynx, Neck, Trachea, Kidney

Method: Use 2-3 points in a session. Puncture with mild stimulation. Treat daily.

2. Hydro-acupuncture

Points: Lianquan (Ren 23), Qiangying (Extra, 2 *cun* lateral to the Adam's apple)

Method: Insert a gauge 5 hypodermic needle into Lianquan (Ren 23) to a depth of 0.5 cm. After the needling sensation is obtained, inject 2 ml of normal saline solution into the point. Treat daily. Or insert a gauge 6 hypodermic needle into Qiangying (Extra) towards the Adam's apple to a depth of 1.5 cm. After the needling sensation is obtained, inject 3 ml of 1% procaine hydrochloride solution into the point. Treat daily.

Remarks: Acupuncture therapy is quite effective in the treatment of acute hoarseness, but poor in the treatment of chronic hoarseness.

REFERENCES:

1. Observed results of acupuncture in treating 115 cases of functional loss of voice

282

Points: a) Tiantu (Ren 22) used for 33 cases; b) Hegu (L.I. 4) for 10 cases; c) Lianquan (Ren 23) for 8 cases; d) bilateral Hegu (L.I. 4) and Tiantu (Ren 22) for 46 cases; e) Lianquan (Ren 23) and Tiantu (Ren 22) for 15 cases; f) Hegu (L.I. 4) and Lianquan (Ren 23) for 3 cases

Method: Apply strong stimulation and reducing method. Voice will be restored as the patient feels stifling sensation in the local area or deep insertion into the trachea giving rise to a loud cough.

Results: Of 115 cases treated, recovery was obtained after 1 treatment in 110 cases. Near recovery was reached in 1 case after multiple treatments. Two cases were cured by electro-acupuncture, and 2 cases were cured by inductance.

(*Source*: Shanghai Journal of Acupuncture and Moxibustion, (4):9, 1987)

2. Clinical observation on ear acupuncture in treating vocal nodules

Principal points: Lung, Large Intestine, Kidney, Urinary Bladder

Supplementary points: Taiyuan (Lu. 9), Lieque (Lu. 7), Hegu (L.I. 4), Zhaohai (K. 6)

Method: Take the ear points as the principal points. For chronic cases, combine the supplementary points. Select bilateral ear points for the treatment. Treat daily. Retain the needles for 30-45 minutes with twice periodic manipulation. Ten treatments constitute one course. The interval between two courses is seven days.

Results: After 1-2 courses' treatments, all the patients recovered their normal voices .The vocal nodules disappeared or only traces remained.

(*Source:* Shaanxi Journal of Traditional Chinese Medicine, 7(11):510, 1986)

3. Observed results of puncturing Renying (St. 9) and Shuitu (St. 10) in treating 50 cases of singers' hypertrophy of vocal cord

Points: Renying (St. 9), Shuitu (St. 10)

Method: Place the patient in a sitting position. To avoid the pulse point of the carotid artery, insert an especially fine filiform needle with "sparrow-pricking" method. Retain the needles for 15-30 minutes. Treat daily. Six treatments constitute one course. Begin another course after a day's rest.

Results: Of 50 cases treated, 14 were cured, 24 showed marked effect and improvement was seen in 12 cases.

(*Source*: Chinese Acupuncture & Moxibustion, (3):17, 1987)

4. Report on acupuncture in treating 22 cases of pharyngoplegia

Principal points: Tiantu (Ren 22), Hegu (L.I. 4), Shaoshang (Lu. 11)

Supplementary points: Tianding (L.I. 17), Yamen (Du 15)

Method: Puncture with reducing method. Retain the needles for 15 minutes with periodic manipulation every five minutes until the appearance of distention and numbness.

Results: Twenty-one cases were cured within 6 treatments, and 1 case was cured after 12 treatments.

(*Source:* Shandong Medical Journal, (8):42, 1964)

116. Toothache

Principal points: Hegu (L.I. 4), Xiaguan (St. 7), Jiache (St. 6), Yifeng (S.J. 17)

Method: Puncture Yifeng (S.J. 17) and Hegu (L.I. 4) with moderate stimulation. Retain the needles for 10-15 minutes. If pain remains, add Xiaguan (St. 7) for upper toothache, Jiache (St. 6) for lower toothache. Retain the needle for 10-15 minutes with periodic manipulation. Treat once or twice a day.

Supplementary points:

Toothache due to wind-heat: Waiguan (S.J. 5), Fengchi (G.B. 20)

Toothache due to upward attacking of fire in the stomach: Neiting (St. 44)

Toothache caused by excessive fire due to deficient *yin*: Taixi (K. 3), Rangu (K. 2)

Headache: Taiyang (Extra), inserting slanted downward to a depth of 1.5 *cun*

Fever: Dazhui (Du 14), Quchi (L.I. 11), pricking to let blood out with a three-edged needle

Other therapies:

1. Ear acupuncture

Points: Jaw, Cheek, Upper Apex of Tragus

Method: Use filiform needles with strong stimulation. Retain the needles for 20-30 minutes. Or use needle-embedding for 2-3 days.

2. Hydro-acupuncture

Points: Hegu (L.I. 4), Taiyang (Extra), Xiaguan (St. 7), Jiache

(St. 6)

   Method: Select Hegu (L.I. 4) and Taiyang (Extra) for upper toothache. Choose Xiaguan (St. 7) and Jiache (St. 6) for lower toothache. According to the routine procedure of hydro-acupuncture, inject 0.5-1 ml of 0.5% procaine hydrochloride solution into each point. Injection starts from Hegu (L.I. 4) on the healthy side or affected side, or bilateral sides. Treat once or twice a day.

   Remarks: Acupuncture therapy is effective in alleviating the pain of toothache. But the cause of the pain must be determined and treated by other means.

REFERENCE:

   Observed results of acupuncture and moxibustion in treating 57 cases of toothache
   Points:
   Upper toothache: Quanliao (S.I. 18), Neiting (St. 44)
   Lower toothache: Jiache (St. 6), Hegu (L.I. 4)
   Fire due to *yin* deficiency: Taixi (K. 3)
   Method: After the needling sensation obtained, retain the needles for 30 minutes with periodic manipulation, rotating once every 10 minutes. Then apply moxibustion with a moxa stick on the points or the local region. Use the "sparrow-pricking" method until pain is completely checked. Treat twice every day.
   Results: Of 57 cases treated, 49 were cured, 6 showed improvement and no effect was evident in 2 cases.
   (*Source:* Shanghai Journal of Acupuncture and Moxibustion, (3):47, 1987)

117. Nasosinusitis

   Principal points: Yingxiang (L.I. 20), Yintang (Extra), Lieque (Lu. 7), Hegu (L.I. 4)
   Method: Use filiform needles with moderate stimulation, and reducing method. Retain the needles for 15-20 minutes. Treat daily or once every other day, and 10-15 treatments constitute one course.
   Supplementary points:
   Bitter taste in the mouth and hypochondriac pain: Foot-Linqi (G.B. 41), Xingjian (Liv. 2)

One-side headache: Fengchi (G.B. 20)
Frontal sinusitis: Shangxing (Du 23), Zanzhu (U.B. 2)
Maxillary sinusitis: Nose-Juliao (St. 3)
Ethmoid sinusitis: Quanliao (S.I. 18)
Impairment of smelling: Tongtian (U.B. 7), Tianzhu (U.B. 10)
Other therapies:
1. Ear acupuncture
Points: Lung, Internal Nose, Lower Apex of Tragus, Forehead, Shenmen
Method: Puncture with strong stimulation. Retain the needles for 20-30 minutes. Treat daily or use needle-embedding method.
2. Needle-embedding method
Points: Zanzhu (U.B. 2), Taiyang (Extra), Sizhukong (S.J. 23), Yangbai (G.B. 14), Dazhui (Du 14), Yuyao (Extra)
Method: Use filiform needles to puncture into the subcutaneous region. Puncture Dazhui (Du 14) downward to a depth of 1-2 cm. Join Yangbai (G.B. 14) to Yuyao (Extra). After the needling sensation obtained, withdraw the needle a bit and leave the needle 1 cm in length in the point. Join Taiyang (Extra) to Sizhukong (S.J. 23). After the needling sensation is obtained, withdraw the needle a bit and leave the needle 0.5 cm in length in the point. Then fix the embedding needles with adhesive tape. Retain the needles for 20 hours. If the disease is not cured, try again.
3. Plum-blossom needle
Points: Jiaji points (Extra) on the neck, Fengchi (G.B. 20), Yingxiang (L.I. 20), Ashi points (on temporal region, and forehead)
Method: Tap with a plum-blossom needle until the local skin becomes reddish in color. Treat daily.
4. Moxibustion
Points: Yintang (Extra), Baihui (Du 20), Shangxing (Du 23), Yingxiang (L.I. 20)
Method: For a chronic case, use moxibustion with 5-7 small moxa cones at each point. Treat daily.
5. Wrist-and-ankle acupuncture
Points: Upper 1, bilateral
Method: Use the routine manipulation in wrist-and-ankle acupuncture.
Remarks: Acupuncture and moxibustion have certain effect to the treatment of nasosinusitis. The courses can be shortened if antibiotics

are combined.

118. Rhinitis

Principal points: Yingxiang (L.I. 20), Yintang (Extra), Hegu (L.I. 4)

Method: When inserting at Yingxiang (L.I. 20), point the tip of the needle towards the ala nasi, and let the needle sensation extend to the nose cavity. Puncture Yintang (Extra) with the tip of the needle downward to a depth of 1 *cun*, then slant to the two sides of the nose, letting the needle sensation extend to the nose cavity. Apply moderate stimulation at Hegu (L.I. 4). Retain the needles for 15-30 minutes with periodic manipulation. Treat daily or once every other day.

Supplementary points:

Acute rhinitis due to invasion by exogenous wind and cold: Fengchi (G.B. 20), Lieque (Lu. 7). Add moxibustion after puncturing.

Acute rhinitis due to invasion by exogenous wind and heat: Quchi (L.I. 11), Waiguan (S.J. 5)

Chronic rhinitis: Feishu (U.B. 13), Taiyuan (Lu. 9), Zusanli (St. 36). Add moxibustion after puncturing or use warm needles.

Atrophic rhinitis: Shangxing (Du 23), Taiyang (Extra), Nose-Heliao (L.I. 19). Apply shallow insertion at Taiyang (Extra), and Shangxing (Du 23) to cause slight bleeding.

Atrophic rhinitis with dryness in the nose: Taiyuan (Lu. 9), Taixi (K. 3)

Allergic rhinitis: Fengchi (G.B. 20), Feishu (U.B. 13), Taiyuan (Lu. 9). Add moxibustion after puncturing.

Severe headache: Taiyang (Extra)

Other therapies:

1. Ear acupuncture

Points: Internal Nose, Forehead, Lung, Lower Apex of Tragus

Method: Use filiform needles with moderate stimulation. Retain the needles for 20-30 minutes with periodic manipulation of twirling and rotating. Treat daily or once every other day.

2. Moxibustion

Point: Feishu (U.B. 13)

Method: Use moxibustion with a moxa stick for 20-30 minutes in a session. Treat once or twice a day

3. Hydro-acupuncture

Points: Yingxiang (L.I. 20), Hegu (L.I. 4)

Method: Use one point in a treatment. The two points was used in turn. Inject 0.2-0.5 ml of Vitamin B₁ complex into the point. Treat once every other day.

Remarks: Acupuncture and moxibustion have certain effect on various rhinitis strains, but are quite effective in the treatment of allergic rhinitis.

REFERENCES:

1. Primary report on acupuncture in treating allergic rhinitis

Principal points: Yingxiang (L.I. 20), Hegu (L.I. 4)

Supplementary points:

Headache: Baihui (Du 20), Yintang (Extra), Yangbai (G.B. 14), Fengchi (G.B. 20), Zanzhu (U.B. 2). Select 1-2 points in a session.

Method: Gently puncture with twirling or rotating until there is a needling sensation of distention, soreness or numbness. Retain the needles for 20 minutes. Treat daily or once every other day.

Results: Of 15 cases in the group treated, 7 cases were cured, marked effect was seen in 6 cases and improvement in 2 cases.

(*Source:* Chinese Otorhinolaryngology Journal, (2):95, 1957)

2. Observed results of deep insertion at Yingxiang (L.I. 20) in treating 10 cases of chronic rhinitis

Point: Yingxiang (L.I. 20)

Method: Apply 35-40 degree insertion to a depth of 0.2-0.5 *cun.* Let the tip reach the anterior and superior border of the inferior nasal concha. Retain the needle for 40 minutes. Treat daily.

Results: The effective rate was 100 percent.

(*Source:* Chinese Acupuncture & Moxibustion, (5):16, 1984)

3. Therapeutic result analysis on ear acupuncture in treating 44 cases of chronic rhinitis

Principal points: Internal Nose, External Nose, Intertragicus, Lower Apex of Tragus, Lung

Supplementary points:

Cough: Ear-asthma

Headache: Shenmen

Method: Apply standard needling techniques.

Results: Of 44 cases treated, 15 were cured, marked effect was evident in 10 cases, improvement was seen in 15 cases and no effect was experienced in 4 cases. The total effective rate reached 91.1 percent.

288

(*Source:* Shanghai Journal of Acupuncture and Moxibustion, (2):34, 1983)

119. Epistaxis

Principal points: Shangxing (Du 23), Yingxiang (L.I. 20), Hegu (L.I. 4), Dazhui (Du 14)

Method: Use a three-edged needle to cause slight bleeding at Dazhui (Du 14) and Shangxing (Du 23). Puncture Hegu (L.I. 4) with moderate stimulation. For acute epistaxis, retain the needles for 3-5 minutes with periodic manipulation until bleeding is checked. For chronic recountered epistaxis, treat daily. Retain the needles for 20-30 minutes.

Supplementary points:

Excessive heat in the lung meridians: Shaoshang (Lu. 11), causing bleeding with a three-edged needle

Excessive heat in the stomach: Neiting (St. 44)

Upward attack of fire of the liver: Taichong (Liv. 3)

Deficient *yin* of the liver and kidney: Taixi (K. 3), Taichong (Liv. 3)

Failure of the spleen in controlling the blood: Yinbai (Sp. 1), Sanyinjiao (Sp. 6). Add moxibustion after puncturing.

Fever: Quchi (L.I. 11)

Invasion by exogenous wind and heat: Fengchi (G.B. 20)

Other therapies:

1. Ear acupuncture

Points: Internal Nose, Lung, Lower Apex of Tragus, Forehead

Method: Use filiform needles with moderate stimulation. Retain the needles for 20-30 minutes after 1-2 minutes rotating. Treat daily.

2. Moxibustion

Point: Fengfu (Du 16)

Method: Use moxibustion with a moxa stick until the bleeding is completely checked. This method is suitable for acute epistaxis. Or apply a garlic paste at Yongquan (K. 1), bilaterally, for 1-3 hours. This is a folk prescription for the treatment of epistaxis. Its therapeutic result is better.

Remarks: Epistaxis refers to a symptom which may be caused by various factors. The first-aid measure is to check bleeding by blocking the nasal cavity. If this fails, acupuncture and moxibustion can be adopted for treatment. Generally speaking, a good therapeutic result to check bleeding can be obtained. In addition to acupuncture treatment, other therapeutic measures should be adopted according to the primary cause.

REFERENCES:
   1. Observed results of acupuncture in treating 30 cases of epistaxis
   Point: Xingjian (Liv. 2)
   Method: Apply contralateral needling with insertion to a depth of 1 *cun*. Retain the needle for 3-5 minutes.
   Results: Of 30 cases treated, 24 cases showed marked effect, 5 cases showed some improvement and 1 case showed no effect.
   (*Source:* Chinese Acupuncture & Moxibustion, (6):5, 1984)
   2. Observed results of moxibustion at Yongquan (K. 1) in treating a case of epistaxis
   Point: Yongquan (K. 1)
   Method: Apply moxibustion with a moxa stick for three minutes.
   Results: It was cured at once.
   (*Source:* Shanghai Journal of Acupuncture and Moxibustion, (2):19, 1986)

120. Temporomandibular Joint Syndrome

   Principal points: Xiaguan (St. 7), Jiache (St. 6), Shangguan (G.B. 3), Ermen (S.J. 21), Hegu (L.I. 4)
   Method: Straightly insert at Ermen (S.J. 21) to a depth of 1 *cun*, with the patient's mouth open. Try to let the needling sensation extend to the cheek. And with the mouth closed, puncture Xiaguan (St. 7) with the tip of the needle pointing to the posterior to a depth of 1 *cun*. The needling sensation should extend to the whole temporomandibular joint. Insert at Shangguan (G.B. 3) to a depth of 0.5-1 *cun* with the needling sensation dispersing. When needling Jiache (St. 6), point the tip of the needle slantly upward, and let the needling sensation radiate to the cheek. Needle Hegu (L.I. 4) with strong stimulation. Retain the needles for 20-30 minutes with periodic manipulation. As to temporomandibular joint syndrome without fever, apply warm needle or moxibustion with a moxa stick to the local area. Treat daily or once every other day. Ten treatments constitute one course.

Supplementary points:

Traumatic injury: Ashi point

Headache: Fengchi (G.B. 20), Taiyang (Extra)

Oscillating sound with the mouth opening and closing due to loose ligament: Quanliao (S.I. 18), combining warm needle or moxibustion with a moxa stick

Other therapies:

1. Hydro-acupuncture

Point: Xiaguan (St. 7)

Method: Place the patient in a sitting position with one side of the head resting on the table or in recumbent position. Inject 1 ml of 0.5 mg dexamethasone mixed with 1 ml of 0.5% procaine hydrochloride solution into the point according to the routine procedure of hydro-acupuncture. Treat once every 3-5 days. Five treatments constitute one course. Stop injecting, if no effect has been proved after two courses of treatment.

2. Electro-acupuncture

Points: Xiaguan (St. 7), Jiache (St. 6), Hegu (L.I. 4)

Method: After the needling sensation is obtained, connect the needles with an electro-stimulator. Use continuous or sparse-dense pulsation and set the frequency to a level the patient can tolerate. Treat once every other day. Each session lasts 15-30 minutes.

Remarks: The illness is very common in clinics. A satisfactory result can be obtained by acupuncture and moxibustion in the treatment of temporomandibular joint syndrome at an early stage. As to a chronic case or a case with manifestations of cold and deficiency, it is better to combine moxibustion for the treatment.

REFERENCES:

1. Observed results of ear acupuncture in treating functional disorders of the temporomandibular joint

Point: At tubercle lateral to the curve of auricular cartilage on the antitragus, which is the spot between Pt. Ear-asthma and Pt. Parotid Gland.

Method: Treat once every two days. Three treatments constitute one course.

Results: The total number of cases was 30. After treatment, 14 cases were cured (pain, oscillating sound, and motor impairment of the mouth disappeared). Improvement after 2-5 treatments was seen in 16 cases (one of the three symptoms remained).

(*Source:* Shanghai Journal of Acupuncture and Moxibustion, (1):33, 1985)

2. A summary of electro-acupuncture in treating 23 cases of temporomandibular joint syndrome

Points: Xiaguan (St. 7), Jiache (St. 6)

Method: Connect Jiache (St. 6) with the positive electrode, and Xiaguan (St. 7) with the negative electrode. Select the points on the affected side. Use the frequency at 180 times per minute. The treatment should last 30 minutes. Treat twice a week.

Results: All cases were cured after 1-4 treatments.

(*Source:* Journal of Traditional Chinese Medicine, 24(3):51, 1983)

3. Primary analysis of clinical therapeutic result on acupuncture in treating 145 cases of temporomandibular joint syndrome

Points:

Lateral pterygoid muscle hyperfunction, spasm or injury: Waiguan (S.J. 5) on the affected side

Injury on the region posterior to the joint: Ermen (S.J. 21)

Medial pterygoid muscle spasm: Jiache (St. 6), the superior of maxillary angle, the posterior and medial side of the anterior portion of mandibular ramus

Method: After the needling sensation is observed, withdraw the needles. Treat once every other day.

Results: The therapeutic result can be obtained in 2-6 treatments. A cure was obtained in 133 cases (91.72 percent), improvement was seen in 6 cases, (4.14 percent), and no effect was evident in 6 cases (4.14 percent).

(*Source:* Chinese Journal of Stomatology, 17(1):53, 1982)

121.Urticaria

Principal points: Quchi (L.I. 11), Xuehai (Sp. 10), Geshu (U.B. 17), Sanyinjiao (Sp. 6), Zusanli (St. 36)

Method: Before or during the episode, puncture the points with strong stimulation and retain the needles for 30-60 minutes with manipulation every 5-10 minutes. However, provide quick thrusting to children without any retention. Usually treat daily, but twice daily for those with excruciating itching.

Supplementary points:

Chills and fever: Dazhui (Du 14), Hegu (L.I. 4)

Severe redness and feverishness of the rashes: Weizhong (U.B. 40) with bleeding method by a three-edged needle

The disease occurs in the throat, giving rise to edema of the mucosa and resulting in dyspnea: Fengfu (Du 16), Fengchi (G.B. 20), Shaoshang (Lu. 11)

Abdominal pain, diarrhea, and vomiting: Neiguan (P. 6), Tianshu (St. 25)

Deficiency of both *qi* and blood with frequent recurrence: Qihai (Ren 6), Pishu (U.B. 20)

The episode comes 2-3 days prior to menstruation, but disappears automatically after the bleeding is finished, and irregular menstruation is associated: Ganshu (U.B. 18), Qimen (Liv. 14), Guanyuan (Ren 4)

If the severe dysmenorrhea is present: moxi Guanyuan (Ren 4)

Other therapies:

1. Ear acupuncture

Points: Urticaria, Lung, Lower Apex of Tragus, Shenmen, Intertragicus

Method: Select 3-4 points each time and produce strong stimulation. Retain the needles for 30-60 minutes, but manipulate intermittently. Treat daily. To treat a chronic case, needle-embedding method can be employed. Change the needles once every 3-4 days and alternate ears.

2. Cutaneous acupuncture

Points: Fengchi (G.B. 20), Quchi (L.I. 11), Xuehai (Sp. 10), Fengshi (G.B. 31), Jiaji points (Extra) from the second to the fifth thoracic vertebrae and from the first to the fourth sacral vertebrae

Method: Tap with a cutaneous needle to cause slight bleeding. Treat daily or once every other day.

3. Head acupuncture

Points: Sensory Area, Blood Vessel Dilation and Constriction Area, Leg Motor and Sensory Area

Method: Insert the needles by routine operation of head acupuncture, then rapidly rotate the needles for 2-3 minutes in each point and retain the needles for 20-30 minutes, but manipulate every ten minutes.

4. Moxibustion

Points: Hegu (L.I. 4), Yangchi (S.J. 4), Xingjian (Liv. 2), Jiexi (St. 41)

Method: Apply indirect moxibustion with ginger, three cones each time at each point, once or twice daily, until the symptoms disappear completely. Chronic cases need 2-5 treatments.

5. Cupping

Point: Shenque (Ren 8)

Method : Place the patient in a supine position. Perform cupping at Shenque (Ren 8) and remove the cup after 3-5 minutes. Repeat the same method twice more. This constitutes one session. Complete one session daily and one course consists of three sessions.

6. Wrist-and-ankle acupuncture

Points: Upper 1, Lower 1, all bilateral

Method: Apply routine operation of wrist-and-ankle acupuncture.

Remarks: Acupuncture and moxibustion have good effect in treating this disease, especially acute urticaria, the effect of relieving the itching and resolving the rashes is notable. To treat chronic and refractory cases, the above-mentioned methods can be incorporated. It is essential to find the etiological factors, so the treatment can deal with the etiology and the recurrence can be avoided or reduced.

REFERENCE:

Observed results of the treatment of 132 cases of chronic urticaria with acupuncture

Points: Xuehai (Sp. 10), Quchi (L.I. 11), Sanyinjiao (Sp. 6)

Method: Perform acupuncture and retain the needles for 20 minutes. Treat once every other day, and 30 treatments constitute one course.

Results: Of 132 cases treated, 104 cases were cured (no relapse occurred after one-month observation), making up 78.5 percent, and the treatment ranged from 5-10 times; and 22 cases were improved, making up 17 percent; no effect was seen in 6 cases, making up 4.5 percent.

(*Source:* Shanghai Journal of Chinese Medicine and Medica Materia, (9):22, 1964)

122. Eczema

Principal points: Quchi (L.I. 11), Xuehai (Sp. 10), Ashi point (local region of the skin lesion)

Method: Use surrounding method in the local region of the skin lesion with needles thrust in certain number of loci according to the area of the skin lesion. To treat acute cases, perform strong stimulation in all the points and retain the needles for 30 minutes, manipulating every 5-10 minutes. To treat chronic cases, produce moderate stimulation and retain the needles for 20-30 minutes. Treat daily, and 10 treatments constitute one course.

Supplementary points:

Chronic cases: Zusanli (St. 36), Sanyinjiao (Sp. 6)

Other therapies:

1. Moxibustion

Points: Ashi points (local region of the skin lesion)

Method: Perform mild moxibustion with a moxa stick to produce flushing of the skin, once or twice daily, or at the time the eczema starts to itch.

2. Collateral-needling with cupping

Points: Ashi points (local region of the skin lesion)

Method: This method is appropriate to the patients with chronic eczema. Tap the local region of the skin lesion heavily with the cutaneous needle to cause bleeding from the focus of the lesion, then perform cupping over it. Treat daily or once every other day.

3. Ear acupuncture

Points: Lung, Lower Apex of Tragus, Intertragicus, Shenmen, and points corresponding to the affected area

Method: Select 2-3 points each time and produce moderate stimulation with filiform needles. Retain the needles for 60-120 minutes, manipulating several times. Treat daily and 10 treatments constitute one course. Needle-embedding method can be also employed. Require the patient to press the needles for a few minutes whenever the itching starts.

Remarks: Eczema is a refractory skin disease, and is susceptible to recurrence. Acupuncture therapy has fair effect in treating this disease. Attention should be laid more on the moxibustion.

Moxibustion and ear acupuncture are fairly effective to alleviate the itching, thus beneficial to those with excruciating itching. Mental stimulation as well as the stimulation by scratching should also be avoided.

REFERENCE:
    Observed results of the treatment of 21 cases of infantile eczema
    Points: a) Hegu (L.I. 4), Sanyinjiao (Sp. 6); b) Quchi (L.I. 11), Zusanli (St. 36)
    Method: Alternate the two groups of points and perform the reducing method by rotating the needles. Puncture to a depth of 0.5-1 *cun*. Do not retain the needles. Treat once every other day.
    Results: All the cases were cured, scabs fell off completely, and the redness and feverishness as well as the itching of skin entirely disappeared. Five cases were cured with 3 treatments, 14 cases were cured with 6 treatments, and 2 cases with more than 6 treatments.
    (*Source:* Shanghai Journal of Acupuncture and Moxibustion, (1):29, 1985)

123. Neurodermatitis

Principal points: Quchi (L.I. 11), Xuehai (Sp. 10), Ashi points
    Method: Provide surrounding method in the local area of the skin lesion. Needle 4-6 Ashi points around the lesion according to the size of the lesion area, and insert the needles subcutaneously from the base towards the center of the focus. Puncture Quchi (L.I. 11) and Xuehai (Sp. 10) with moderate or strong stimulation and retain the needles for 20-30 minutes. Treat daily or once every other day, and 10 treatments constitute one course. When the skin lesion is resolved, one more course should be continued in order to consolidate the effectiveness.
    Supplementary points:
    Blood deficiency and dryness of wind: Sanyinjiao (Sp. 6), Geshu (U.B. 17)
    Disease on the neck: Lieque (Lu. 7), Weizhong (U.B. 40)
    Disease in the elbow: Ximen (P. 4), Laogong (P. 8)

Disease in the popliteal fossa: Yinmen (U.B. 37), Kunlun (U.B. 60)

Disease in the medial aspect of the thigh: Sanyinjiao (Sp. 6)

Disease on the upper eyelid: Touwei (St. 8), Baihui (Du 20)

Sleeplessness due to the itching: Zhaohai (K. 6), Shenmen (H. 7)

Other therapies:

1. Cutaneous acupuncture

Points: Ashi points

Method: After applying routine skin sterilization in the local region, tap the area of the skin lesion from the center to the border until causing slight bleeding. Perform moxibustion with a moxa stick over the area to bring on full congestion in the local region, or provide cupping instead. Treat daily or once every other day. Ten treatments constitute one course and there is a 3-5 days' interval between every two courses.

2. Ear acupuncture

Points: Lung, Liver, Brain, Shenmen, Lower Apex of Tragus

Method: Select 2-3 points each time. Provide moderate or strong stimulation, and retain the needles for 30-60 minutes. Treat daily and 10 treatments constitute one course.

3. Moxibustion

Point: Ashi points

Method: Provide suspending moxibustion with a moxa stick over the skin lesion from the border towards the center, 20-30 minutes each time. Treat once or twice daily.

4. Electro-acupuncture

Points: Quchi (L.I. 11), Xuehai (Sp. 10), Sanyinjiao (Sp. 6), Hegu (L.I. 4), Ashi points

Method: Select 2-4 points each time. Needle Ashi points from the border of the base towards the center of the focus. Set frequency at 200 times per minute, and the intensity according to the patient's tolerance. Connect with electricity for 20-30 minutes each time. Treat daily and 10 treatments constitute one course.

5. Hydro-acupuncture

Points: Quchi (L.I. 11), Xuehai (Sp. 10), Sanyinjiao (Sp. 6), Fengshi (G.B. 31), Ashi points

Method: Select two pairs of points each time, and inject 2-4 ml of 0.5% novocain plus 50 mg of Vitamin B_1 or 2-4 ml of 0.5%

novocain plus 25 mg of diphenhydramine hydrochloride into each point, by means of routine operation of hydro-acupuncture. Select 3-4 Ashi points around the skin lesion. Obliquely insert the needle towards the center of the focus, and inject 0.5 ml of the liquid into each Ashi point. Inject the other points with 1 ml of the liquid. Treat once every 2-3 days, and five treatments constitute one course.

Remarks: The above methods have certain effect in the treatment of this disease, but the most effective one is the combination of cutaneous acupuncture and moxibustion with a moxa stick. To treat the refractory cases, several methods can be integrated.

Require the patient to avoid mental overstrain and stimulation, and warn against irritant food.

REFERENCES:

1. Observed results of 71 cases of neurodermatitis treated with surrounding method by electro-acupuncture.

Points: Local area of the skin lesion

Method: Insert gauge 28 filiform needles, 2-3 *cun* in length, from the border towards the center of the focus in 4 loci, and connect with a Model G-6805 electro-acupuncture apparatus. Set the intensity to a continuous wave, 500-600 times per minute, but adjust according to the patient's tolerance. Retain the needles for 15-20 minutes. Treat daily or every other day, and 10 treatments constitute one course.

Results: Of 71 cases treated, 59 cases were cured, 10 showed improvement, and 2 showed no evidence of any effect.

(*Source:* Chinese Acupuncture & Moxibustion, 5:(19), 1987)

2. Observation on the therapeutic effect of 41 cases of neurodermatitis with plum-blossom needling

Points:

1) Localized neurodermatitis:

a. The head, face and neck are affected: tender region and cord-like substances on both sides of the cervical vertebrae, the focus, and Quchi (L.I. 11), Hegu (L.I. 4), Taiyuan (Lu. 9)

b. The arm is affected: tender region and cord-like substances on both sides of the fourth and fifth thoracic vertebrae, the focus, and Neiguan (P. 6), Quchi (L.I. 11), Feishu (U.B. 13), Xinshu (U.B. 15)

c. The leg is affected: cord-like or vesicular substances in the lumbosacral region, the focus, and Xuehai (Sp. 10), Zusanli (St. 36), Shenshu (U.B. 23)

d. The abdominal region and perineum are affected: tender region, nodules and cord-like substances on both sides of the tenth-twelfth thoracic vertebrae, in the lumbosacral region, the focus, and Pishu (U.B. 20), Shenshu (U.B. 23), Guanyuan (Ren 4), Sanyinjiao (Sp. 6), Zusanli (St. 36)

2) Disseminated neurodermatitis: Both sides of the spine, mainly from the third to the twelfth thoracic vertebrae, tender area, nodules and cord-like substances in the lumbar region, the focus, and Fengchi (G.B. 20), Quchi (L.I. 11), Xuehai (Sp. 10), Zusanli (St. 36)

3) Points to consolidate the effect: Both sides of the spine, mainly Feishu (U.B. 13), Xinshu (U.B. 15), Pishu (U.B. 20), Taiyuan (Lu. 9), Zusanli (St. 36), and the focus

Method: Tap with a plum-blossom needle and adjust the stimulation according to the patient's constitution. Treat once every other day and 15 treatments constitute one course.

Results: Of 41 cases treated, 22 cases were cured, 15 showed marked effect, 3 saw some improvement, and 1 failed. The total effective rate was 97.6 percent.

(*Source:* Jiangsu Chinese Medical Journal, 7(8):30, 1986)

124. Acne

Principal points: Hegu (L.I. 4), Quchi (L.I. 11), Lingtai (Du 10), Weizhong (U.B. 40)

Method: Produce moderate stimulation with filiform needles and use reducing method. Retain the needles for 20-30 minutes. Treat daily or once every other day, and 10 treatments constitute one course.

Supplementary points:

Lung-heat: Chize (Lu. 5), with reducing method

Excessive fire in liver and gall bladder: Xingjian (Liv. 2), with reducing method

Excessive fire of stomach: Jiexi (St. 41), with reducing method

Long-lasting acne: Xuehai (Sp. 10), and bleeding at Weizhong (U.B. 40)

Other therapies:

1. Pricking method

Points: Ashi points

Method: Require the patient to sit with the body leaning forward and find several red spots on the back. After routine sterilization of the skin, use a three-edged needle to prick the red spots to the bottom, about 3 mm in depth, then raise the tip of the needle to make a small incision in the skin. Use thumbs and index fingers to press around the needle hole to cause slight bleeding which is then cleaned with a dry cotton ball. Treat once weekly and 3-5 treatments constitute one course.

2 Ear acupuncture

Points: Intertragicus, Brain, Occiput, Upper Portion of Back of Auricle, Stomach and corresponding parts of the acne

Method: Employ filiform needles to produce moderate stimulation, and then retain the needles for 20-30 minutes. Treat once every other day. The needle-embedding method is also applicable.

3. Wrist-and-ankle acupuncture

Points: Upper 1 and 2, bilateral

Method: Apply the routine operation of the wrist-and-ankle acupuncture.

Remarks: Acupuncture has fair effect in treating acne, but pungent, spicy or other irritable food should be avoided during the treatment.

REFERENCES:

1. Observation on the clinical therapeutic effect of 144 cases of acne treated with acupuncture

Principal points: Quchi (L.I. 11), Hegu (L.I. 4)

Supplementary points:

Wind-heat affecting lung meridian: Dazhui (Du 14), Feishu (U.B. 13)

Wind-heat affecting lung and spleen: Zusanli (St. 36)

Disharmony of Chong and Ren meridians: Sanyinjiao (Sp. 6)

Method: Treat the simple acupuncture group with even method and retain the needles for 20 minutes; treat the electro-acupuncture group with a Model G-6805 electro-acupuncture apparatus, connecting with the needles for 20 minutes. Use an intermittent wave. Treat both groups daily and 20 treatments constitute one course.

Results: The simple acupuncture group included 57 cases, of these 30 were cured, 25 showed marked effect and 2 failed. The electro-acupuncture group had 87 patients, 76 were cured and 11 showed marked effect.

(*Source:* New Journal of Traditional Chinese Medicine, 18(5):36, 1985)

2. Clinical observation on 80 cases of acne treated with ear acupuncture

Principal points: Lung, Kidney
Supplementary points:
Purulent blister: Heart
Excessive sebum: Spleen
Constipation: Large Intestine
Dysmenorrhea: Liver, Intertragicus

Method: Swiftly thrust with filiform needles, 0.5 *cun* in length, but do not penetrate the cartilage. Retain the needles for 15-30 minutes, manipulating 3-6 times in between. Treat daily and 30 treatments constitute one course.

Results: Of 80 cases treated, 62 cases were cured, 11 showed marked effect, and 7 failed. The total effective rate was 91.3 percent.

(*Source:* Journal of Traditional Chinese Medicine, 28(6):18, 1987)

125. Herpes Zoster

Principal points: Ashi points, and Jiaji points (Extra) on the affected side at the corresponding section of the herpes

Method: Provide surrounding method at 4-8 Ashi points, 1 cm from the verge of the skin lesion, i.e., select one point from each end of the herpes, and puncture 1-3 points on each side according to the length of the zoster lesion. Thrust filiform needles, 1-2 *cun* in length, horizontally towards the center of the lesion, and retain the needles for 20-30 minutes. After the needles are withdrawn, press the holes to cause slight bleeding. Puncture the Ashi points in pairs, one on each side. Reduce with strong stimulation Jiaji points (Extra) on the affected side at the corresponding level of the skin lesion and retain the needles for 20-30 minutes, during which perform mild moxibustion with a moxa stick over the local area of the skin lesion. Treat daily and seven treatments constitute one course.

Supplementary points:

The skin lesion on the face and neck: Fengchi (G.B. 20), Waiguan (S.J. 5), Hegu (L.I. 4)

The lesion on the upper limbs: Quchi (L.I. 11), Hegu (L.I. 4)

The lesion on the chest and costal region: Zhigou (S.J. 6), Yanglingquan (G.B. 34)

The lesion on the back and abdomen: Weizhong (U.B. 40), Taichong (Liv. 3), Xiaxi (G.B. 43)

The lesion on the lower limb: Sanyinjiao (Sp. 6), Taichong (Liv. 3)

Severe pain: Geshu (U.B. 17), Xuehai (Sp. 10), or the tender spot in the local region with needling and moxibustion

Other therapies:

1. Cutaneous acupuncture

Points: Ashi points

Method: Apply circular tapping 1 cm away from the verge of the herpes three times to cause subcutaneous congestion. Treat daily. When the herpes is resolved but the pain remains in the local region, perform the tapping on the painful area with a cutaneous needle to produce slight bleeding, and provide moxibustion with a moxa stick after needling. Treat daily and five treatments constitute one course.

2. Hydro-acupuncture

Points: Jiaji points (Extra) on the affected side at the corresponding section of the herpes, and Ashi points

Method: Mix 100 μg of Vitamin B_{12} with 5-7 ml of 1% procaine. Obliquely puncture the Ashi points on both end of the herpes towards the center while perpendicularly needling Jiaji points (Extra). Inject 1 ml of the liquid into each point by means of routine operation of hydro-acupuncture. Inject daily.

3. Ear acupuncture

Points: Liver, Gall Bladder, Shenmen and corresponding parts of the skin lesion

Method: Produce strong stimulation with filiform needles. Retain the needles for 30 minutes. Treat daily. The needle-embedding method is also applicable.

302

Remarks: Acupuncture has quick and fair effect in treating this disease.

REFERENCES:
1. Observed results of 60 cases of herpes zoster treated with plum-blossom needling

Points: The focus, and Jiaji points (Extra) at the corresponding section of the herpes on the affected side

Method: After routine sterilization, employ a plum-blossom needle to tap the herpes and the surrounding skin, thrust the herpes to release the fluid, and produce a flushing of the skin around the focus. Jiaji points (Extra) may be needled for some patients. Administer oral medication of Bolus of Gentiana to purge the liver-fire to those with remarkable symptoms of damp-heat in liver and gall bladder.

Results: Of 60 cases treated, 30 cases were cured, 24 showed marked effect, 4 experienced some improvement, and 2 failed. The total effective rate was 96.7 percent.

(*Source:* Chinese Acupuncture & Moxibustion, 5(10), 1987)

2. Observed results of rotary moxibustion in treating 120 cases of herpes zoster

Point: The focus of the herpes

Method: Perform moxibustion with a moxa stick circling around over the focus.

Results: All the cases were cured and the treatment took an average of 2.21 days. The analgesic effect appears from between 5 minutes and 24 hours.

(*Source:* Shaanxi Journal of Traditional Chinese Medicine, 9(5):214, 1988)

126. Tinea

Principal points:
Skin lesion of the hand: Hegu (L.I. 4), Neiguan (P. 6)
Skin lesion of the foot: Bafeng (Extra), Yongquan (K. 1), Kunlun (U.B. 60)
Skin lesion of the head: Quchi (L.I. 11), Rangu (K. 2)
Method: Provide moderate stimulation with filiform needles,

and apply penetrating method from Hegu (L.I. 4) to Laogong (P. 8) and from Neiguan (P. 6) to Waiguan (S.J. 5) for a skin lesion of the hand; from Kunlun (U.B. 60) to Taixi (K. 3) for a skin lesion of the foot. Retain the needles for 20-30 minutes, and manipulate by lifting, thrusting and rotating every 5-10 minutes. After withdrawing the needles, offer mild moxibustion with moxa sticks over the area of the skin lesion until the itching disappears. Treat daily and 10 treatments constitute one course.

Supplementary points:

Blood deficiency: Sanyinjiao (Sp. 6), Zusanli (St. 36), with reinforcing method

Heat of blood: Quchi (L.I. 11), Weizhong (U.B. 40), with bleeding method

Stagnation of blood: Xuehai (Sp. 10), Geshu (U.B. 17)

Other therapy:

Hydro-acupuncture

Points:

Tinea manuum: Neiguan (P. 6), Hegu (L.I. 4)

Tinea pedis: Sanyinjiao (Sp. 6), Taixi (K. 3)

Method: Inject 1 ml of 0.25% procaine solution into each point by means of the routine operation of hydro-acupuncture. Treat once every other day and seven treatments constitute one course.

Remarks: The above-mentioned methods have certain effect in treating tinea.

REFERENCE:

Observation on the clinical effect of 100 cases of scald-head treated with acupuncture

Points: Quchi (L.I. 11), Rangu (K. 2), Ganshu (U.B. 18), Shenshu (U.B. 23), Zusanli (St. 36)

Method: Needle bilateral Quchi (L.I. 11) and Rangu (K. 2), once daily and one course of treatment consists of seven days. Combine Ganshu (U.B. 18), Shenshu (U.B. 23), and Zusanli (St. 36) to those who are not cured after 2-3 courses.

Results: Among 100 cases, there were 45 cases of tinea favosa, 33 cases of tinea alba, 12 cases of black dot tinea and 10 cases of kerion. After 1-5 courses, 83 cases were cured, 15 cases improved and 2 cases remained unchanged.

(*Source:* Journal of Traditional Chinese Medicine, 25(1):57,

127. Verrucae

I. Verruca vulgaris

Principal point: Ashi point (in the middle of the "mother wart," i.e., the primary one or the biggest one)

Method: Use a thick filiform needle 0.5 or 1 *cun* in length, and insert with the right hand swiftly into the bottom of the mother wart from the mid-point while the left hand grasps tightly the base of the wart to alleviate the pain caused by the needling. Lift, thrust and rotate the needle in large amplitude for 30 times, then the needle hole is enlarged by shaking the needle and the needle is swiftly taken out to give rise to a few drops of blood, which can then be checked by applying pressure. If the wart is considerably large or elliptic, insert one more needle at the junction of the wart and the skin, along the maximal diameter, to penetrate the wart, and perform the same manipulating method as above. Treat once every other day. The mother wart and the rest will fall off after a few treatments.

Supplementary points:

There are a number of warts or they are diffusely spread over the body: Feishu (U.B. 13), Quchi (L.I. 11), Fengshi (G.B. 31), Xuehai (Sp. 10), retaining the needles for 20-30 minutes

Other therapies:

1. Moxibustion

Points: Ashi points (warts proper)

Method: After applying routine sterilizing technique on the focus, inject an anesthetic solution of 1% procaine. While this takes effect, put a moxa cone as big as the wart at the top of the wart, and ignite until it burns up. Then clear away the ash, and hold the wart with forceps, remove it with a few shakes. Use a small knife to scrape gently the base of the wart. After some time, apply a 2% gentian violet or 5% ammoniated mercury ointment on the wound, which is bound with gauze. Usually one cone is sufficient to remove the wart but two cones can be performed when the wart is too big and deeply rooted. The wound will be healed in about three days and usually no scars will be left except the occasional deep lesion.

2. Ear acupuncture

Points: Lung, Brain, Intertragicus, and the corresponding part of the body

Method: Produce moderate stimulation with needles. Do not retain or retain the needles for only 10 minutes. Select two points each time and alternate all the points. Treat daily and 10 treatments constitute one course.

II. Verruca plana

Principal point: Ashi point (the middle of the mother wart), Fengchi (G.B. 20), Quchi (L.I. 11), Hegu (L.I. 4), Xuehai (Sp. 10)

Method: The needling method in the mother wart is the same as for verruca vulgaris. Moderately stimulate the remaining points and retain the needles for 20-30 minutes. Treat once every other day.

Supplementary points:

Those on the face and forehead: Taiyang (Extra), Yangbai (G.B. 14)

Those on the dorsum of hand, forearm, and scapular region: 1-2 points from the adjacent meridians in the affected area

Other therapies:

1) Ear acupuncture

Points: Lung, Large Intestine, Occiput, Shenmen, Brain, Intertragicus, and the corresponding parts of the body

Method: Embed 2-3 points with intradermal needles which are retained for 1-3 days. Ten treatments constitute one course.

2) Cutaneous acupuncture

Points: Both sides of the cervical and thoracic vertebrae, the first line of the urinary bladder meridian on the nape and upper back, and Ashi points (local region of the warts)

Method: Tap the meridian on the nape and back from up to down three times with moderate stimulation to produce flushed skin. In the area of skin lesion, apply strong stimulation by heavy tapping to cause slight bleeding. Treat once every other day.

III. Infectious molluscum

Principal points: Ashi points (warts proper)

Method: After applying routine sterilization on the skin of the local region, use a three-edged needle to prick out the top of the wart, and squeeze out the cheese-like content. Apply 2.5% iodine

306

tincture to the wound. If there are a number of warts, give the treatment by groups.

Remarks: Acupuncture and moxibustion have quick and positive effect in treating various verrucae. Usually verruca vulgaris and verruca plana will fall off soon after the treatment. The treatment is painless and scarless if the technique is applied properly and skillfully.

REFERENCE:

Observed results of the treatment of verruca vulgaris with moxibustion

Points: The affected regions

Method: Utilize a 1% procaine solution for a local anesthesia, applying for 2-3 minutes. Put a moxa cone as big as the wart on top of it and ignite. After burning up, hold the wart with forceps and shake by force, then remove it. Gently scrape the residual of the base with a small knife. Apply the sunder wound with a 2% gentian violet or 5% ammoniated mercury ointment and then bind with gauze.

Results: More than 100 cases were treated and all were cured. Usually 1 cone is sufficient to remove the wart. The wound will be healed in three days, and no scars will be left. The recurrent rate is approximately 10 percent. If the wart tissue is deeply rooted, this treatment is not appropriate.

(*Source:* Chinese Dermatology Journal, 10:(4):273, 1964)

128. Leukoderma

Principal points: Ashi points

Method: Select 4-6 Ashi points 0.5-1 cm away from the verge of the skin lesion and use filiform needles to thrust subcutaneously towards the center of the skin lesion to make an encircling puncture. Retain the needles 20-30 minutes. Treat daily, and 10-15 treatments constitute one course.

Supplementary points:

The skin lesion on the face and head: Hegu (L.I. 4), Quchi (L.I. 11)

The skin lesion on the chest: Shanzhong (Ren 17)

The skin lesion on the upper limbs: Quchi (L.I. 11)

The skin lesion on the lower limbs: Xuehai (Sp. 10), Sanyinjiao (Sp. 6)

Disharmony of *qi* and blood: Xuehai (Sp. 10), Sanyinjiao (Sp. 6), Zusanli (St. 36), using the even method

Deficiency of liver and kidney: Ganshu (U.B. 18), Shenshu (U.B. 23), Mingmen (Du 4), Taixi (K. 3), Sanyinjiao (Sp. 6), employing reinforcing method

Obstruction of the stagnated blood: Xuehai (Sp. 10), Geshu (U.B. 17), Sanyinjiao (Sp. 6), applying reducing method

Other therapies:

1. Plum-blossom needling plus moxibustion

Points: Ashi points

Method: Tap on the local area of the skin lesion with a plum-blossom needle, and give mild stimulation in the central part of the lesion and strong stimulation on the margin of the lesion. The needling is finished when the local region has begun to bleed slightly. Then perform suspending moxibustion with a moxa stick for 5-10 minutes. Treat once every other day, and one course consists of five treatments.

2. Moxibustion

Points: Ashi points

Method: Use about five moxa cones for moxibustion. Put the cones on the dorsal mid-point of the proximal interphalangeal joint of both hands. Treat daily or once every other day.

3. Bleeding technique in combination of cupping

Points: Ashi points

Method: Utilize the three-edged needle to prick the central area of the skin lesion in a leopard spot way, then apply cupping on the area to suck out the blood. Treat once or twice weekly. The method is more devoted to the obstruction of the stagnated blood.

4. Ear acupuncture

Points: Intertragicus, Lower Apex of Tragus, End of Inferior Helix Crus, Occiput, and the corresponding region of the skin lesion

Method: Select alternately 2-3 points on one ear in each treatment. Embed needles for 5-7 days.

Remarks: In the treatment of leukoderma, some patients acquire effectiveness with above-mentioned methods. In most cases, several methods are used simultaneously in clinic.

REFERENCE:

Observation on the therapeutic effect of 26 cases of leukoderma treated with acupuncture

Points: Xiaxia (Extra, located at the junction of the middle one-third and inferior one-third of the lateral border of the biceps brachii), and Dianfeng (Extra, located at the transverse crease of the distal interphalangeal joint of the middle finger)

Method: Bleed the points with a three-edged needle. If the bleeding is scant, use cupping at the bleeding site. Treat once weekly on alternate sides. Following each application of needling, give moxibustion with three cones at Dianfeng (Extra), one side alone, and no blister should be caused.

Results: Of 26 cases treated, 2 cases were cured, 11 showed marked effect, 10 were improved and 3 were unchanged. The effectiveness became distinguishable at the time between two weeks and six months after the treatment began.

(*Source:* Journal of Clinical Dermatology, 10(1):12, 1981)

129. Alopecia

Principal points: Ashi points (around the alopecia), Fengchi (G.B. 20), Geshu (U.B. 17) Sanyinjiao (Sp. 6)

Method: Apply surrounding method around the local area of the alopecia. Insert four needles horizontally from up to down, and left to right respectively towards the center of the alopecia areata. When the area of the alopecia is large, thrust more needles around it. Provide the other points with moderate stimulation and retain the needles for 15-20 minutes. Treat daily or once every other day. Mild moxibustion with a moxa stick can be combined over the area of alopecia during the retention of needles.

Supplementary points:

Palpitation and insomnia: Neiguan (P. 6), Shenmen (H. 7)

Deficiency of blood: Zusanli (St. 36), Pishu (U.B. 20)

Deficiency of liver and kidney: Ganshu (U.B. 18), Shenshu (U.B. 23), Taixi (K. 3)

Stagnation of *qi* and blood: Taichong (Liv. 3), Xuehai (Sp. 10)

Other therapies:

1. Cutaneous-acupuncture

Points: Ashi points (the focus of the alopecia)

Method: In the initial stage of the alopecia areata, when the skin of the focus is luminous, and no new hairs grow, perform heavy tapping with a cutaneous needle to cause slight bleeding. When sparse hairs are visible in the local region, gentle tapping is necessary. Treat once every other day, and 10 treatments constitute one course.

2. Moxibustion

Points: Ashi points (the focus of the alopecia)

Method: Perform moxibustion with a moxa stick over the area of the alopecia, to cause flushing of the skin. Treat daily.

3. Hydro-acupuncture

Points: Xinshu (U.B. 15), Feishu (U.B. 13), Geshu (U.B. 17), Pishu (U.B. 20), Fengchi (G.B. 20), Dazhui (Du 14), Mingmen (Du 4), Quchi (L.I. 11)

Method: Select 2-3 points each time, alternating the above-mentioned points. Inject 0.5-1 ml of 100-200 μg of Vitamin B_{12} solution into each point. Treat daily, and 10 treatments constitute one course. There is a 5-7 days' interval between two courses.

Remarks: Acupuncture therapy is fairly effective in treating alopecia. Especially body acupuncture and cutaneous acupuncture are more markedly effective, thus they are used alternatively in clinic. After tapping with the cutaneous needle, use fresh ginger to rub the local area, or perform moxibustion with a moxa stick, so the effect can be enhanced.

The duration of treatment for this disease is long, so confidence and patience are essential. The patients should be convinced to release themselves from the mental misgivings and to avoid any unfavorable emotional stimulation. Meanwhile, sleep should be guaranteed.

REFERENCES:

1. Observed results of 82 cases of alopecia treated with electric plum-blossom needling

Points: The focus of the alopecia, Fengchi (G.B. 20), the spine from the cervical to the sacral vertebrae

Method: Tap the focus of the alopecia to cause slight bleeding.

Treat for 10-15 minutes each time.

Results: Of 82 cases treated, 91.5 percent were completely cured and 8.5 percent showed some improvement.

(*Source:* Chinese Acupuncture & Moxibustion, (1):25, 1982)

2. Observed results of acupuncture using "three head-points" for treating 108 cases of alopecia

Principal points: Fanglao (Extra, 1 *cun* posterior to Baihui, Du 20), Jiannao (Extra, 1 *cun* below Pt. Fengchi, G.B. 20)

Supplementary points:

Severe alopecia on the temporal region: Touwei (St. 8)

Itching on the head: Dazhui (Du 14)

Excessive secretion of sebum: Shangxing (Du 23)

Method: Reinforce the principal points, and retain the needles for 15-30 minutes. Treat daily or once every other day, and 10 treatments constitute one course. The treatment should be given for several months or half a year.

Results: Of 108 cases treated, 70 cases (81.5 percent) were cured, 38 (18.5 percent) showed improved and the total effective rate reached 100 percent. Among 70 cases suffering from alopecia areata, 55 were cured, and 15 were improved. Among 38 cases suffering from alopecia seborrhoeica, 32 were cured and 6 were improved.

(*Source:* Jiangsu Chinese Medical Journal, 3:(6), 1982)

130. Folliculitis

Principal points: Ashi point (the focus), Shenzhu (Du 12), Lingtai (Du 10)

Method: Perform indirect moxibustion with garlic on the focus once or twice daily. Bleed Shenzhu (Du 12) and Lingtai (Du 10) with a three-edged needle.

Supplementary points:

Those on the head, face and upper limbs: Hegu (L.I. 4), Quchi (L.I. 11)

Those on the back and lower limbs: Zusanli (St. 36), Weizhong (U.B. 40)

Method: Use filiform needles with moderate stimulation. Retain the needles for 15-30 minutes or not at all.

Remarks: Acupuncture, moxibustion and bleeding have fair therapeutic effect in treating this disease, but do not directly needle the focus so as to prevent the diffusion of the infection.

REFERENCES:
1. Observed results of 17 cases of multiple furuncles on the nape treated with acupuncture
Points and method:
1) Insert a special-made round-sharp needle, 2 *cun* in length and 2 mm in diameter, perpendicularly at the sixth thoracic vertebra, and then thrust subcutaneously down to the seventh thoracic vertebra. Retain the needle for 30 minutes.
2) Utilize filiform needles 2.5 *cun* in length to bring on strong stimulation in bilateral Hegu (L.I. 4), and then withdraw and thrust the needle horizontally under the skin towards the index finger, with the tip of the needle going through the matacarpophalangeal joint. Retain the needle for 30 minutes and rotate every 10 minutes. Treat twice weekly, and 3-10 treatments constitute one course.
Results: Of 17 cases treated, 13 were cured, 3 were improved and 1 failed.
(*Source:* Journal of Beijing College of Traditional Chinese Medicine, (1):39, 1984)
2. Observed results of the treatment of 80 cases of furuncle with moxibustion
Point: The apex of the focus
Method: Perform mild moxibustion with a moxa stick to produce flushing of the skin and to slightly raise the skin temperature. Treat for 30 minutes daily.
Results: Of 80 cases treated, 54 cases of nonsuppurative furuncle were resolved with 2-3 treatments. Among 26 cases of initial suppurative furuncle, 10 cases were resolved or absorbed after 3 treatments, and 16 cases, which were drained of pus by incision, were cured with the application of moxibustion after the incision.
(*Source:* Shanghai Journal of Acupuncture and Moxibustion, 7(2):19, 1988)

131. Heloma

1. Red-hot needling

Points: Ashi points

Method: After sterilizing the local region, heat a needle to red-hot and swiftly insert into the center of the base of the heloma. Penetrate the horny layer and thrust the needle into the root of the heloma, then swiftly remove as soon as the patient feels pain. After withdrawing the needle, press the hole with a cotton ball soaked in iodine tincture, and cover the hole with adhesive plaster. Usually a mild case needs only one treatment and after a week, the heloma will automatically fall off. With a severe case treat once again after one week's rest.

2. Moxibustion

Points: Ashi points

Method: Apply direct moxibustion at the focus with moxa cones which are slightly smaller than the area of the heloma. Each heloma needs 3-5 cones once. Treat daily or once every other day. Usually approximately 10 treatments are necessary for the tissue of the heloma to be burned dry and turned into necrosis. It will then automatically fall off.

Remarks: Fair therapeutic effect can be obtained in the treatment of heloma with red-hot needling and moxibustion.

REFERENCE:

Observed results of the treatment of 65 cases of heloma with acupoint injection

Points: Taichong (Liv. 3), Taixi (K. 3), on the affected side

Method: Inject 0.2 mg of adrenalin hydrochloride and 1 ml of 2% novocaine solution into each point. Treat once every six days.

Results: The cure rate was 89.23 percent and the failure rate was 10.77 percent. Of 65 cases treated, 49 cases were cured with 1-5 injections, 9 cases with 5-8 injections, and 7 cases were failed.

(*Source:* Chinese Acupuncture & Moxibustion, 4(9), 1982)

132. Acute Lymphangitis

Principal points: Ashi point (the proximal end of the red line),

313

and the Xi-Cleft point of the meridian in the affected area

Method: First puncture Ashi point, then the Xi-Cleft point of the meridian, which the red line passes through or is near, and then thrust the points close to the red line or on both sides of it. Retain the needles for 15-30 minutes and treat once or twice daily.

Supplementary points:

High fever: Shixuan (Extra) with bleeding method, or Quchi (L.I. 11)

The lower limbs affected: Yinlingquan (Sp. 9), Jimen (Sp. 11)

The upper limbs affected: Chize (Lu. 5), Quze (P. 3)

Other therapies:

1. Bleeding method

Points: The twelve Jing-Well points (bilateral Lu. 11, L.I. 1, H. 9, S.I. 1, S.J. 1, P. 9), the Xi-Cleft point of the meridian in the affected area, and Ashi point

Method: Use a three-edged needle to thrust the meridian through which the red line passes to cause bleeding, and bleed the red line from the initial to the terminal points at a distance of 1-2 cm. Also provide bleeding around the focus of the infection at several points. Needle five loci in the form of plum-blossom at the Xi-Cleft point of the meridian which the red line passes through or is near, and allow the bleeding to form drops as big as a bead. Simultaneously, press with your hand the place 2-3 cm away from the proximal side of the Xi-Cleft point.

2. Ear acupuncture

Points: Shenmen, Lower Apex of Tragus, Brain, Occiput, and the corresponding parts of the infection

Method: Select 2-3 points each time, provide moderate or strong stimulation, and retain the needles for 30-60 minutes. Treat once or twice daily.

3. Moxibustion

Points: Ashi points (the part of the red line)

Method: Provide mild moxibustion with a moxa stick. Slowly move the stick from the proximal end down to the distal of the red line for 15-20 minutes to produce a comfortable feeling of heat for the patient.

Remarks: Acupuncture therapy has anti-inflammatory and analgesic effect in the treatment of this disease, thus the effect is satisfactory. To treat severe cases, medication should be incorporated.

REFERENCE:
   Observed results of 18 cases of acute lymphangitis treated with red-hot needling
   Points: The local areas of the disease
   Method: Perform red-hot needling at 3-5 spots on the red line. After the needling, sterilize the spots with alcohol, apply with berberine ointment and fix with the antiseptic dressing.
   Results: The cure rate was 100 percent.
   (Source: New Journal of Traditional Chinese Medicine, 20(3):34, 1988)

133. Scrofula

   Principal points: Ashi point, Bailao (Extra), Zhoujian (Extra), Jianjing (G.B. 21), Quchi (L.I. 11), Binao (L.I. 14)
   Method: Employ filiform needles to thrust the lymph node from the sides to the bottom, and lift, thrust, twirl and rotate after the insertion. Insert at Bailao (Extra, 2 *cun* above Dazhui, Du 14, and 1 *cun* lateral to Du meridian) to a depth of 0.3-0.5 *cun*; horizontally needle Zhoujian (Extra, at the tip of the olecranon when the elbow is flexed) downward for 0.5-1 *cun*; puncture Jianjing (G.B. 21) perpendicularly for 0.5-0.8 *cun*; and thrust Binao (L.I. 14) towards Quchi (L.I. 11) for 3-4 *cun*. Produce moderate or strong stimulation at all points, and retain the needles for 10-20 minutes. Treat daily or once every other day. Mild moxibustion with a moxa stick can be simultaneously combined over the points.
   Supplementary points:
   Cervical scrofula: Shousanli (L.I. 10)
   Nuchal scrofula: Yifeng (S.J. 17), Zhigou (S.J. 6), Foot-Linqi (G.B. 41)
   Stagnation of *qi* and accumulation of phlegm: Yanglingquan (G.B. 34), Fenglong (St. 40)
   Internal heat resulting from *yin* deficiency: Dazhui (Du 14), Jianshi (P. 5), Sanyinjiao (Sp. 6), Taixi (K. 3)
   Deficiency of both *qi* and blood: Pishu (U.B. 20), Qihai (Ren 6), Zusanli (St. 36), Sanyinjiao (Sp. 6)
   Excessive night sweating: moxi Yinxi (H. 6), Houxi (S.I. 3)

Other therapies:

1. Red-hot needling

Points: Ashi points (the focus of the swelling)

Method: After sterilization of the skin in the local region, use novocain for local anesthesia. Using the left hand, fix the swollen lymph node, and using the right hand, hold a gauge 28 needle, 1 *cun* in length, over an alcohol burner until it is red-hot. Swiftly insert the needle into the center of the lymph node and rapidly withdraw. Thrust 1-3 nodes each time, but ensure the insertion is not too deep, just reaching the center of the node. After needling, cover the surface of the node with antiseptic gauze. If the lumps are stuck together, the red-hot needling can be applied all around the lumps at a distance of 1-2 cm. If the area is larger, the middle of the nodes can also be thrust. The site of the red-hot needling should be changed. Treat once weekly.

2. Pricking method

Points: Ashi points (tuberculosis spots)

Method: The tuberculosis spot can be found on both sides of the spine, above the inferior angle of the scapula, where red, millet-sized spots slightly rise from the skin of which the color does not fade under pressure. When the disease is located on the left, the spots should be found on the right, and vice versa. After sterilization of the skin, employ a thick needle to prick out the epidermis of the spots and needle further inside to remove several dozen of the white fiber-like matters. At this moment, the patient will feel slight pain but no blood will come out. After removing all the fibers, cover the spot with antiseptic gauze and fix with plaster. Treat once every 1-2 weeks.

3. Cutting method

Points: Ganshu (U.B. 18), Geshu (U.B. 17)

Method: After sterilizing the skin in the local region, provide local anesthesia. Make a 0.5-cm-long incision at each point, deep inside the skin, then remove a small amount of subcutaneous fat. Cover the incision with antiseptic gauze and fix with plaster. Treat once weekly or fortnightly, using a pair of points each time.

4. Moxibustion

Points: Ashi points (focus of the swollen node)

Method: Use the lateral recumbent position, and place a slice of garlic 3 mm thick on the lymph node. Then put moxa cones on

316

the slice and apply moxibustion until the garlic slice is burned dry. After the therapy, blisters may appear. Apply gentian violet externally, or use gauze to cover the blisters. Provide treatment once in 20-30 days.

Remarks: Acupuncture and moxibustion are fairly effective in treating this disease. What needs mentioning is the application of red-hot needling, which can obtain notable effect, but the insertion must never be too deep. Medication and surgical measures should be combined in cases of suppuration or ulceration. If the ulceration is long-lasting and difficult to heal, mild moxibustion can be provided with moxa sticks over the focus or around it, 5-10 minutes each time, once or twice daily, so the healing can be accelerated.

REFERENCE:

Observed results of 211 cases of scrofula treated with cutting method at Ganshu (U.B. 18)

Point: Ganshu (U.B. 18)

Method: After locating the point accurately and doing routine antisepsis on the skin, apply 1-2% procaine for a local anesthesia. Cut the skin of the point location to make a 1-1.5 cm incision, deep inside the layer of the muscle. Use a specially made pricker to cut 10-20 muscle fibers. Smear the incision with iodine tincture and cover with antiseptic gauze. Exert pressure and use a flexible fabric bandage to fix the gauze. Attention should be paid that your left hand holds up the pricked area to prevent the bleeding when the right hand is manipulating the specially made pricker. Cut the point on the affected side.

Results: All the cases obtained effectiveness, the rate of cure was 93 percent and the marked effective rate was 7 percent.

(*Source:* Chinese Acupuncture & Moxibustion, (3):45, 1987)

134. Malaria

Principal points: Dazhui (Du 14), Taodao (Du 13), Jianshi (P. 5), Houxi (S.I. 3)

Method: Treatment is better to be given 1-2 hours before an attack. Generally speaking, first puncture Dazhui (Du 14) with lift-thrust reducing method to strengthen the needling sensation. Try to

317

let the sensation extend downward. Puncture all the other points with strong stimulation. Retain the needles for 20-30 minutes with periodic manipulation. Treat once or several times a day. Continue the treatment for 2-3 days.

Supplementary points:

Fever: The twelve Jing-Well points (bilateral Lu 11, S.I. 1, L.I 1, S.J. 1, H. 9, P. 9), Weizhong (U.B. 40), pricking to cause bleeding

Coma: Renzhong (Du 26), Zhongchong (P. 9), with strong stimulation

Severe vomiting: Neiguan (P. 6), Zhongwan (Ren 12)

Abdominal pain and diarrhea: Tianshu (St. 25), Qihai (Ren 6), Zusanli (St. 36)

Chills: Zhiyang (Du 9), Zusanli (St. 36), puncturing with reinforcing method and combining moxibustion with a moxa stick or indirect moxibustion with ginger, 5-7 moxa cones for each point.

Chronic malaria due to exhaustion of *qi* and blood: Ganshu (U.B. 18), Pishu (U.B. 20), Zusanli (St. 36), Sanyinjiao (Sp. 6), puncturing with reinforcing method, and combining moxibustion

Other therapies:

1. Ear acupuncture

Points: Lower Apex of Tragus, Brain, Intertragicus, Liver, Spleen

Method: Choose bilateral points on ears. Treat 2-6 hours before an attack. Puncture with strong stimulation. Retain the needles until 1-2 hours after the expected time of the attack. Apply periodic rotation 2-3 times. Treat daily for three days.

2. Cupping

Points: Dazhui (Du 14), Taodao (Du 13)

Method: Apply cups an hour before an attack. Retain the cups for 5-10 minutes. Treat daily.

3. Cutaneous acupuncture

Points: Dazhui (Du 14), pathway of the Du meridian on the back, lumbar and sacral region, Jiaji points (Extra) T5-S4, Jianshi (P. 5), Hegu (L.I. 4), Taichong (Liv. 3), Taixi (K. 3)

Method: Prick to cause bleeding at Dazhui (Du 14) before the attack. Then repeatedly tap the other portions and points.

Remarks: Acupuncture and moxibustion are quite effective in the treatment of quotidian malaria, tertian malaria and quartan malaria. As to malignant malaria, they have certain effect too. A severe case of malignant malaria should be treated with a combination of medications.

REFERENCE:

1. Observed results of acupuncture in treating 126 cases of malaria

Points: a) Dazhui (Du 14), Neiguan (P. 6); b) Taodao (Du 13), Jianshi (P. 5)

Method: Alternate the two groups of points. Treat two hours before an attack. After the needling sensation is obtained, retain the needles for 30 minutes with periodic manipulation once every five minutes. Treat once or twice a day. Three days of treatment constitute one course.

Results: Of 126 cases treated, 11 cases (8.7 percent) obtained cure (the symptoms controlled in 72-96 hours, malarial parasite report showed negative in 120 hours), improvement was seen in 40 cases (31.7 percent), (the symptoms controlled in 72-96 hours, but malarial parasite report showed positive) and no effect was evident in 75 cases (59.5 percent).

(*Source:* Journal of Hunan College of Traditional Chinese Medicine, 7(3):37, 1987)

135. Epidemic Encephalitis B

Principal points: Zhongchong (P. 9), Fengchi (G.B. 20), Fengfu (Du 16), Yongquan (K. 1), Quchi (L.I. 11)

Method: During acute stage, puncture the above-mentioned points with repeated manipulations. Apply reducing method of rotating at Fengchi (G.B. 20) and Fengfu (Du 16), while applying reducing method of combination of lifting, thrusting, rotating and twirling to the other points. Retain the needles for 30-60 minutes. Treat 1-3 times a day depending upon the severity of the illness. But even method should be applied to epidemic encephalitis B at recovery stage, and its sequelae. With children or babies, shallow insertion with needles rapidly thrusting in and out is advisable.

Supplementary points:

Fever: Dazhui (Du 14), Hegu (L.I. 4), puncturing with reducing method and retaining needles

Lose of consciousness: Hegu (L.I. 4), Renzhong (Du 26), Baihui (Du 20), pricking to cause bleeding at Hegu (L.I. 4) and Zhongchong (P. 9), puncturing Renzhong (Du 26) with upward slanted insertion to a depth of 1 *cun*, and applying repeated manipulation

Convulsion: Taichong (Liv. 3), Dazhui (Du 14), Yanglingquan (G.B. 34), applying repeated manipulation with strong stimulation

Shock: Renzhong (Du 26), Suliao (Du 25), using strong stimulation and retaining needles. Add Guanyuan (Ren 4), Shenque (Ren 8) and Zusanli (St. 36) with indirect moxibustion with ginger, 10 cones each point. Moxibustion with a moxa stick can be used instead.

Low fever, profuse sweating at the recovery stage: Taodao (Du 13), Jianshi (P. 5), Fuliu (K. 7), Zusanli (St. 36)

Aphasia: Yamen (Du 15), Tongli (H. 5), Lianquan (Ren 23)

Eyes staring forward: Jingming (U.B. 1), Xingjian (Liv. 2)

Paralysis on the upper limbs: Dazhu (U.B. 11), Jianyu (L.I. 15), Shousanli (L.I. 10), Hegu (L.I. 4), applying repeated manipulation with strong stimulation

Paralysis on the lower limbs: Huantiao (G.B. 30), Fengshi (G.B. 31), Yanglingquan (G.B. 34), Kunlun (U.B. 60), applying repeated manipulation with strong stimulation

Deficient *qi* and blood: Zusanli (St. 36), Ganshu (U.B. 18), Pishu (U.B. 20), puncturing with reinforcing method, or applying moxibustion

Other therapies:

1. Ear acupuncture

Points: Heart, Liver, Central Rim, Brain, corresponding points on the paralysis region

Method: Puncture gently with shallow insertion. Retain the needles for 30 minutes. Electro-acupuncture may be also used.

2. Head acupuncture

Points: Motor Area, Sensory Area, Leg Motor and Sensory Area, bilateral

Method: Apply deep insertion with 10-20 minutes' continuous manipulation. Treat daily or once every other day.

Remarks: Acupuncture and moxibustion therapies have certain effect in treating epidemic encephalitis B. But other medications should be adopted. For the recovery stage and its sequelae, massage therapy can be combined. Ask the patient to strengthen the functional exercise.

REFERENCE:

Report on acupuncture in treating 11 cases of aphasia in the sequelae of viral encephalitis

Points: a) Yamen (Du 15), Shanglianquan (Extra), Tiantu (Ren 22), Neiguan (P. 6); b) Yamen (Du 15), Zengyin (Extra), Tongli (H. 5)

Method: Treat daily. Use Group A for two treatments, then use Group B. Ten treatments constitute one course. The interval between two courses is 7-10 days. Sometimes, add Yongquan (K. 1) after failure by using the above-mentioned points. Or prick Jinjin-Yuye (Extra) to cause bleeding with a three-edged needle when motor impairment of the tongue exists. Retain the needles in the points except Yamen (Du 15) for 15-20 minutes with periodic manipulation.

Results: All the 11 cases were cured within 3-30 treatments.

(*Source:* Jiangxi Journal of Traditional Chinese Medicine, (4):54, 1983)

136. Carboxyhemoglobinemia

Principal points: Baihui (Du 20), Neiguan (P. 6), Taiyang (Extra)

Supplementary points:

Mild and moderate cases of the poisoning: Touwei (St. 8), Fengchi (G.B. 20), Hegu (L.I. 4)

Severe poisoning with coma: Renzhong (Du 26), Shaoshang (Lu. 11), Shixuan (Extra), Yongquan (K. 1)

Method: For mild cases of the poisoning, perform strong stimulation at the points, and retain the needles for 20-30 minutes, rotating intermittently. To treat the severe cases, give intense and rapid stimulation with swift rotating and thrusting of the needle.

Withdraw needles after the patient regains consciousness.

Other therapies:

1. Bleeding method

Points: Shixuan (Extra), Quze (P. 3)

Method: Prick Shixuan (Extra) with a three-edged needle and then bind the upper arm of the patient tightly to congest the veins. Bleed Quze (P. 3) with a three-edged needle or injection needle, usually on one side, but on both sides for severe cases.

2. Moxibustion

Points: Baihui (Du 20), Shenque (Ren 8), Qihai (Ren 6), Suliao (Du 25), Zusanli (St. 36)

Method: Apply heavy suspending moxibustion with moxa sticks until the patient's limbs become warm.

Remarks: The patients suffering from carboxyhemoglobinemia must first be moved out away from the source, and to a place with fresh air and good ventilation, and then provided with emergency treatment. Warmth must be kept in winter.

Acupuncture and moxibustion have good effects in relieving the symptoms for the mild and moderate cases, but comprehensive measures must be taken to rescue the severe cases and acupuncture can also be combined.

Cases of hronic poisoning or sequela from acute poisoning can be treated with the method of body acupuncture, moxibustion, ear acupuncture, electro-acupuncture, or hydro-acupuncture, and effectiveness can also be obtained.

REFERENCE:

Preliminary report on 58 cases of carboxyhemoglobinemia treated with acupuncture

Points and method:

1) Tense syndrome:

Mild cases: Puncture Renzhong (Du 26), Chengjiang (Ren 24), Shaoshang (Lu. 11), and the patient will regain the consciousness immediately.

Severe cases: Supplement Suliao (Du 25), Yintang (Extra), Jiache (St. 6), Zhongchong (P. 9), Shaochong (H. 9), and Yongquan (K. 1), but reduce all with strong stimulation, and after the needling, press Tianrong (S.I. 17) heavily with the middle finger, then perform massage on the neck, the shoulder axillary fossa and cubital fossa. Pinch the olecranon, pull fingers, heavily pinch the big tendon below the hypochondriac region, and then pinch the tendons of Weizhong (U.B. 40), Kunlun (U.B. 60), and Taixi (K. 3). After the massage, put Lying-Dragon Pellets into the nose to cause sneezing. If the patient does not come to, heavily press Tianrong (S.I. 17) again.

2) Flaccid syndrome:

Mild cases: Needle Renzhong (Du 26), Yintang (Extra) and Shaoshang (Lu. 11), and the patient will regain consciousness immediately.

Severe cases: Supplement Suliao (Du 25) with needling, and Shenque (Ren 8), Qihai (Ren 6) and Baihui (Du 20) with moxibustion. If the patient fails to regain consciousness, perform massage and force hot drink into the patient's mouth. In case of absence of breathing and pulse, artificial respiration and other methods should be employed.

Results: Of 58 cases treated, 18 cases came back immediately with needling at Renzhong (Du 26) and Shaoshang (Lu. 11); 25 cases with Chengjiang (Ren 24) and Suliao (Du 25) supplemented, 9 cases with Zhongchong (P. 9), Yintang (Extra) and Hegu (L.I. 4) supplemented by needling but Shenque (Ren 8) supplemented by moxibustion, in combination with massage, Lying-Dragon Pellets, and ginger-juice drippings in eyes; and 6 case with needling at Huiyin (Ren 1) and artificial respiration.

(*Source:* Journal of Anhui College of Traditional Chinese Medicine, (2):55, 1959)

137. Heatstroke

Principal points: Quchi (L.I. 11), Dazhui (Du 14), Renzhong (Du 26), Neiguan (P. 6)

Method: Produce moderate or strong stimulation with filiform needles which will be retained for 10-20 minutes for the mild cases, but continuously manipulate to bring about strong stimulation for the severe cases.

Supplementary points:

High fever: Shixuan (Extra), Quze (P. 3), Weizhong (U.B. 40), all bled with three-edged needles

Convulsion of limbs: Yanglingquan (G.B. 34), Hegu (L.I. 4), Chengshan (U.B. 57)

Excessive sweating, cold limbs and hardly palpable pulse: Shenque (Ren 8), Guanyuan (Ren 4), Qihai (Ren 6), Taiyuan (Lu. 9)

Severe thirst with profuse drinking preferable: Bleeding Jinjin-Yuye (Extra)

Other therapies:

1. *Sha*-scraping method (a fairly effective folk method for treating mild cases of heatstroke)

Use a smooth pottery spoon sipped with vegetable oil or clean water to scrape the paraspinal muscles, the nape of the neck, the chest and the intercostal space, the shoulder, the arms, the cubital fossa and the popliteal fossa, to make the skin purplish or dark-red.

2. Ear acupuncture

Points: Ear Apex, Shenmen, Heart, Lower Apex of Tragus, Occiput

Method: Apply strong stimulation with filiform needles, then rotate for five minutes and retain for 20 minutes thereafter. Bleed Ear Apex. Some points can be supplemented according to the specific symptoms, e.g., Pt. Forehead for headache.

Remarks: Modern medical measures should be incorporated in severe cases.

138. Dizziness and Vertigo

Principal points: Fengchi (G.B. 20), Touwei (St. 8), Yintang (Extra), Neiguan (P. 6)

Method: First puncture Neiguan (P. 6). Then insert at Fengchi (G.B. 20) to a depth of 0.5-1 *cun*, and let the needling sensation extend to the temple. Then needle Touwei (St. 8) and Yintang (Extra). Retain the needles for 20-30 minutes.

Supplementary points:

Hyperactivity of *yang* of the liver: Taichong (Liv. 3), Xiaxi (G.B. 43), Shenshu (U.B. 23), Ganshu (U.B. 18)

Deficient *qi* and blood: Zusanli (St. 36), Pishu (U.B. 20), Qihai (Ren 6), Baihui (Du 20)

Phlegm-damp obstructing in the middle *jiao*: Fenglong (St.

40), Zhongwan (Ren 12)

Other therapies:

1. Head acupuncture

Points: Vertigo and Hearing Area, bilateral

Method: Puncture according to the routine procedure of head acupuncture. Treat daily and 5-10 treatments constitute one course.

2. Ear acupuncture

Points: Kidney, Shenmen, Occiput, Internal Ear, Brain

Method: Choose 2-3 points in a session. Puncture with moderate stimulation. Retain the needles for 20-30 minutes with periodic manipulation. Treat daily and 5-7 treatments constitute one course.

3. Hydro-acupuncture

Points: Hegu (L.I. 4), Taichong (Liv. 3), Yiming (Extra), Neiguan (P. 6), Fengchi (G.B. 20), Sidu (S.J. 9)

Method: Choose 2-3 points in a session. Inject 1-2 ml of 5% or 10% glucose solution, or 0.5 ml of Vitamin B_{12} solution, into each point. Treat once every other day.

4. Cutaneous acupuncture

Points: Baihui (Du 20), Taiyang (Extra), Yintang (Extra), Jiaji points (Extra)

Method: Use cutaneous needles to tap with moderate stimulation for 1-2 treatments a day, and 5-10 treatments constitute one course.

Remarks: If the symptoms involve dizziness and vertigo, the primary cause should be found and treated first.

REFERENCES:

1. Observed results of applying camphol on ear points in treating 77 cases of dizziness and vertigo

Points: Shenmen, Central Rim, Brain, Heart, End of Inferior Helix Crus

Method: Choose 2-3 points bilaterally in a session. Apply grain-like camphols with adhesive tape at the points. Change once every two days. Four treatments constitute one course.

Results: Of 77 cases treated, 53 cases were cured without relapse after more than one year. Improvement was seen in 22 cases, no effect in 2 cases. Most of the patients' dizziness and vertigo were reduced after 30 minutes' application. This method is not to be used with a pregnant woman.

(*Source:* Henan Traditional Chinese Medicine, (4):14, 1986)

2. Observed results of embedding vaccaria seeds on ear points in treating 200 cases of dizziness and vertigo

Principal points: Dizziness, Vertigo, Eye

Supplementary points:

Hypertension: Shenmen, Lowering Blood Pressure Groove

Hypotension: Spleen, Elevating Blood Pressure Spot

Neurasthenia: Neurasthenia, Shenmen

Insomnia: Brain

Cervical vertebrae disorder: Cervical Vertebrae, Neck

Tinnitus: Internal Ear, Sanjiao

Nausea or vomiting: Stomach, Middle of Ear

Results: The cure rate reached 76 percent, marked effect rate was 13.5 percent and the improvement rate was 10.5 percent. The total effective rate reached 100 percent.

(*Source:* Chinese Acupuncture & Moxibustion, (6):22, 1987)

3. Clinical study on moxibustion with moxa cones as the main measure applied at Baihui (Du 20) in treating 255 cases of dizziness and vertigo

Point: Baihui (Du 20)

Method: For tinnitus in the left ear, apply moxibustion at 0.5 cm lateral to Baihui (Du 20) on the left side; for tinnitus in the right ear, 0.5 cm lateral to Baihui (Du 20) on the right side; for tinnitus of both ears, in the center of Baihui (Du 20). Apply 50-70 moxa cones at the point in a session. After moxibustion, puncture Zusanli (St. 36) with reducing method.

Results: Of 255 cases treated, a short-term cure was obtained in 201 cases (78.9 percent) and improvement was seen in 54 cases (21.1 percent).

(*Source:* Xinjiang Chinese Medicine and Medica Materia, (4):30, 1985)

4. Observed results of needling Vertigo and Hearing Area of head acupoint in treating 15 cases of dizziness and vertigo

Point: Vertigo and Hearing Area

Method: Rapidly insert the needle into the stimulating area. Continue rotating for two minutes. Retain the needle for 10 minutes, then, rotate the needle again three times. Treat daily or once every other day.

Results: Among 15 cases, 7 cases were cured and improvement

326

was seen in 8 cases.

(*Source:* Shanghai Journal of Acupuncture and Moxibustion, (2):16, 1988)

139. Motion Sickness

Principal points: Hegu (L.I. 4), Neiguan (P. 6), Baihui (Du 20), Fengchi (G.B. 20)

Method: Apply mild and moderate stimulation with filiform needles. Retain the needles for 20-30 minutes and intermittently rotate in between. The needling can be provided prior to getting on board or even just on the occurrence of some mild symptoms.

Supplementary points:

Collapse (accompanied by sudden falling, pallor, cold limbs, feeble breathing, thready and forceless pulse): Renzhong (Du 26), Guanyuan (Ren 4), Qihai (Ren 6), Zusanli (St. 36), with warm-needle moxibustion or mild moxibustion with moxa sticks until the consciousness is regained and limbs become warm

Other therapies:

1. Bleeding method

Points: Zhongchong (P. 9), Neiguan (P. 6), Taiyang (Extra), Fengchi (G.B. 20)

Method: Before getting on board or after the occurrence of symptoms, one or several points can be bled slightly.

2. Ear acupuncture

Points: Brain, Shenmen, Stomach, Heart

Method: Stimulate the points with needles. Retain the needles for 10-20 minutes and rotate intermittently in between. Needle-embedding method can be also used during the journey for the sake of pressing the points at any time.

3. Moxibustion

Points: Neiguan (P. 6), Baihui (Du 20), Shenmen (H. 7), Zusanli (St. 36), Zhongwan (Ren 12)

Method: Apply suspending moxibustion with a moxa stick, 2-3 minutes at each point.

140. Edema

Principal points: Shuifen (Ren 9), Qihai (Ren 6), Sanjiaoshu (U.B. 22), Zusanli (St. 36)

Method: Use filiform needles with moderate stimulation. Retain the needles for 20-30 minutes. If the edema is deficient and cold in nature, add moxibustion. Treat daily.

Supplementary points:

Edema of the face: Renzhong (Du 26)

Edema of the upper limbs: Pianli (L.I. 6)

Edema of the lower limbs: Yinlingquan (Sp. 9), Foot-Linqi (G.B. 41), Shangqiu (Sp. 5)

Exterior symptoms due to invasion by exogenous wind and cold: Hegu (L.I. 4), Feishu (U.B. 13)

Deficient *yang* of the spleen and kidney: Moxi Pishu (U.B. 20), Shenshu (U.B. 23), Pangguangshu (U.B. 28)

Other therapies:

Ear acupuncture

Points: Liver, Spleen, Kidney, Brain, Urinary Bladder, Abdomen

Method: Choose 2-3 points in a session. Puncture bilateral points with moderate stimulation. Treat once every other day.

Remarks: Acupuncture and moxibustion are of certain effect in treating edema, however, they need other medications in combination.

REFERENCE:

Observed results of head acupuncture in treating 25 cases of edema

Principal points: Blood Vessel Dilation and Constriction Area, Motor Area, on the healthy side

Supplementary points:

Stifling sensation in the chest, and abdominal distention: Thoracic Cavity Area, Stomach Area

Method: Place the patient in a prone position. Slantly insert gauge 28 filiform needles 2-3 *cun* in length, along the scalp to a depth of 2-3 *cun*. Retain the needles for an hour with periodic manipulation, once every 10 minutes. Seven treatments constitute one course. Begin another course after three days' rest.

Results: There were 25 cases in this group, 15 male cases and 10 female cases. Among them there were 21 cases with cerebrothrombosis, 3 cases with cerebrohemorrhage and 1 case with cerebroembolism. All 25 cases had the manifestations of edema on the upper or lower limbs, accompanied by stifling sensation in the chest, abdominal distention, insomnia and aphasia. After treatments of less than 3 courses, the total disappearance of edema on the affected limbs resulted in 22 cases, a marked reduction was present in 3 cases and the other manifestations improved to different degrees.

(*Source:* Shanghai Journal of Acupuncture and Moxibustion, (4):30, 1987)

141. Frostbite

I. Localized frostbite

Principal points: Ashi points (around the focus)

Method: Perform surrounding method all around the focus, with needles inserted into several points according to the size of the affected area. Produce moderate or strong stimulation and retain the needles for 30-60 minutes, but manipulate every 5-10 minutes. Treat daily. After the needling, mild moxibustion can be performed with a moxa stick over the focus for 10-20 minutes.

Supplementary points:

The dorsum of the hand is affected: Houxi (S.I. 3)

The dorsum of the foot is affected: Kunlun (U.B. 60)

The auricle is affected: Waiguan (S.J. 5)

II. Generalized frostbite

Points: Dazhui (Du 14), Renzhong (Du 26), Yongquan (K. 1), Hegu (L.I. 4), Zusanli (St. 36)

Method: Provide strong stimulation, and retain the needles for 30 minutes. Treat 2-3 times daily. When shock is present, comprehensive measures of both traditional Chinese and Western medicines should be taken.

Remarks: In case of localized frostbite cured with acupuncture therapy, mild moxibustion with moxa sticks can be provided over the affected area during the next winter, to prevent the recurrence of the frostbite.

142. Drowning

Principal points: Renzhong (Du 26), Chengjiang (Ren 24), Shixuan (Extra), Yongquan (K. 1)

Supplementary points: Baihui (Du 20), Suliao (Du 25), Neiguan (P. 6), Shenque (Ren 8), Zusanli (St. 36), Huiyin (Ren 1)

Method: First puncture the principal points with strong stimulation by means of rapid lifting, thrusting and rotating the needles for 3-5 minutes. After removing the needles, needle the supplementary points with strong stimulation, and retain the needles and intermittently manipulate. Do not needle Shenque (Ren 8), which is performed indirect moxibustion with salt.

Remarks: To treat the drowned, comprehensive measures should be taken. First of all, dirty matters should be removed from the mouth and the nose, and artificial breathing should be administered. Acupuncture therapy is employed only as one of many rescuing measures.

143. Addiction to Smoking

Ear acupuncture

Points: Mouth, Trachea, Lung, Intertragicus, Shenmen

Method: After routine skin sterilization, embed sterilized intradermal needles in the points and fix with adhesive plaster. Change the needles every five days. During the embedding, needles are pressed by the thumb or index finger for one minute whenever the craving to smoke comes.

Remarks: In recent years, there has been an increase of reports on giving up smoking with ear acupuncture. After the needling on ear points, the smoker feels the unpleasant taste similar to that of cigarettes or tobacco in his mouth, and the feeling towards the cigarettes or tobacco becomes bitter and pungent. Coughing due to the irritation of smoking and dizziness after the smoking will appear, so the smokers will have no more desire to smoke. Ear acupuncture can also eliminate "giving-up-smoking syndrome," such as restlessness, after stopping to smoke.

REFERENCES:

1. Observation on the effect of 80 cases of smoking addiction treated with electric ear acupuncture

Points: Shenmen, Smoking 1 (tender spot between Pts. Lung and Trachea), Smoking 2 (tender spot around Pt. Lower Apex of Tragus)

Method: Utilize gauge 28 filiform needles, 1 *cun* in length, to puncture both ears. Connect with a Model G-6805 electro-acupuncture apparatus (direct current, 6 v) after the arrival of *qi*. Select continuous wave, set the frequency at 200 times per minute, and adjust the output of the electricity to between 2 and 3 on the switch button. If the patient has higher tolerance, the electricity can be stronger. The connection lasts for 30 minutes. Treat daily. The average course is 1-3 treatments.

Results: Of 80 cases treated, 38 cases showed marked effectiveness, 22 cases showed positive effects, 11 cases showed improvement and 9 cases failed.

(*Source:* Shanghai Journal of Acupuncture and Moxibustion, (2):29, 1985)

2. Summary of the treatment of 108 smoking cases with acupuncture

Points: Hegu (L.I. 4), Zusanli (St. 36), bilateral

Method: Needle daily in one point each time. Ten treatments constitute one course. After the arrival of *qi*, repeat gentle thrusting, then strong lifting, thrusting and rotating in large amplitude with rapid frequency. Connect the needles with a Model G-6805 electro-acupuncture apparatus. Use a continuous wave, adjust the electricity according to the patient's tolerance, and connect for 15 minutes. After the withdrawal of the needles, insert intradermal needles subcutaneously to 1 cm in the punctured points, keep the needle body perpendicular to the running course of the meridian and fix with adhesive plaster. Retain the needles for one day and require the patient to press the point several times daily for a couple of minutes each time.

Results: Of 108 cases treated, 82 cases (75.4 percent) showed some effect (no desire of smoking, and no longer smoking a month after the treatment is finished), and 26 cases (24.6 percent) failed.

(*Source:* Guangxi Journal of Traditional Chinese Medicine, 9(1):34, 1986)

144. Simple Goiter and Hyperthyroidism

Principal points: Naohui (S.J. 13), Tiantu (Ren 22), Tianding (L.I. 17), Hegu (L.I. 4), Zusanli (St. 36)

Method: Puncture with moderate stimulation and retain the needles for 30 minutes. Treat daily or once every other day. Ten treatments constitute one course.

Supplementary points:

Qi stagnation of the liver: Taichong (Liv. 3), Shanzhong (Ren 17)

Deficient *yin* and excessive fire: Jianshi (P. 5), Taixi (K. 3), Taichong (Liv. 3)

Fire of the liver attacking the stomach: Neiting (St. 44), Taichong (Liv. 3), Fengchi (G.B. 20)

Enlargement of the thyroid gland: Local area of the thyroid gland. Place the patient in a supine position. Insert the needle at the margin of the thyroid gland towards the center of the mass. Generally speaking, Choose 1-2 points around the margin for each treatment. Manipulation should be mild to avoid damage to the blood vessel or nerves. It is advisable to withdraw needles without bleeding.

Stifling sensation in the chest and cough: Shanzhong (Ren 17)

Palpitation: Neiguan (P. 6), Shenmen (H. 7)

Irritability, insomnia: Shenmen (H. 7)

Exophthalmos: Jingming (U.B. 1), Zanzhu (U.B. 2), Sizhukong (S.J. 23), Fengchi (G.B. 20)

Severe hand-shaking: Quchi (L.I. 11), Hegu (L.I. 4)

Lassitude: Qihai (Ren 6)

Other therapies:

1. Ear acupuncture

Principal Points: Thyroid, Intertragicus, Brain, Shenmen

Supplementary points: Hyperthyroidism: Heart, Kidney

Method: Puncture with filiform needles and strong stimulation. Retain the needles for 30 minutes. Treat once every other day, or embed intradermal needles for 1-2 days. Use points on ears in rotation, or embed apply vaccaria seeds with adhesive tape at ear points for five days. Begin another treatment after two days' rest.

2. Cutaneous acupuncture

Points: The local area around the goiter, corresponding Jiaji points (Extra) on the neck

Method: Gently tap the local area until congestion appears. Treat once every other day.

Remarks: Acupuncture is effective in treating simple goiter and hyperthyroidism. It can be combined with other medication.

REFERENCES:

1. Observed results of moxibustion in treating 30 cases of hyperthyroidism

Principal points: Dazhu (U.B. 11), Fengmen (U.B. 12), Feishu (U.B. 13), Fengfu (Du 16), Dazhui (Du 14), Shenzhu (Du 12), Fengchi (G.B. 20)

Supplementary points: Points according to symptoms

Method: Use direct moxibustion, indirect moxibustion, fire needle, or warm needling for certain patients.

Results: Of 30 cases treated, a short-term cure was obtained in 4 cases, marked effect was evident in 11 cases, and improvement was seen in 15 cases. Most cases showed therapeutic result after 2-10 treatments.

(*Source:* Journal of Chengdu College of Traditional Chinese Medicine, 10(1):23, 1987)

2. Long-term therapeutic result observation on acupuncture in treating 50 cases of hyperthyroidism

Principal points: Center of the thyroid gland

Supplementary points:

Exophthalmos: Sizhukong (S.J. 23), Zanzhu (U.B. 2), Jingming (U.B. 1), Fengchi (G.B. 20), Sikuangxue (Extra, four points on the left, right, above, and below the ridge of eye ball)

Palpitation: Neiguan (P. 6), Shenmen (H. 7)

Easily hungry, emaciation, profuse sweating: Sanyinjiao (Sp. 6), Zusanli (St. 36)

Method: Apply the reinforcing or reducing method by lifting and thrusting needle to the center of the thyroid gland, while applying even method to the other points. Puncture with mild stimulation. Do not retain the needles.

Results: All were cured except 2 cases which required operations.

(*Source:* Beijing Traditional Chinese Medicine, (1):45, 1982)

3. Clinical observation on acupuncture in improving vision of hyperthyroid exophthalmos

Points: Shangtianshu (Extra, right above Tianzhu, U.B. 10), Fengchi (G.B. 20), Tongziliao (G.B. 1), Zanzhu (U.B. 2), Hegu (L.I. 4)

Method: Retain the needles for 30 minutes with periodic manipulation every 10 minutes. Apply a combination of lifting, thrusting, twirling and rotating for manipulation to strengthen the needling sensation. Treat twice a week. Two months' treatment constitutes one course. Follow with three courses of treatments.

Results: A marked effect on eye's vision after puncturing or three courses of treatment was evident in 15 eyes, improvement in 27 eyes and no effect in 3 eyes.

(*Source:* Jiangsu Chinese Medical Journal, 7(1):28, 1986)

145. Diabetes

Principal points: Yishu (Extra), Feishu (U.B. 13), Pishu (U.B. 20), Shenshu (U.B. 23), Zusanli (St. 36), Sanyinjiao (Sp. 6)

Method: Use filiform needles to produce mild or moderate stimulation, and retain the needles for 15-20 minutes. Treat daily or once every other day. Ten treatments constitute one course, and there is an interval of 3-5 days between two courses. Yishu (Extra) is used in treating diabetes. It has good effect of controlling the blood sugar and urine sugar, and modern research proved it is able to regulate the secretion of insulin. The point is located on the back, 1.5 *cun* lateral to the lower border of the eighth thoracic vertebra.

Supplementary points:

Thirst and polydipsia: Shaoshang (Lu. 11), Yuji (Lu. 10), Taiyuan (Lu. 9)

Polyorexia and emaciation: Weishu (U.B. 21), Zhongwan (Ren 12), Neiting (St. 44)

Polyuria: Guanyuan (Ren 4), Taixi (K. 3), Shuiquan (K. 5)

Cold limbs due to *yang* deficiency: Mingmen (Du 4), Guanyuan (Ren 4), Qihai (Ren 6), applying mild moxibustion with moxa sticks or moxa cones

Blurring of vision: Zanzhu (U.B. 2), Guangming (G.B. 37),

Fengchi (G.B. 20), Taichong (Liv. 3)

Itching of the genital organ: Qugu (Ren 2), Qihai (Ren 6)

Palpitation: Neiguan (P. 6), Xinshu (U.B. 15), Shanzhong (Ren 17)

Insomnia: Shenmen (H. 7)

Dizziness: Shangxing (Du 23), Fengchi (G.B. 20)

Other therapies:

1. Ear acupuncture

Points: Pancreas, Intertragicus, Kidney, Sanjiao, Thirst point, Stomach, Lung

Method: Select 3-5 points each time and produce mild stimulation with filiform needles. Retain the needles for 20 minutes. Treat once every other day. The intradermal needle-embedding method is also applicable.

2. Cutaneous acupuncture

Points: Paraspinal muscles, mainly 7th-10th thoracic vertebrae

Method: Apply mild or moderate tapping for 5-10 minutes each time. Treat once every other day and 10 treatments constitute one course.

Remarks: The disease is susceptible to the complication of skin infection, thus strict skin antisepsis should be performed in acupuncture treatment.

Acupuncture therapy has satisfactory effect in the treatment of mild and moderate cases but hardly obtains any effectiveness in insulin dependents.

146. Obesity

Principal points: Pishu (U.B. 20), Zusanli (St. 36), Sanyinjiao (Sp. 6)

Method: Utilize filiform needles to produce moderate stimulation, and retain the needles for 20-30 minutes. Repeat manipulation of needles during the retention to strengthen the stimulation. Treat daily or once every other day. Other points can be combined and appropriate moxibustion performed.

Supplementary points:

Hyperactivity of spleen and stomach with excessive food intake: Weishu (U.B. 21), Quchi (L.I. 11), Hegu (L.I. 4), Neiting

(St. 44), with reducing method

Deficiency of spleen and stomach with anorexia: Weishu (U.B. 21), Shenshu (U.B. 23), Qihai (Ren 6), Guanyuan (Ren 4), with reducing method or add moxibustion

Yang deficiency of spleen and kidney with the fatness most distinguishable in hips and thighs: Shenshu (U.B. 23), Mingmen (Du 4), Taixi (K. 3), with reducing method or add moxibustion

Distress in the stomach and polyorexia: Zhongwan (Ren 12), Liangqiu (St. 34)

Constipation associated: Tianshu (St. 25), Zhigou (S.J. 6)

Oliguria and edema: Yinlingquan (Sp. 9)

Abdominal distention: Zhongwan (Ren 12)

Somnolence and amnesia: Renzhong (Du 26), Baihui (Du 20)

Seminal emission, impotence and premature ejaculation: Guanyuan (Ren 4), Zhongji (Ren 3), with reducing method or add moxibustion

Palpitation and shortness of breath: Neiguan (P. 6)

Hyperlipemia: Yanglingquan (G.B. 34), Taichong (Liv. 3), Fenglong (St. 40)

Other therapies:

Ear acupuncture

Points: Stomach, Small Intestine, Kidney, Shenmen, Intertragicus, Spleen

Method: Select 2-3 points each time and after the routine skin antisepsis, embed sterilized intradermal needles and fix with adhesive plaster. In summer, change the embedded needles every four days, and in winter every seven days. Press the needles before meals or when feeling hungry.

Remarks: There are many reports home and abroad on losing weight with acupuncture of which the effect is satisfactory. In the clinic, the needling is combined with needle-embedding method in ear points, or the needle-embedding can be used alone.

REFERENCE:

Clinical observation on 567 cases of obesity treated with ear acupressure

Points: Intertragicus, Ovary, Central Rim, Hunger point, Thirst point, Shenmen, Spleen, Stomach, all bilateral

Method: Press 4-6 points each time, once weekly, five treatments constitute one course.

  Results: Of 567 cases treated, 84 cases showed marked effect (15 percent), 385 cases showed some effect (68 percent), and 98 cases failed (17 percent). The total effective rate was 83 percent.

  (*Source:* Shanghai Journal of Acupuncture and Moxibustion, (2):22, 1984)

Extra Acupuncture Points (I)

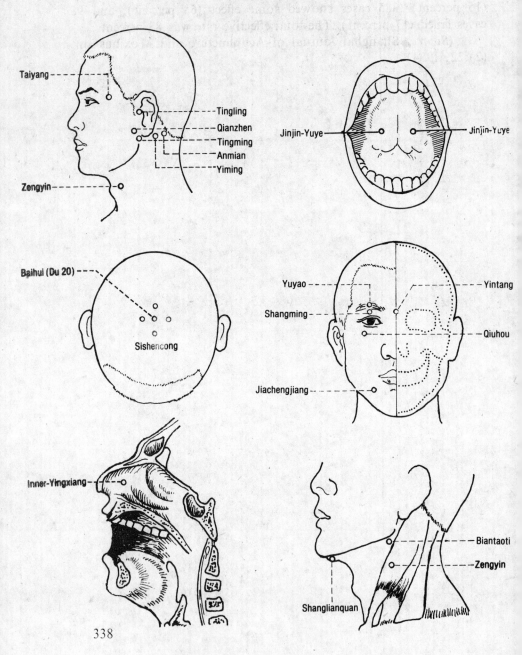

Extra Acupuncture Points (II)

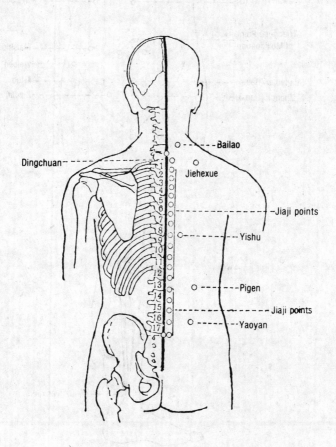

Extra Acupuncture Points (III)

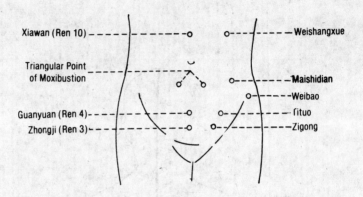

Xiawan (Ren 10) ------------- Weishangxue

Triangular Point
of Moxibustion ------------- Maishidian

------------- Weibao

Guanyuan (Ren 4) ------------- Tituo

Zhongji (Ren 3) ------------- Zigong

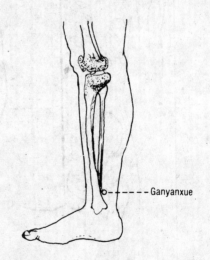

Ganyanxue

Extra Acupuncture Points (IV)

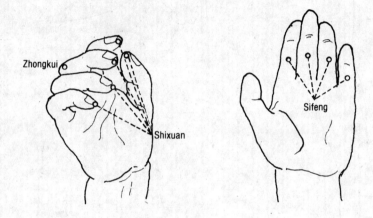

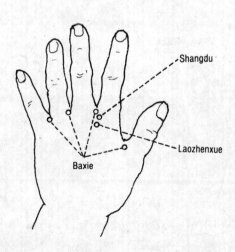

Extra Acupuncture Points (V)

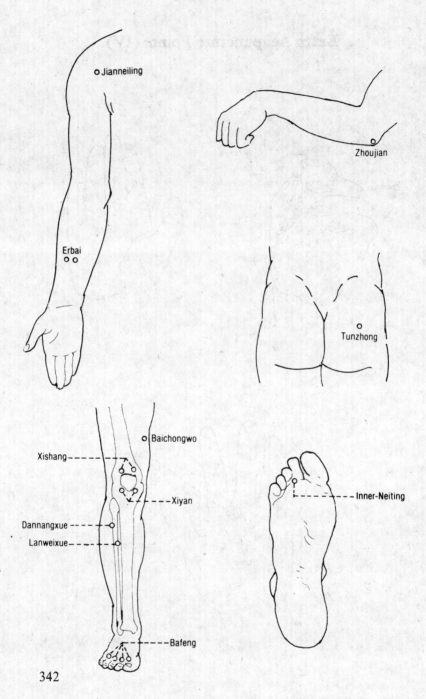

Jianneiling

Zhoujian

Erbai

Tunzhong

Baichongwo
Xishang
Xiyan
Dannangxue
Lanweixue
Bafeng

Inner-Neiting

INDEX OF THERAPEUTIC ACUPOINTS

Feishu (U.B. 13), 181, 182, 183, 184, 185, 186, 187, 188, 189, 200, 250, 281, 287, 305, 310, 328, 334

Feiyang (U.B. 58), 110

Femur-Futu (St. 32), 92, 93, 95, 106

Femur-Juliao (G.B. 29), 130

Femur-Zhongdu (G.B. 32), 92

Fengchi (G.B. 20), 60, 61, 66, 73, 81, 83, 88, 89, 98, 101, 105, 117, 119, 138, 143, 181, 182, 236, 251, 254, 255, 258, 260, 261, 262, 263, 264, 267, 269, 270, 273, 275, 277, 282, 284, 286, 287, 289, 291, 293, 302, 306, 309, 310, 319, 321, 324, 325, 327, 332, 335

Fengfu (Du 16), 133, 289, 293, 319

Fenglong (St. 40), 61, 76, 81, 101, 137, 138, 140, 152, 182, 183, 184, 185, 188, 214, 227, 229, 236, 249, 250, 315, 324, 336

Fengmen (U.B. 12), 130, 182, 184, 188, 249, 250

Fengshi (G.B. 31), 65, 66, 70, 88, 92, 93, 106, 248, 293, 297, 305, 320

Foot-Linqi (G.B. 41), 273, 275, 285, 315, 328

Foot-Zhongdu (Liv. 6), 179

Fujie (Sp. 14), 195

Fuliu (K. 7), 91, 320

Fushe (Sp. 13), 222

Futu (St. 32), 248

Fuyang (U.B. 59), 248

Ganshu (U.B. 18), 66, 76, 77, 88, 90, 98, 107, 147, 148, 151, 159, 160, 167, 168, 175, 178, 179, 191, 206, 210, 219, 220, 221, 227, 229, 230, 247, 260, 261, 262, 263, 264, 270, 277, 293, 308, 309, 316, 318, 320, 324

Gaohuangshu (U.B. 43), 183, 185, 186, 188, 189

Geguan (U.B. 46), 77

Geshu (U.B. 17), 70, 76, 77, 78, 101, 107, 109, 130, 133, 137, 140, 147, 148, 149, 151, 160, 183, 188, 189,

206, 207, 254, 258, 262, 270, 292, 296, 302, 304, 308, 309, 310, 316

Gongsun (Sp. 4), 101, 152, 160, 166, 178, 197, 214

Guanchong (S.J. 1), 270

Guangming (G.B. 37), 260, 261, 262, 264, 270, 334

Guanyuan (Ren 4), 59, 64, 77, 98, 101, 104, 131, 138, 140, 149, 154, 156, 157, 158, 160, 162, 166, 178, 188, 189, 191, 194, 195, 197, 198, 199, 201, 202, 203, 204, 205, 206, 207, 210, 211, 212, 213, 221, 222, 226, 227, 229, 236, 239, 242, 243, 245, 250, 293, 320, 324, 327, 334, 336

Guilai (St. 29), 197, 199, 207, 210, 211, 212, 222, 227, 243, 245, 246

Hand-Wangu (S.I. 4), 95, 130

Hand-Zhongzhu (S.J. 3), 60, 94, 95, 141, 275, 277

Head-Wangu (G.B. 12), 277

Hegu (L.I. 4), 60, 61, 64, 65, 66, 73, 80, 81, 82, 83, 88, 89, 90, 94, 95, 101, 102, 106, 121, 130, 138, 139, 141, 144, 145, 146, 152, 153, 156, 164, 167, 168, 171, 181, 182, 187, 194, 200, 201, 206, 210, 217, 233, 235, 236, 239, 244, 245, 248, 249, 251, 252, 254, 256, 260, 262, 264, 267, 269, 273, 275, 276, 277, 278, 280, 282, 284, 285, 287, 288, 289, 290, 291, 293, 294, 297, 299, 302, 303, 304, 306, 307, 311, 318, 320, 321, 324, 325, 327, 328, 329, 332, 335

Henggu (K. 11), 243

Houding (Du 19), 60

Houxi (S.I. 3), 60, 65, 79, 94, 95, 101, 106, 110, 118, 121, 130, 236, 247, 315, 317, 329

Huantiao (G.B. 30), 65, 67, 70, 71, 88, 90, 96, 101, 109, 130, 132, 248, 320

Huiyin (Ren 1), 198, 203, 330

344

Inner-Neiting (Extra), 77, 154, 160, 163, 239

Jiache (St. 6), 64, 65, 73, 80, 81, 82, 83, 89, 236, 244, 245, 251, 252, 284, 290, 291

Jiachengjiang (Extra), 73

Jiaji points (Extra), 66, 70, 71, 76, 91, 94, 95, 99, 106, 108, 130, 131, 142, 174, 186, 238, 242, 248, 252, 270, 286, 293, 301, 302, 318, 325, 333

Jianjing (G.B. 21), 116, 230, 233, 247, 315

Jianli (Ren 11), 104, 160, 215, 239

Jianliao (S.J. 14), 65, 94, 120, 121, 247

Jianneiling (Extra), 117

Jianshi (P. 5), 98, 104, 105, 137, 238, 247, 281, 315, 317, 318, 320, 332

Jianwaishu (S.I. 14), 117, 119

Jianyu (L.I. 15), 65, 66, 67, 88, 90, 94, 106, 108, 117, 120, 121, 125, 130, 139, 247, 320

Jianzhen (S.I. 9), 89, 90, 94, 95, 121

Jianzhongshu (S.I. 15), 117

Jiaosun (S.J. 20), 251, 278

Jiaoxin (K. 8), 195

Jiehexue (Extra), 189

Jiexi (St. 41), 65, 91, 96, 106, 111, 130, 248, 294, 299

Jihexue (Extra), 189

Jimen (Sp. 11), 143, 314

Jinggu (U.B. 64), 119

Jingmen (G.B. 25), 195

Jingming (U.B. 1), 101, 254, 257, 260, 261, 263, 267, 269, 271, 320, 332

Jinjin-Yuye (Extra), 66, 152, 324

Jiuwei (Ren 15), 105

Jueyinshu (U.B. 14), 98, 137, 140, 189

Jugu (L.I. 16), 247

Juliao (G.B. 29), 248

Juque (Ren 14), 77, 137, 176

Kongzui (Lu. 6), 189, 249

Kunlun (U.B. 60), 65, 70, 96, 107, 111, 130, 135, 248, 258, 297, 303, 320, 329

Lanweixue (Extra), 163, 164

Laogong (P. 8), 64, 296

Laozhenxue (Extra), 118

Liangmen (St. 21), 77, 154, 160, 166, 248

Liangqiu (St. 34), 95, 111, 130, 248, 336

Lianquan (Ren 23), 65, 66, 83, 89, 101, 104, 276, 277, 280, 282, 320

Lieque (Lu. 7), 60, 94, 119, 121, 128, 181, 182, 200, 236, 249, 252, 281, 285 287, 296

Ligou (Liv. 5), 104, 197, 206, 213, 224

Lingdao (H. 4), 247

Lingtai (Du 10), 152, 299, 311

Mingmen (Du 4), 90, 95, 98, 133, 147, 156, 178, 191, 195, 197, 201, 204, 206, 207, 210, 211, 239, 246, 260, 308, 310, 334, 336

Mouth-Yinjiao (Du 28), 173

Naohui (S.J. 13), 332

Naoshu (S.I. 10), 130

Neck-Futu (L.I. 18), 66, 276, 282

Neiguan (P. 6), 59, 77, 78, 89, 95, 98, 99, 101, 102, 104, 137, 140, 143, 144, 152, 154, 156, 158, 159, 160, 161, 162, 163, 164, 166, 167, 168, 175, 176, 178, 188, 195, 201, 203, 210, 214, 217, 219, 230, 236, 237, 239, 247, 249, 250, 254, 261, 262, 270, 293, 303, 304, 309, 318, 321, 323, 324, 325, 327, 330, 332, 335, 336

Neiting (St. 44), 65, 73, 130, 158, 164, 166, 171, 175, 239, 257, 281, 284, 289, 332, 334, 335

Nose-Heliao (L.I. 19), 281, 287

Nose-Juliao (St. 3), 73, 83, 286

Pangguangshu (U.B. 28), 98, 107, 194, 195, 202, 328

Pianli (L.I. 6), 328

Yuji (Lu. 10), 94, 95, 278, 281, 282, 334

Yunmen (Lu. 2), 189

Yuyao (Extra), 255, 257, 286

Zanzhu (U.B. 2), 65, 73, 77, 80, 83, 257, 258, 260, 261, 262, 263, 264, 265, 267, 286, 332, 334

Zhangmen (Liv. 13), 156, 160, 168, 178

Zhaohai (K. 6), 130, 135, 229, 261, 281, 282, 297

Zhibian (U.B. 54), 70, 71, 106, 172

Zhigou (S.J. 6), 75, 81, 107, 162, 164, 168, 171, 178, 183, 188, 195, 210, 211, 248, 249, 302, 315, 336

Zhishi (U.B. 52), 109, 110, 133, 189, 197, 201, 203, 204, 275

Zhishu (Extra), 173

Zhiyang (Du 9), 137, 152, 167, 168, 178, 318

Zhiyin (U.B. 67), 73, 215, 217

Zhizheng (S.I. 7), 119

Zhongchong (P. 9), 59, 235, 318, 319, 320, 327

Zhongfeng (Liv. 4), 194

Zhongfu (Lu. 1), 189, 250

Zhongji (Ren 3), 65, 104, 107, 149, 154, 190, 191, 194, 195, 197, 202, 203, 204, 207, 210, 213, 224, 226, 227, 229, 242, 243, 336

Zhongliao (U.B. 33), 229

Zhonglushu (U.B. 29), 158

Zhongwan (Ren 12), 77, 81, 98, 101, 147, 152, 153, 154, 156, 158, 159, 160, 161, 162, 163, 166, 171, 175, 176, 178, 195, 214, 237, 238, 239, 244, 250, 318, 325, 327, 334, 336

Zhoujian (Extra), 315

Zhouliao (L.I. 12), 125

Zigong (Extra), 225, 226, 229

Zulinqi (G.B. 41), 230

Zusanli (St. 36), 59, 61, 65, 66, 70, 76, 77, 79, 81, 87, 89, 90, 91, 95, 96, 98, 99, 101, 104, 106, 108, 131, 139, 141, 144, 146, 147, 148, 149, 151, 152, 153, 156, 157, 159, 160, 161, 162, 163, 164, 166, 167, 168, 174, 178, 179, 183, 185, 188, 189, 195, 197, 201, 203, 204, 206, 207, 210, 211, 213, 214, 217, 218, 219, 220, 222, 225, 226, 227, 229, 230, 233, 236, 237, 238, 239, 240, 242, 244, 246, 247, 250, 257, 258, 260, 261, 262, 263, 264, 270, 273, 275, 287, 292, 295, 304, 308, 309, 311, 315, 318, 320, 322, 324, 327, 328, 329, 330, 332, 334, 335

图书在版编目（CIP）数据

针灸治疗选穴手册：英文/耿俊英著.
—北京：新世界出版社，1995. 1
ISBN 7-80005-181-1

Ⅰ．针…

Ⅱ．耿…

Ⅲ．针灸疗法-穴位-手册-英文

Ⅳ．R245-62

针灸治疗选穴手册

耿俊英　著

*

新世界出版社出版

（北京百万庄路 24 号）

北京大学印刷厂印刷

中国国际图书贸易总公司发行

（中国北京车公庄西路 35 号）

北京邮政信箱第 399 号　邮政编码 100044

1995 年（英文）第一版

ISBN 7-80005-181-1

04200

14-E-2924P